Melancholy Madness

Cover image obtained from IMSI's Master Photos Collection, 1895 Francisco Blvd East,
San Rafael, CA 94901-5506, USA

First published in 2003 by Mercier Press
Douglas Village, Cork
Email: books@mercierpress.ie
Website: www.mercierpress.ie

Trade enquiries to CMD Distribution
55A Spruce Avenue
Stillorgan Industrial Park
Blackrock, County Dublin
Tel: (01) 294 2560; Fax: (01) 294 2564
E-mail: cmd@columba.ie

© Michelle McGoff-McCann 2003
ISBN 1 85635 424 5
10 9 8 7 6 5 4 3 2 1

A CIP record for this title is available
from the British Library

Cover design by mercier vision

Printed in Ireland by ColourBooks, Baldoyle
Industrial Estate, Dublin 13

MELANCHOLY MADNESS
A CORONER'S CASEBOOK

MICHELLE McGOFF-McCANN

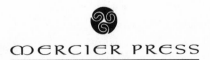
MERCIER PRESS

To my husband, Ryan
'And once again we come forth to dance amongst the stars'

Contents

ACKNOWLEDGEMENTS

I am grateful, not only to Jimmy Wells for his good judgement in saving Waddell's casebook in the nick of time from a burning pyre, but to the man to whom he gave the book, his nephew, the late Mr James McCrory (1925–1999) formerly of Hillsborough, Co. Down. James McCrory's son and daughter-in-law, Allister and Angela McCrory, and his loving wife, Violet, speak of how James cared for the old faded brown book, taking it out of its case on occasion to read some of its stories of tragedy; likely contemplating the fate of those recorded on its pages. I have been fortunate enough to gain their permission to look through its faded pages and share its stories.

It is a pleasure to thank the many persons who helped me create this work although it is likely to be impossible to thank them all here. My many thanks to the librarians and museum staff as well as those organisations and agencies who helped guide me to their many publications, documents and collections: The National Archives of Ireland, Dublin: Senior Archivist, Tom Quinlan and his staff who helped me find the right materials and have allowed me permission to print the wonderful collection of photographs from the Penal Records; Queen's University Belfast, specifically those at the science, medical and main libraries; The National Library, Dublin; Trinity College Library, Dublin; Valuation Office, Dublin; The National Photographic Archive, Temple Bar, Dublin; The Public Record Office of Northern Ireland, Belfast; The Linen Hall Library, Belfast; Ulster-American Folk Park, Omagh; Local History Library, Armagh; Enniskillen Library, Enniskillen, Co. Fermanagh; Ulster Folk and Transport Museum, Holywood, Co. Down; Registrar's Office, Deaths, Births and Marriages, North-Eastern Health Board, Monaghan – Mary Lenehan and Suzanne Cronin; Central Statistics, Cork – Gary; Lisburn Linen Museum, Lisburn – Brenda Collins; The National Union of Journalists, Dublin; and the staff at the Co. Monaghan libraries, Clones and Monaghan. Special thanks to Faber and Faber, London, for kindly granting me permission to reproduce a letter by John Butler Yeats.

To those I interviewed for more personal information about their knowledge of history and family: William Joyce Topley and Thomas Norman Topley; Professor Clarke, Royal Victoria Hospital; Molly Skeath; Tommy Crow; Nora Campbell; David O'Daly; my friends and clients at Solas Resource Centre; Des Fitzgerald; and especially to Theo McMahon and Maire O'Neill who first introduced me to the photocopies of the coroner's casebook and allowed me to use their private collection of microfilm to begin my research. Additionally, for his generosity and offering his camaraderie in research, thanks to the Revd Mr David Nesbitt and his wife Elsie.

For contributing their professional ideas, information and time: Dr Martin Watters, North Monaghan Coroner for all his candour and in-depth discussion regarding the nature of the coroner's office; Dr Brian Farrell, Dublin City Coroner for his support and critique of the duties of the coroner's office in the nineteenth century and sharing his work from his publication, *Coroners: Practice and Procedure* (Dublin, 2000); Dr Myrtle Hill, lecturer in the Institute of Lifelong Learning and head of the department of Women's Studies at Queen's University, Belfast, for her expertise and review of women's issues in the nineteenth century; Dr Denis A. Cusack, University College Dublin for contributing research; Brian

Kennedy, Curator, Ulster Folk and Transport Museum, Co. Down for explaining the intricacies involved in building the railway; forensic researcher, Cristy Ettenson, New York City.

To those who read drafts of the book, in whole or in part, and offered me their comments, I am especially grateful.

To Patrick McCabe for his support, advice and most of all, for understanding the goals and objectives of this book. He is a generous and talented man.

Warm thanks to Mercier Press for their interest and patience with this publication.

I am fortunate to have surrounded myself with a supportive family and close friends who have continued to encourage and support this endeavour throughout the past few years: my husband, Ryan McCann, Mom, Mayor Nancy Hurley, Dad, Mr Kevin McGoff and my brother, Kevin McGoff, Linda Koerbel McGoff, Thomas Hurley, Kathy McGoff, Barbara, Jason, Jeff and Jacqui McCann, Geraldine Skeath, Henry Skeath, Jen Levy, Teresa Mushik, Blaithin and Tiarnach Ronaghan, Paula Nolan and Stephen Quinn, Kathy Quinn and Tony Sherry, Adrian Quinn, Caroline Quinn and Fil Barry Quinn, Bernadette Williams and the Williams family, Dennis Hunt, Geraldine Rooney, Catherine Mulligan, Amanda Brady, Helen Fitzpatrick, Alice O'Neill, Olivia Duffy, Michael Kavanagh, Thomas Shanahan, Grace Maloney, Patricia McElwaine, Seamus Casey and the Casey family of the Black Valley, Co. Kerry, Christine Jobson, Clodagh and Bernadette (Rush) McKenna, Peadar and Margaret McGeough, Kathleen Ward and Packy Ward, John Williams, Ann McCabe, Shane McNamee and Jill, Tony Quinn and Grace, Jason Williams, Larry Meegan, and my extended McGoff, Monroe, Roach, Hall, Byrnes, McCann, Skeath and McGeough families, my friends in San Francisco, California and those many people in the community in Monaghan town who have been good to me. Additionally, my gratitude to those who are no longer with us, Professor Milton Kessler, Binghamton University, Robert Bridges and Caroline Prospect of Binghamton, New York.

Thanks to all of you.

MICHELLE McGOFF McCANN
August 2003

Chronicling the Soul along 'the Permanent Way'

'A ball through the heart might end my pain.' I don't know if those were the exact words spoken by Nathaniel Beatty, a twenty-six-year-old man who had been married for just two months in Kilmore West in 1861, not so very long before his wide-eyed bloated face broke the surface of the water in a well very close to his home; or if the cause of death was a broken heart. All we have to go on are the bald, prosaic facts and some rumours regarding an 'unhappy union'.

Equally I am not privy to the innermost workings of a certain John Treanor's mind when he, having fallen asleep while working on a tall building some sixty feet up from the ground, and being rescued by two fellow workers, decided some time later to climb back onto the roof, thereby hastening his untimely demise. Not long afterwards, Treanor was discovered by a William Grimley, impaled by railing spikes through the bowels and chest, on an otherwise unremarkable evening in the small town of Monaghan in the first month of the year 1872.

Did the gatekeeper of the Irish Northern Railway, his fallen body limp upon the tracks of 'the Permanent Way' (the name given to the railway track) yearn for that same ball of steel as the life ebbed from his body, the eyes turning in his head as he moaned: 'Will no person lift me?' before Ann Sheenan arrived to cradle his head, perhaps to recite the Act of Contrition into the dying man's ear?

Such postulations, obviously, must belong in the realm of speculation, for who can claim to begin to be familiar with the arterial complexities that map the inner republic of any human soul; particularly when the subject walked the earth almost a century and a half ago?

The past, wrote William Faulkner, being far from irrelevant, is not even *past*. It seems pointless, even frivolous, to point this out in an age when vast armies once again are being massed in desert sands as they were in the days of Horace, Virgil and Ovid. But one could perhaps be forgiven for suggesting that society in the past twenty years or so, and nowhere more so than in Ireland, has become so taken with materialism and disposable culture that this inevitable, enduring truth has been, if not forgotten, then overlooked. Life changes but it does not change in the slightest. Perhaps even as I write, a broken-hearted soldier awaits someone to cradle his head, the 'eyes turning in his head', the sun, as it must, burning down upon this particular 'permanent way', another very familiar journey indeed. Except that, on this trip, the train doesn't stop at Bundoran.

But, if we accept this, however strained metaphor for the itinerary that is our lot, its never-meeting tracks stretching far into infinity, there can be no better guide for us than the extraordinary character that is William Charles Waddell, whose life's work within these pages is compiled and further investigated by Michelle McCann, who brings a modern sensibility to bear on some of his findings.

I cannot praise this book highly enough. And I think it would be a great pity if it were to be perceived as some workmanlike exercise in a purely local history, of which there are many. All of them valid in their own way. For surely, as Patrick Kavanagh, a better man than ever I'll be, pointed out – all history must be local.

Inevitably, *Melancholy Madness* concerns itself with the habits and mores of the latter part of the nineteenth century. But more than anything, I think of it as a fabulous detective story, with more than a whiff of fogbound chilling Gothic. It is as though Edgar Allan Poe, Charles Maturin, Arthur Conan Doyle and a number of their more modern counterparts (such as Cracker played by Robbie Coltrane, for example), had joined forces to produce from a necronomicon of old, an enduring, entertaining, incisive illumination of human behaviour which happens to be set in Co. Monaghan, in the exotically named townlands of Tydavnet, Aghabog, Clontibret, Latton and Lacken.

For that is what one gleans as chapter after chapter unfolds this feeling of exoticism, of life lived in some faraway place that is vaguely troubling, familiar, a country one has visited in a half-forgotten dream. Except that when you've finished the book, you feel you know it inside out, which of course you do, as you ought to, because you've been reading about yourself. You look into the mirror one day to see your great-grandfather looking back out, into the future and out of the past, in the words recorded by William Waddell every day of his thirty-two years in the county.

In the strict scheme of things, William Waddell wasn't a detective, even if that's how he appears to me, tentatively shining his pencil of light as he cautiously negotiates the Monaghan darkness, our innermost longings that lie swathed in shadow. Whenever death had occurred, it was his job to hold an inquest to determine its cause. To this end he would work with police, clergy, physicians and grieving relatives, interviewing witnesses, ordering autopsies and samples of tissue for analysis, as well as organising juries to evaluate the evidence.

In all, William Charles Waddell investigated the circumstances surrounding the deaths of almost 900 persons who perished in nineteenth-century Co. Monaghan, recording his findings and experiences in a most remarkable casebook, which Michelle McCann has drawn on, thereby in her own right creating yet another remarkable work which ought to be required reading not only for students of the period but for anyone interested in human behaviour and the mysteries that attend this journey we make, from the beginning to the end, to the end of the beginning, from A to Z along this 'permanent way'.

The material is magnificently organised, broken up into a series of immensely readable chapters, each dealing with a particular aspect of Waddell's work – whether infanticide, suicide, dangers in the home, death by misadventure, strange and unusual occurrences, etc.

Time and again one uncovers little nuggets: the book can be read in sequence or viewed as an eccentric 'lucky dip' in which yet another aspect of social and psychological behaviour is revealed. For many years I had been fascinated by the story of 'the Sleepwalking Nun', which was current when I was a student in Monaghan, and apparently, still is. Where did it come from I would wonder and why in this particular form? Its *raison d'être* is simply and concisely explained here and one's heart cannot but go out to the unfortunate sister herself and the generous, protective souls who dreamed up the tale as a means of protection, both for her and the community.

I'm not going to tell you any more about them here. You'll have to read the book to find out for yourself.

Michelle McCann has done us all a great service in discovering William Waddell's casebook – I had certainly never heard of it before – and employing her fine sense of editing and scholarship in distilling the material within to present it to the general reader.

Melancholy Madness is Robert Louis Stevenson with a dash of Rosa Mulholland. It is James Clarence Mangan with a goodly portion of Patrick Kavanagh. It is Charles Kickham with Charles Maturin. *The Hungry Grass* bleeds into *The Hound of the Baskervilles*. It is entertaining, erudite and perceptive. It is scholarly and wise, accurate and fastidious; and many other things I don't have the time to name.

But, more than anything, it is a work of love for a place and the people who make it unique, whose private history more than deserves to be written. Within these pages, it most certainly has been, with a rare and commendable eloquence.

PATRICK McCABE

This book began as my imagination and interest peaked having read through, over and over, the catalogue of sad tales of death recorded by coroner William Charles Waddell. While contemplating just exactly how these tales might be presented for others to read, one of the darkest days in history took place: 11 September 2001. It was then that I was again reminded of the significance of the last moments of life. It is the stories leading up to that moment, those details included in a coroner's inquest, that are the most poignant for those left behind. The need for these facts is an ontological curiosity that we all share. It is more than the wanting and needing to understand how death occurred – particularly in sudden, unusual, unexplained or suspicious ways – it is a quest for answers to help us understand our own lives and, under some unfortunate circumstances, to get justice for the dead.

I called this book *Melancholy Madness*, having read one particular inquest, that of a young woman named Jane Divine. The only facts recorded in the brief account of her death were that she was twenty-two-years-old, a servant to James Fiddes, Esq. and that she was in a physically weak state due to English Cholera, which, when combined with her inherited trait of 'melancholy madness', accounted for her drowning herself in Holywood lake. I was stunned. What was this melancholy madness she suffered from? My first inclination was to define her medically, clinically. She suffered from depression. But what were the factors contributing to this state of mind, those which drove her to commit suicide? Was it truly mental illness or a chemical imbalance – as we classify such persons today – or rather, were there other possible reasons for her fateful decision?

I became a sociologist, a historian. I knew that women in Victorian times were considered biologically inferior to men, unable to handle such issues as love affairs, spousal arguments, grief and ultimately 'emotions'. Further research showed that servants were often subjected to the unwanted attentions of the master and his other male visitors and were usually isolated from friends and family. Now I became a detective for the dead, the buried, the forgotten. The possibilities for her suicide became endless and Jane Divine weighed heavily on my mind. I found myself creating scenarios, piecing together the few details of her inquest with academic research, information from novels of the time and my own creations of what happened that fateful day in 1872. I was hooked.

William Charles Waddell, Esq, was a man whose life was dedicated to recording and investigating death. He had the unfortunate task of working as a coroner during the Great Famine; he watched the massive population decline due to emigration and ultimately saw the darkest effects that these events had on those persons who remained in the country. Waddell was on the front-line of brutality, viewing and inspecting the bodies of murdered infants; the bruises and open wounds of wives beaten to death; men murdered in passionate rages, hit in the head with rocks, slaughtered with knives or cut down with guns. He also visited the homes where death occurred under suspicious circumstances, within families, where it was likely that the murderer was interviewed and stared Waddell in the face while telling their fabricated tale of the last moments of their victim's demise.

These were tumultuous times in a country that saw much death, sadness and trouble. Waddell's casebook is a valuable collection of stories from a county, but more so of the country. These atrocities did not just happen in Co. Monaghan, they were occurring all over Ireland. This collection is special because it is an uninterrupted record of his travels, from townland to townland, mangled corpse to breathless body. It tells not only the stories of death, but the life and experiences of a nineteenth century Irish coroner.

Cataloguing and investigating death is an unusual task and was even more so in a time before formal protection and preservation of the corpse; when the general populace adhered to strict customs and rituals of waking and burial; and when there was disharmony between the law and the public, who distrusted this intrusion of their privacy in their time of mourning. However, we can now gain much remarkable information from these inquests about how people lived – their diet, clothing, chores and duties in the home, work on the railway and in the mills, alcohol consumption, social activities, marriage patterns, family strife and violence, games played by children, religious and political activities, the treatments, herbs and medicines given to the sick and dying and old names for locations within the county.

When reading *Melancholy Madness*, my hope is that readers will be intrigued by the facts presented but will also gain more understanding about the lives and deaths of the people in these pages. Some of you may find some new insight into understanding your own Irish ancestors and may remember a whispered story or secret, that, although dismissed, may now be revisited and reconsidered as a version of the truth. And for those who just like a good mystery or murder novel, take these facts presented in the coroner's casebook and develop your own theories as to why some of these unfortunate souls went to a world beyond ours – from time to eternity.

MICHELLE MCGOFF-MCCANN

CHAPTER ONE

THE CORONER AND HIS CASEBOOK
INQUESTS, INVESTIGATIONS AND AUTOPSY

'You see,' he explained, 'I consider that a man's brain originally is like a little empty attic, and you have to stock it with such furniture as you choose. A fool takes in all the lumber of every sort that he comes across, so that the knowledge which might be useful to him gets crowded out, or at best is jumbled up with a lot of other things so that he has a difficulty in laying his hands upon it. Now the skilful workman is very careful indeed as to what he takes into his brain-attic.'

Sir Arthur Conan Doyle, A *Study in Scarlet*

The Casebook of Coroner William Charles Waddell is an exceptional collection of historical information capturing the circumstances surrounding the death of almost 900 persons who perished in nineteenth-century Co. Monaghan. By examining this text, we are able to get a clearer picture of both life in post-famine Ireland as well as the duties and responsibilities of the coroner. Waddell was not a medical man, but a gentleman acting as an investigator, solicitor and judge. Working with police, clergy, physicians and grieving relatives, he held a formal investigation to determine the cause of death of the deceased and considered the possibility of guilt or liability of a suspect who may have contributed to the final moments of the deceased. Waddell was responsible for interviewing witnesses, ordering post-mortem examinations as well as organising juries to evaluate the evidence. Autopsies conducted by country doctors were often mere observations of the dead corpse, or crude and quick dissections. Depending upon the state of the body, many cadavers must have been quite gruesome to onlookers – regardless of their years of experience.

The cases covered in the coroner's career and the procedures by which Waddell obtained a cause of death help to create a profile of the man as well as a window into the procedures and reactions of those who contributed to gaining justice and closure for the deceased and their families.

DEATH INVESTIGATION
W. C. Waddell and the Office of Coroner in Ireland

The role of the modern coroner is to inquire into the circumstances of sudden, unexplained, unnatural and suspicious death. A coroner is an independent office holder with responsibility under the law for the medico-legal investigation into such deaths.[1] It requires an evaluation of forensic information, such as autopsy or special analysis of organs and tissues, in addition to the testimony of witnesses with information, all of which can help reach a verdict. Although the coroner is often the first public official to hold a formal investigation into a death, contrary to public perception, he is not permitted to consider civil or criminal liability, let alone to determine such matters.[2] He must simply establish facts. Without the coroner, public suspicion and doubt might be cast on every death that required further investigation by a judicial or public enforcement authority. The coroner's role, by its very nature, protects the integrity of the deceased and in many cases, spares the relatives the pain of public mistrust and uncertainty.

The first coroner in Ireland is believed to have been appointed in the thirteenth century. Initially, the office was founded to limit the powers of the royal sheriff whose additional activities as a financial and judicial official had caused great resentment in and around Dublin.[3] By appointing a coroner, the sheriff would not be able to make as much money in the preliminary procedures prior to going to trial. Not only was the office of coroner created to limit one person's ability to profit from the investigation surrounding death, but also to uncover the truth. If a person were to profit greatly from say, a murder investigation, an inquest and a criminal trial, such as in the case of the royal sheriff, it is likely there would be more cases recorded and an increased possibility of corruption.

Over the centuries, reforms were made to maintain the integrity of the office. By the nineteenth century, although changes were made, corruption and extortion did exist. At a time when liability might be considered by the coroner and his jury, suspects contributing to the death could be held for an indefinite time in local jails until petty and assizes juries might consider more evidence. Coroners could be pressured by the local political climate and sway a jury towards a predetermined verdict. Salary and travelling expenses were increased, but some offices around Ireland had fallen into disrepute. It was during this time, from 1829 and 1908, that nine acts dealing specifically with the office of coroner were passed.[4] The coroner was now empowered to order the performance of a post-mortem examination and to summon a qualified medical practitioner to attend an inquest for the purpose of providing a more accurate, expert and *credible* opinion into the cause of death.[5] With the Coroner's Act of 1846, coroners' districts were defined in each county in Ireland in an attempt to cover each area of the country as completely as possible. At a time when communications and transport were limited, when news travelled by word of mouth and horse and cart, these districts were designed to ensure proper coverage.

William Charles Waddell, Esq., was appointed to the office of coroner on 24 April 1846. Not only was he starting his career as the only coroner for the entire county, it was also the early years of the Great Famine in Ireland. Soon realising that an impossible task had been set before him, he appealed to the county for the appointment of a second coroner to cover the southern region of Monaghan. Hugh Swanzy, Esq., was chosen for the position and working out of Castleblayney, covered the southern half of Co. Monaghan. Waddell's region is most easily described as the northern half of Co. Monaghan, where he was to carry out his duties of investigating, recording and determining the cause of unnatural, sudden and suspicious deaths.[6]

Waddell lived in the townland of Lisnaveane in the parish of Tullycorbet, a landholding of almost fifty acres, where he rented to several tenants.[7] He was born in 1798 as one of five children of James Waddell and Susanna Hope and his family was well-known in Co. Monaghan. William's grandfather, Alexander Waddell was a leader of the Volunteers and his brother, Hope Waddell, was a noted Presbyterian missionary and scholar.[8] W. C. Waddell was also a devout Presbyterian. It is likely he was selected to become coroner owing to his reputation as a gentleman, as well as for being a large landholder who resided within the district to be covered. It was not until the latter part of the century that the coroner was required to be a physician, barrister or solicitor. Therefore Waddell was considered a man who could be relied upon to faithfully attend the cases presented before him and to see that a proper verdict of death was reached.

He kept a casebook which he maintained in three volumes that spanned his thirty-two-year career from 1846 to 1878. Volume one (1846–1855) covering 408 deaths in Co. Monaghan during the famine, is now missing.[9] Volume two, containing 861 inquests and inquiries into death from January 1856 to March 1876, is the casebook referred to throughout *Melancholy Madness*.[10] Volume three covered the brief period from April 1876 until a few months before Waddell's death in 1878. This volume is presumed missing or destroyed.

The inquests recorded in Waddell's casebook follow a particular format. Except for those entries in his casebook that are mere *inquiries* – notes taken to record a notice of death or a short investigation when an inquest was not deemed necessary – all the inquests are numbered.[11] An inquest is given two numbers, for example 4.290 or 4 (290). The first number (i.e. 4) is the number given to the inquest to distinguish it from one assizes to another. When an assizes was held, Waddell would submit his expenses for the inquests to the grand jury for receipt of his salary and reimbursement. The second number (i.e. 290) is the number of the inquest in relation to the entire book – a running total. In the margins of the book, at the side of each inquest, he recorded costs incurred for each. He kept careful record of various expenses that ranged from grave-digger's fees to expenses for chemical analysis. It was vital for Waddell to keep accurate records in order to keep track of his expenses, fees and payments and he offered details under certain circumstances to justify the costs. The beginning of each inquest verifies the identity of the body, where the inquest took place and on what date. For example, 'In the townland of Cooldarragh in the parish of Drumsnat, an inquest was held on view of the body of Philip Coyle'. Next, the depositions of witnesses who provided information as to the events surrounding the death are recorded. These persons were usually relatives, neighbours, physicians and anyone with additional evidence. At the end of each inquest, a verdict of death was determined. For example: 'The verdict was death from apoplexy accelerated by previous habits of intoxication and a free indulgence of spirits.'[12]

Carrying out the duties of the office of coroner was challenging, burdensome and sometimes exhausting for Waddell. Throughout his thirty-two-year career as coroner he investigated and organised inquests into the deaths of over 1,300 persons. His job was not an easy one. Viewing abandoned infants left by the roadside, their bodies half-scavenged by animals or the bloated bodies of the unfortunate and disturbed floating in canals and rivers are images not easily erased from the mind and memory. Besides viewing the lifeless shells of the destitute and starving, the poor and uneducated, the political and the religious, the educated and gentrified, old and young, grandparents and babies, as well as the victims and their violators, the duties of the coroner can more accurately be described as 'services for the living'. One might imagine the importance of his presence when investigating the sudden death of a young woman dying in childbirth with her sobbing family standing around her body asking the doctors and coro-

Page from the coroner's casebook. Each inquest was recorded and numbered with various expenses such as gravediggers' fees and miles travelled, written along the margin.

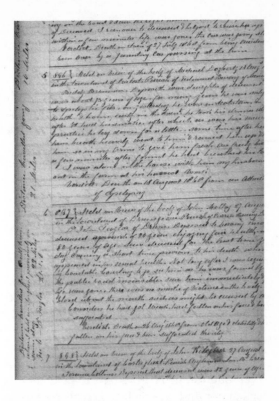

ner, 'What went wrong?' When investigating the circumstances surrounding a possible political murder, he might be confronted by an angry mob demanding to know if the deceased met his fate at the hands of foul play and who might be considered a suspect. Doctors and jury members were not always eager to participate and some high profile cases, such as the murder of an Orangeman or Fenian, required a strict adherence to procedure without allowing tempers and political beliefs to influence proceedings. Ultimately, when the coroner embarked upon an inquest, he travelled in a wake of doubt, suspicion and caution; yet by maintaining order and strict professionalism, an accurate verdict of death might be reached, instilling confidence in the public and allowing the living and the dead to rest in peace.

CONDUCTING AN INQUEST
Responsibility to a Curious and Suspicious Public

The duty of a coroner is to uncover the truth about the circumstances concerning the death of the deceased in cases of unnatural, suspicious or sudden death. The coroner must ensure that all the facts are 'fully, fairly and fearlessly investigated'.[13] He or she must determine: 1. the identity of the deceased; 2. the place of death; 3. time of death; and 4. how the deceased came by his death. These four objectives can best be remembered by asking 'who? where? when? and how?' The necessity of answering these four questions has remained the same throughout the past century. Of course, the ability to determine an exact time of death has become more accurate over the past two centuries as modern forensic techniques developed. Determining how a person died has become more precise with the development of new techniques in criminal investigation and forensic science.

Inquests are inquiries conducted by the coroner, with or without a jury, where the facts surrounding a death are evaluated and a verdict as to the cause of death is determined. Its purpose is to establish the facts and place those facts on public record.[14] A contemporary coroner is first informed of the death by police and then makes arrangements for the body to be sent for a post-mortem examination. Depending upon the circumstances of the death, an inquest might not take place for several weeks or months. More than a century earlier, Waddell would have been informed of a sudden or suspicious death by the local constabulary immediately or as soon as possible. Having been notified, he had two days to hold an inquest. This was a short amount of time especially in complicated cases, such as suspicion of murder. If he failed to do so, any two local magistrates in the district could conduct the inquest themselves. In complicated cases, Waddell might begin an inquest for the purposes of having the body examined, laying it to rest and then adjourning until a later time as evidence and witnesses were gathered.

An inquest had to be initiated within two days of death primarily owing to the strict adherence to Irish traditional rituals of waking and burying the dead. Some practices regarding the dead are believed to go back as far as the megalithic age. Customs involved washing and preparing the body and lying the deceased in a coffin or bed or 'waking' table (which was usually the kitchen table). This was followed by visiting relatives, friends and neighbours coming to the home to pay their respects. Contrary to the serious nature of such an event, wakes were more like parties. A *good* wake was one to be remembered, and involved storytelling, drinking, dancing and games played in celebration of the deceased's life. It was important not to leave the body alone in case the spirit had not yet left it. A code of behaviour was carefully executed when removing the dead from the house in procession to the graveyard for burial. Such rituals as bringing the body out of the house 'feet-first' and turning over the chairs, table or bed where the body had lain were important so as to avoid another death. This particular belief was prevalent in Ulster and any shortcuts taken or interruptions in such tradition were believed to be a sign that another death would occur shortly after.[15] With such superstitious practices surrounding a dead body, an investigation such as an inquest conducted by a coroner and a jury comprising strangers would have been regarded with suspicion. On more than one occasion Waddell would have met resistance. In fact, in one instance he was driven from the scene of the inquest. He warned those present that they would be committing an offence by not allowing him to hold the inquiry and perform his duties. It was said that they arrived at his residence the next day, begged his forgiveness and assured him they would participate in the inquiry.[16]

With preliminary information from the constabulary, the coroner proceeded to the location of the body and interviewed witnesses to determine the cause of death and if an inquest should be held. If Waddell deemed an inquest necessary, he informed the sub-inspector of police in the district to summon a sufficient number of persons to attend and be sworn as jurors. Jurors were selected from a list of residents in the district who paid not less than £4 annually to the relief of the poor and were householders residing in the county. It was the coroner's duty to issue summonses to every witness required to be present.

A post-mortem examination was not always required and it was Waddell's responsibility to assess this. Autopsies were carried out by local country doctors but any further tests, specifically chemical analysis, tissues and fluids were sent to Belfast. Professor John Hodges of Queen's University (1815–1899) conducted all toxicology tests for Waddell during his years as the coroner. Hodges was educated at Trinity College, Dublin, Glasgow University and the University of Giessen in Germany. He was a lecturer in Medical Jurisprudence at Queen's University in Belfast and was dedicated to the science of chemistry. He analysed the samples requiring the detection of metallic and non-metallic poison, usually when murder by such was suspected.[17]

When an inquest begins, it is run in a format similar to that of a court trial with the coroner reigning as the judge with a jury who listen to the evidence. In our contemporary society, criminal and civil liability is not determined in this court. However, in the nineteenth century, not only could Waddell's verdicts be used later at petty and

assizes courts to prove liability but he was also able to remand suspects to jail in suspicious cases until a verdict of death had been reached. Over the years, owing to many cases of improper imprisonment
and lack of evidence, this practice was abandoned. The only issue
decided upon in the coroner's court today is the cause of death. Once
the verdict is reached in the coroner's court, it is then up to the family members (regarding civil liability) or the justice and criminal
system to prosecute any persons suspected of causing or bringing
about the death of the deceased.

'An inquest is a public forum to find out how someone died, but
has another purpose as well – to allay public suspicion. It is for the
dignity of the person themselves and for the entire society, so they
don't think anything is covered up,' says Dr Martin Watters, MD of
Emyvale. Watters is the acting coroner for the northern region of Co.
Monaghan, the same position and territory as W .C. Waddell one hundred and sixty years earlier. The current caseload in the district of
North Monaghan of between thirty to forty cases per year matches
that of Waddell between the years 1856 and 1876.

Dr Watters explains that he conducts his inquests either in his
office in Emyvale or at the courthouse in Monaghan town. 'Some
people think because the inquests are held here in Emyvale in the
evening time after normal business hours this is secretive and adds an
element of mystery ... but really it's for the convenience of the participants.' Inquests are held after 5p.m. in the evening. Most persons
work between 9a.m. and 5p.m. and evening hours are more suitable
for those people attending. During the nineteenth century, Waddell
held inquests at any time of day or evening depending upon what
time he arrived on the scene and how quickly medical examination
could be made and witnesses and a jury gathered. The inquest was
most often held in a local residence in the townland where the body
was at the time of death, sometimes in a public office or building or
else it took place at the Monaghan courthouse. The courthouse was
often convenient for various reasons such as travel for participants,
more space to accommodate a larger crowd, or in some high profile
cases, a suspect was remanded in the jail pending the outcome of the
inquest and a criminal trial.

Investigating Death at State Institutions
Similar in scope to today's cases, the general public viewed inquests
and the duties surrounding the coroner's office with a watchful eye.
These were deaths that required further explanation and many had a

possibility of foul play. When a death of unnatural, suspicious or sudden nature occurred at a public facility, such as the jail, asylum or workhouse, the coroner was occasionally requested to attend and investigate. Prisoners at the jail most often died from disease and if the coroner was brought in, these deaths might be regarded as suspicious. Such an inquest was conducted to determine whether the prisoner 'died by the ill usage of the gaoler'. There are only a handful of inquests from the Monaghan jail. The first is recorded in 1856 and the last in July 1868.

From the Poorhouse to the Jail: Death Behind Bars
The Death of William Harvison, Monaghan Jail, February 1867
William Harvison was a pauper in the Monaghan Poorhouse. During his stay there it became clear that his violent nature was a danger to others. He was uncontrollable and a local magistrate was contacted to have him removed to the Monaghan jail. John Temple, the attending doctor at the jail, told the coroner that William Harvison had been admitted on 7 February 1867 as a dangerous lunatic for further examination. Having observed his behaviour for six days, he was committed as an inmate.

The evening after William's committal to the jail, turnkey James Campbell saw the new prisoner eating his supper heartily and in good health. Within ten minutes, while sitting on a bench in his cell, William apparently keeled over and never spoke again. Campbell told the coroner that 'he'd returned and found the prisoner lying on the floor of his room quite dead'. With no other information presented or evidence contradicting the turnkey, the inquest into the death of William Harvison was concluded. The verdict reached was death from natural causes.[18]

Another institution surrounded by great suspicion was the Monaghan District Lunatic Asylum. From the time of its opening in 1869, many persons entered its walls only to exit in a casket. The coroner attended the asylum quite regularly to investigate the deaths occurring there. Asylums, which will be discussed in more detail in chapter 3, were considered to be places of disgrace and shame and were filled with disease. In fact, in 1875 Waddell conducted a record 71 inquests – the majority were just *inquiries* recording a visit to the asylum. Most of the entries in the casebook for the asylum that year were just a record, documenting only the death:

> On this 2nd day of November 1875, [I] attended at Monaghan Asylum to enquire into the death of Catherine Dobson, an inmate of the said asylum

from 4 August 1869 to this day, being 6 years and 3 months and the period of her illness previous to her disease was 2 years and the cause of her death. Disease of the kidneys and the heart.

When disease was not believed to be the cause of death, more detail was required with respect to the manner in which the body was found and the nature of the illness of the patient. Again, something similar to 'death by ill usage by the gaoler' would need to be determined or ruled out when conducting an inquest at the asylum.

Suffocating in the Sheets?
The Death of Thomas McCormick, Monaghan Asylum, January 1871
Dr John Robertson first received Thomas McCormick as a patient into the lunatic asylum on 16 June 1869. He was suffering from epilepsy. The doctor attended him daily over the next six months but Thomas was becoming worse. One morning in January 1871, Dr Robertson got word that one of the attendants heard Thomas in a fit. The attendant, Edward Cosgrove, went to the patient and attended to him until the fit passed off. He then settled the man comfortably before leaving.

The next morning at 7a.m., Cosgrove opened the door of the room and found Thomas lying on his face and dead. Dr Robertson deposed, 'Frequently epileptic patients when in a fit turn on their face and begin turning the bed clothes. That is what happened in this case, and the attendant settled the clothes and made deceased comfortable. I consider he had a fit between the one in the night and being found dead at 7a.m.'

Edward Cosgrove, the attendant to Thomas McCormick, explained how at 2 o'clock in the morning before the death he heard the patient having a fit. Cosgrove went in, 'I settled the bed clothes and then left having fulfilled my instructions.' Joseph Brown, an assistant attendant, was also present during Thomas' epileptic fit. He said, 'We found him lying partly out of bed and put him back into it. We settled his bed clothes comfortably and then left, the fit being over.'

Cosgrove added, 'I attended him as carefully as if he had been my Father.'

The jury seeing no cause to believe there was any foul play or any evidence, concluded that death resulted from suffocation from having turned on his face during an epileptic fit 'to which he had long been subject'. Thomas McCormick was 40 years of age.[19]

When death occurred at a county workhouse, depending upon the circumstances, it was of little consequence. Only three such inquests were recorded in the twenty-year time span of volume two of the coroner's casebook. Since the workhouse was an institution that an adult person could *voluntarily* leave, unlike the jail or asylum where they were confined until released, it might be assumed that less suspicion followed these deaths. Many in the workhouse were destined to die within its walls. Such institutions were disease-ridden and it was likely that many who entered would not return. These were the poor, unwanted and the destitute who found some relief either temporarily or permanently. It is apparent in each of the poorhouse inquests, that the deceased persons suffered from pre-existing conditions prior to their death.

Children were at great risk in the workhouse, usually dying from a combination of starvation and lack of proper care. At one inquest held by Waddell in 1855 (referred to in *The Northern Standard*) the jury concluded that the nurses at the Clones Union workhouse should be charged with culpable neglect and noted that the officers had not discharged their duties in a vigilant manner. Two children, Richard Gillespie and Jane Armstrong were both said to be 'very emaciated' by a Dr Henry, but he would not commit himself to what he believed caused their death.[20] It appears that authorities were reluctant to accuse employees of the workhouse when intent and proof might be lacking for further investigation.

Bleeding Sores and Injuries
The Death of Elizabeth Smith, Clones Workhouse, January 1860
The four-year-old child of Ann McManus had been unable to walk for eight months. The girl had a 'very severe discharge' oozing from her right thigh resulting from a large lump which had formed in her groin. On 18 January 1860, while both mother and daughter were residents of the Clones Workhouse, a fatal accident occurred. Ann was holding her daughter Elizabeth on her knee and nursing her, as was her usual routine. Two other women, Mary McDonald and Sally Slowey, were present. Having fed her child, Anne stood up to go for a pail of water and set the sickly child down on the table as the girl was unable to stand. The mother then asked Mary if she would mind taking her child. As she was assured the woman would keep an eye on the girl, the mother left the room. However, when Mary went to put the child in her arms, the child gave a 'hitch' turning from her, lost her balance and fell to the ground. Sally quickly caught her and ran

to carry her to her mother. She later explained that while running with the child, her apron had become stained with blood that was pouring from the little girl.

Shocked and horrified, Ann took Elizabeth to the master and matron of the workhouse, who in turn contacted Dr Henry. He was in attendance within an hour after the fall. Sadly, the child died within twenty-four hours after the accident. The verdict was death on Thursday, 19 January 1860 from the effects of a fall off a table on which she had been sitting and which proved fatal in consequence of her extreme delicacy of health and emaciated state of body.[21]

TAKING DEPOSITIONS
The Stories Surrounding the Death

Most of the witnesses at Waddell's inquests were the grieving relatives and friends who were present before, and at the time of, the death. They were usually allowed to simply tell their story, the way they saw or experienced the event, guided by questions asked by the coroner. Although the questions asked at an inquest are not transcribed in the casebook, they were sometimes recorded and published in newspapers. Jurors, physicians and solicitors are often quoted asking questions of witnesses, although it was Waddell in charge of the proceedings who was ultimately responsible for extracting the necessary information from the witnesses and steering the jurors towards a verdict. 'Anyone can ask questions at an inquest. The coroner is responsible for making sure all evidence is revealed and brought to light to answer the four primary questions – who? where? when? and how? – but all present have the opportunity to ask questions of the witnesses and of the pathologist in regard to the physical evidence,' explains Dr Watters. This appears to have been true at Waddell's inquests as well. It is important to note, however, that inquest procedures in regard to asking questions of witnesses vary between districts, counties and cities.

It is the coroner's duty to consider only the facts when reviewing evidence in the depositions to uncover the cause of death. In some cases, Waddell concluded that an inquest was not required having interviewed several witnesses. Although sometimes circumstances surrounding a death appeared suspicious, it was the coroner's duty to decide that if the evidence was too circumstantial, it did not warrant any further exploration.

Inheritance and Suspicion
The Death of Mary Nesbitt, Annagose, Aghabog Parish, March 1869
The coroner arrived at the townland of Annagose in the parish of
Aghabog on 15 March 1869 to investigate the death of Mary Nesbitt. When the death was reported to him, she had died three days
earlier and her body was already buried. Yet, some in the family and
neighbourhood were suspicious of foul play. Waddell was told her
death might have been 'hastened' and some of the family wanted an
inquest to be held and her body raised from the ground. Having made
the necessary inquiries, he did not consider that any further investigation was necessary.

A month later in April, Waddell received a letter from James Nesbitt of Corkish, son of the late Mary Nesbitt, speaking of the circumstances surrounding the death of his mother. In the letter he stated
that he and other members of his family were of the opinion that
their mother had been murdered. He described how his mother had
received some punch from her daughter-in-law the day before her
death. The family suspected there was poison in it. James also wrote
that he and other members of the family would make affidavits swear-
ing to this allegation.

This letter raised new questions about how Mary Nesbitt died and
meant Waddell needed to take a closer look at the case yet again. He
met with the Sergeant of Police and then spoke with the Revd Henry
Cowan, the minister of Newbliss Presbyterian church, and discussed
the letter and the circumstances surrounding the death of the old
woman. In their long conversation, Mr Cowan explained that he had
seen Mary repeatedly and the last time he spoke with her was just a
few days before her death. He told the coroner that she spoke very
highly of her daughter-in-law's kindness. Mr Cowan considered that
the anger of the remainder of the family was 'more spite because
Mary had left everything to her daughter-in-law's husband'. Since it
appeared to Waddell that one son was envious that his brother had
gained all of the inheritance and meant only to make trouble, there
was no further inquiry into the suspected murder.[22]

One must wonder if the Revd Mr Cowan and the coroner were
correct. Was the Nesbitt family so jealous of the gift of inheritance
that they would make such an accusation against the inheriting members and request that the coroner dig up their dead and buried mother? In many of the stories and evidence throughout Waddell's casebook, it is possible that the answer to this question is 'yes'. Not only
were money and property motives for murder; they were also the

basis for family division, which in truth, is still a characteristic of contemporary society. By not accepting the death of a loved one or the financial gain or loss as a result of their death, grieving or jealous family members look for other means to punish the living for their perceived injury. Yet, one might continue to contemplate this case based upon our lack of information. Did the Revd Mr Cowan present such compelling and clear explanations for the dispute in the Nesbitt family that the coroner immediately stopped his investigation? Or did Waddell not have enough evidence to warrant disinterring the body, conducting a possibly costly investigation? Such situations are presented in an open forum for judgement in many of the inquests presented throughout the casebook. Each must make up his/her own mind as to what appears to be the 'truth' given our lack of evidence in most cases.

An inquest is not a pleasant experience. Although from time to time there are high profile cases, heated arguments and some drama, it should not be compared to a highly publicised criminal trial. Most often there are relatives present who are devastated at the loss of the deceased. Some are grieving at the loss of their loved one, crying and quite emotional. It is with a careful and sensitive nature that the coroner asks questions of the witnesses while attempting to keep order and maintain a proper and dignified proceeding. This was especially necessary when children served as witnesses discussing the death they experienced first hand. They were required to discuss the circumstances surrounding the death. Listening to their tiny voices revealing the harsh realities of how a death in the family occurred must have been difficult.

Tiny Voices Tell the Story
The Death of Pat Sherry, Knockballyroney, Tedavnet Parish, January 1870
The coroner arrived to the Sherry home in Knockballyroney in the parish of Tedavnet to conduct an inquest on the body of Pat Sherry, an eleven-year-old boy who was found dead by his nine-year-old sister. His mother, Isabella, gave her explanation for the events on the day of the tragedy:

'For some time past, Pat complained of pains in his bowels and also about his heart. On the morning of 20 January 1870, I gave him some senna and salt which relieved him so much that he said he felt quite well. He then took his breakfast heartily,' she said. 'I went to a neighbour's house for about an hour with Pat accompanying me a short distance of the journey. When the time came for him to return home, *he asked me not to stay long.*' She concluded, 'On my return, I found my child on his back on the kitchen floor, dead.'

One of Pat's sisters, a little girl nine years old, told the jury that when her brother returned, he put out one of the cows and then went to clean out the byre. When she went out to see him a short while later, she found him lying on the ground with the spade he was using to shovel the dung beside him. Pat was dead. Assisted by her two brothers, aged five and seven years of age, she carried the corpse of their brother into the house. The small children then sat around the body and waited for their mother to return home.

Dr Woods examined the body. The verdict was death from inflammation of the bowels – aged 11 years.[23]

'... AND THE VERDICT IS ...'

A verdict of death is the statement at the end of an inquest including the name of the person who died, when they died, where and the cause of their death. Of the 861 inquests recorded by Waddell, most death occurred as a result of accidents. These accidents include drowning, burning, choking, farming and industrial accidents, victims being struck by lightning and other fatal occurrences due to negligence or misadventure, many of which involved alcohol.

Drowning deaths were the leading cause of accidental fatality. Men and boys underneath the surface unable to pull themselves back from the depths, elderly women retrieving pails from the well, and many children playing or running errands near rivers, lakes, streams, canals, wells and water-filled flax and bog holes were too quickly taken from this earth. Some drowning deaths describe the victim as having been 'of weak mind'; that they were showing signs of 'insanity' or suffering from a form of mental anguish. Although such verdicts reflected 'accidental' drowning deaths, it can be assumed that some were suicides. An accurate recording of such a death was a difficulty for the coroner if evidence could not conclusively prove that the deceased took their own life, as well as for the victim's families who did not want to bring shame on their loved one or the surviving family members. One example is that of Judith Fox, a sixty-year-old woman who was described as having 'recently become of melancholy and weak mind'. She had left her home in the middle of the night and was found the next morning drowned in a flax-hole. The verdict of her death was from accidentally falling into a pool of water and thereby

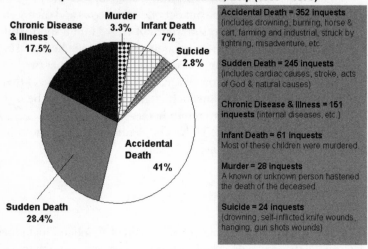

Verdicts of Death
Inquests of William Charles Waddell, Esq. (1856 – 1876)

Chronic Disease & Illness 17.5%

Murder 3.3%

Infant Death 7%

Suicide 2.8%

Accidental Death 41%

Sudden Death 28.4%

Accidental Death = 352 inquests (includes drowning, burning, horse & cart, farming and industrial, struck by lightning, misadventure, etc.

Sudden Death = 245 inquests (includes cardiac causes, stroke, acts of God & natural causes)

Chronic Disease & Illness = 151 inquests (internal diseases, etc.)

Infant Death = 61 inquests Most of these children were murdered.

Murder = 28 inquests A known or unknown person hastened the death of the deceased

Suicide = 24 inquests (drowning, self-inflicted knife wounds, hanging, gun shots wounds)

Percentages tallied from 861 inquests recorded by Waddell between the years 1856 and 1876

drowning.[24] Her death was documented as an accidental drowning either because it was not conclusively proven that she acted upon her own will or Waddell modified the language of the verdict for the surviving members of the family. If deaths such as these were to be considered suicides, the actual percentage of suicide would probably be higher than the total recorded.

Other accidental fatalities might be considered suspicious cases and 'open' on the books of public opinion even in the present day. These inquests were vague and lacked a convincing and definitive cause of death, often owing to a lack of evidence. Usually, the coroner could not determine whether the death occurred as the result of violence or due to the nature of death. Being inconclusive, these deaths were not recorded as manslaughter or murder since it could not be determined if the beating or violence caused the death. The case of Thomas Hughes illustrates how a neutral verdict of accidental death was established rather than that of murder. It was suggested that Hughes was possibly attacked by Francis Steele Jr after a night of drinking in the pub. Hughes was found drowned in a bog hole by his friends later in the night. The post-mortem examination showed that he had indeed received a blow to the head which hastened his death after falling into the water and drowning in the bog hole; yet it could not be determined if the blow was caused by another person or if he possibly hit his head on the ice before falling. One detail that was only mentioned in passing was that the water was 28 inches deep and there was a primary suspect, Francis Steele Jr, overheard threatening Hughes earlier in the evening. Hughes' death was recorded as an accidental drowning. The verdict was death on the night of 4 February 1856 from injuries sustained or inflicted previous to falling or being thrown into the pool of water in which he was found, but under what circumstances sustained or by whom inflicted there was not evidence produced to the jury to show.[25]

Sudden death includes all cardiac causes and heart attacks, stroke, acts of God, and natural causes. The verdict of natural causes appears to have been used when a conclusive physical verdict could not be determined, but the coroner and his jury concluded that the death did *not* occur as a result of actions of another party. One man, Henry Jackson of Rockcorry, had drunk heavily one evening and passed out at his home. Dr Moore performed a post-mortem examination and found a decolourisation over the man's entire body and a slight abrasion on the upper lip. His face was 'very livid and had blood coming from his nostrils'. The doctor concluded he had suffocated on his own bodily fluids. The verdict was death from suffocation but of natural causes. Although no one was blamed for causing Jackson's death, the jury expressed their regret that more care was not paid to Jackson by those around him in his state of intoxication.[26]

Sudden deaths were also investigated if other chance or suspicious circumstances took place soon before or after the death of the deceased. For example, when Rebecca Phillips was found dead, lying peacefully in her bed with her arms covering her chest, the coroner determined there was no need for a post-mortem examination. It looked as if she had died in her sleep. The only apparent reason for an inquest into her death was because, the day she died, Rebecca had travelled to Cootehill to pick up a small annuity left to her by her late husband, Richard Phillips. Considering that someone might have wanted the money and there could potentially have been foul play, an inquiry was made into her death. The verdict was that death came to her on the morning of 27 February 1858 from natural causes and not by any act of violence perpetuated by any person.[27]

Death from chronic illness and disease includes various types of ailments such as cholera, typhus, dysentery, consumption and other plagues and afflictions prevalent in the nineteenth century. Illnesses including 'failure of the nervous system', general debility, paralysis and epilepsy are also included. It appears that deaths of this nature were recorded by Waddell because they too were sudden, and unusual circumstances dictated that their long-standing disease or illness may or may not have been the cause of death.

In many cases those dying of disease and chronic illness expired at institutions such as the jail, workhouse or asylum and were required to be formally investigated. However, not all deaths at institutions were covered by the coroner. Again, death by chronic illness and disease was investigated only if it was sudden, or appeared unnatural and under suspicious circumstances.

Fighting a Cough and her Husband until her Last Breath
The Death of Isabella Keelan, Monaghan town, July 1858
Pat Keelan was the stepson of Isabella Keelan, a seventy-year-old woman described as being of very infirm health and much afflicted by a severe cough which often rendered her unable to rise in the morning or finish dressing herself. When Pat arrived home for dinner one day in July 1858, he found Isabella sitting at the fire having been in a fight with his father. The elderly couple had been arguing. Her husband had made some answer that so exasperated her that she threw a tin of water in his face. Pat endeavoured to make the peace but was not very successful. Shortly after the argument, while Isabella sat in front of the open hearth, brooding over the heated exchange between herself and her husband, she fell forward into the flames. Pat and his father rushed forward and carried her to the door for some air to revive her. Some spirits were sent for and in the meantime, water was sprinkled on her face. But Isabella never woke up. Dr Coote arrived and examined the body of the old woman. He found no marks of injury whatever on her person and was of the opinion that the death arose from 'internal disease hastened by extreme excitement ... the scene which took place immediately before her death would be quite sufficient so to excite her'.[28]

Infant deaths have been recorded separately since their results might distort the statistics. Most of these newborns were murdered because they were children born to unmarried mothers. Many of these children were unwanted and disposed of in various ways including being dropped in fields and by the side of the road, buried under rocks and bushes, placed in streams, rivers and canals and hidden along the banks. Other methods of disposal included suffocation and head trauma shortly after birth at the hands of the mother or with the help of midwives. If the murder statistics reflected infant death, the total percentage of murders would exceed 9%. [See chapter two for more information on infant death.]

Murder victims in Waddell's casebook had been subjected to beatings, stabbings, gunshot wounds, forced drowning, head trauma from stones and other crude instruments, poisoning and neglect. Family members and neighbours fighting over land and property, political agendas, domestic strife, alcohol-related violence and neglect were just some of the motives behind the killings. Elderly neglect was one area difficult to prove and prosecute later in criminal court. Only in the case of George Lee was a suspect named in the verdict of death. Dr Moore determined that Lee was not properly taken care of by his daughter and granddaughter. Lee, an elderly blind man, had been subjected to starvation and slept on the floor in a scant pile of straw without as much as a blanket to cover him while he lay next to an open window. The verdict was death from insufficiency of food, exposure to the severity of the weather and culpable neglect on the part of his daughter, Elizabeth Donaghoe.[29]

Stone throwing, a pastime of many young children in the nineteenth century, caused a handful of deaths. Such deaths occurred as a result of game playing and misadventure and were not considered as murder but as accidental deaths. However, when riots broke out amongst adults and stones were thrown with the intention of causing injury, any consequent death was treated as murder. Two groups of men were in a fight after a dance in the parish of Killeevan as they made their way home. At the end of the affray, Thomas McCarvle lay dead, bleeding from the head. Dr Moorehead determined that he'd been hit by a blunt, jagged instrument such as a stone which had been submitted into evidence. McCarvle had an extensive fracture from his temporal bone that extended down to his ear. None of the parties could be proved to have caused the injuries as none of the witnesses could accurately report the event. The verdict was 'death from injuries sustained but how sustained or by whom inflicted the jury have not had evidence to show them'.[30]

The objective of any inquest is to get as accurate an account of death as possible, which sometimes meant stating the name of the person responsible for the murder. Michael Mooney was killed by his in-laws in a heated dispute over a field. The verdict stated that the deceased came to his death from certain injuries inflicted by Francis and John Mulligan in a scuffle arising out of a dispute connected with the land.[31] After the coroner's jury named a suspect or culpable party, local authorities were responsible for gathering evidence needed to prosecute in a criminal trial. One significant difference between the nineteenth-century coroner and those of today is that Waddell would have had authority to remand suspects in a possible murder, to be kept by police until the verdict of death was reached. Suspects were also allowed to be held without any formal charges for an indefinite amount of time. It is important to note that the accused had not yet been formally charged with any crime and evidence was often lacking at this early stage in the investigation. Suspects are recorded often in newspapers as being present at the inquests although never providing any testimony on their own behalf. This must have been an uncomfortable situation for surviving family members to set their eyes upon the possible killer, but also for those suspects who were innocent of any crime.

In the case of suicides, which were carried out in several ways: hanging, self-inflicted gunshot wounds, knife wounds and drowning, family members might request that the verdict be changed to 'death by misadventure', 'death by strangulation' or even 'death by natural causes' to protect the reputation of the deceased and prevent shame being brought upon the family. Most modern coroners report that providing the most accurate description of death is the most important issue at hand. It is an uncomfortable and difficult position for all parties, but most will conclude an inquest with an accurate verdict explaining the exact cause of the death of the deceased, especially in cases describing that death resulted from suicide. From reviewing Waddell's verdicts, it appears he may have been under pressure to lessen the actual cause of death or to be vague in his description of some suicides. It is a reasonable assumption considering that coroners today are also challenged by surviving family members in cases of suicide.

WILDE TALES
Concealing the Truth or Protecting the Innocent?

In recording his inquests, Waddell frequently transcribed different spellings of various names: Kieff instead of Keefe, Mcgloan or Maglone rather than McGlone, Donnelly for O'Donnell. For a modern day researcher attempting to determine the spelling of a name, it is safe to assume that the correct spelling can be determined by its phonetic pronunciation. At a time in Irish history when many of the lower classes did not know how to read or write, the spelling of the name of the de-

ceased was irrelevant to the bereaved. The dead were recorded simply for the record and for the Crown to keep track of their expenses.
However, sometimes a name was deliberately misspelled to protect
the family name and the reputations of those involved. One such example is the inquiry into the deaths of Mary and Emily Wilde, the
illegitimate daughters of Sir William Wilde, prominent surgeon and
scholar as well as the father of literary genius, Oscar Wilde. Sir William wrote to Waddell requesting that not a lot of attention be drawn
to the cases and that only an inquiry into the deaths be conducted,
not formal inquests. His request was granted. Additionally, Mary and
Emily Wilde's deaths were recorded in his casebook as 'Wylie' rather
than Wilde so as not to draw attention to the sensitive matter of their
illegitimacy. [See chapter five for the burning deaths of Mary and
Emily Wilde].

Although the concealment involved little but a name change
and a less public forum for discussion, would it not be fair to question
if one should alter the legal documents of death even once – might
they repeat the same offence if enough pressure was applied in other
situations? Were there other inquests in which Waddell did not record an inquest accurately as he was under pressure? Ultimately, a verdict of death was only as reliable as the investigation, evidence, coroner and jury that decided upon it. It is here we begin to get an idea
of Waddell's nature and standing as a gentleman. The death of the girls
appears straightforward. They died as a result of a tragic accident. He
doesn't appear to have compromised the investigation in any way and
certainly not the verdict of death. It was simply the courteous and
proper thing to do, especially given the sensitive nature of the job he
had to perform. Waddell was human. He made his decision based on
the personal request of the girls' father as well as accepting what it
meant to be a *gentleman* in the Victorian age. This case and others
like it, prompt the inquisitive mind of the contemporary reader to
examine the details recorded and question those that are absent from
the coroner's casebook. It is important to raise questions and attempt
to uncover the answers when the evidence presented does not appear
to best answer *how* the deceased died.

EXAMINING THE PHYSICAL EVIDENCE
Doctors and Autopsies

Doctors conducting autopsies in the nineteenth century were not ex-
perts in the field of pathology or forensic medicine. Most were local

country doctors who were called upon to perform post-mortem examinations to determine the cause of death. This procedure varied depending upon the practitioner and the circumstances of the inquest.

A thorough post-mortem examination would be similar to that of today, following a routine procedure. Before the autopsy begins, the body is weighed and measured. The corpse must be placed on a table where it is allowed to drain and secrete fluids. The body is positioned with a 'body block' under the back of the body that pushes the chest forward and the arms and neck fall backwards to allow a series of incisions to be made more easily. The first cut is down the front of the torso from the base of the neck down to the pubic bone. Next a cut is made from the front of each shoulder to the bottom of the breastbone. This is known as the 'Y' incision. The incision is deep enough to cut through all layers of skin to expose all the internal organs. The skin is then peeled back with the top flap of the 'Y' falling over the face. The ribs are sawn off to expose the internal organs surrounding the chest. All the major internal organs are removed from the body and weighed. It is at this stage that any irregularities in the appearance or odour of the internal organs or tissues are scrutinised. The extent to which this stage of examination was carried out in Ireland in the post-famine era depended upon the skills of the practitioner and the conditions under which the body was being evaluated. Many of the post-mortem examinations in Waddell's casebook were not as thorough as described above.

There were two different types of examinations of cadavers by country doctors. When a physician was called to testify at an inquest, he often gave evidence of having conducted an external examination of the body. For example, Dr Reid deposed to having examined the body of Peter Moorehead, a victim of drowning. He stated that there were no marks of injury and from its appearance and the evidence adduced, he considered his death to have resulted from drowning while in a state of intoxication.[32] Dr Reid's assessment of the body was a result of observation rather than completion of an autopsy. In contrast, when a post-mortem examination was ordered, details of the state of the wounds and dissection were available in the transcript of the inquest. Most began with an exterior examination of the corpse, identifying and commenting on items such as surroundings, clothing, posture, or any marks on the body that were visible. Although a routine inspection of the body would include the primary cut opening the thorax and abdomen, along with a tactile inspection of the lungs, heart, diaphragm, peritoneum, colon, liver, intestines, spleen, pelvis,

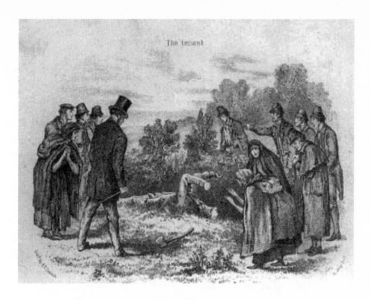

A dead body is found in the countryside.
(Trench, Realities of Irish Life, 1868)

retroperitoneal structures, thoracic cavity, diaphragm, omentum and pericardium and then a full examination of all the major organs of the body including heart, brain, sex organs, kidneys, etc. Each varied depending upon the doctor's experience and the circumstances of the inquest. Surprisingly, of the many deaths recorded in the coroner's casebook, it appears that *only sixty-eight post-mortem examinations were performed* over the twenty years from 1856 to 1876. Their descriptions and details range from pulling back the scalp for further investigation of a head wound or a complete examination of the internal organs. In the event of an exhumation, the post-mortem was recorded as having taken place while the corpse lay in the casket at the gravesite. It is unclear if only the necessary details were recorded for post-mortems or if the procedure was dictated by what the practitioner was looking for in regard to the cause of death.

Clarifying the Cause of Death
The Death of Richard Steenson, Drumcall, Ematris Parish, February 1875
In the neighbourhood of Drumcall a man named Steenson died under what had been considered suspicious circumstances. On Friday morning in February of 1875, he was on a hunt with four other companions. The men then drank in a roadside public house, two glasses and a half of whiskey to each man. When the men separated, Steen-

son was believed to have taken a pint of whiskey with him to continue drinking. The next morning, Steenson was found insensible in
the yard of a stranger's house at a considerable distance from the road
and never regained consciousness. He died on Saturday evening. A
report soon spread that the deceased met with foul play and the police
began an investigation. Some men were even arrested as suspects.[33]

Although many witnesses testified, it was still unclear what motive anyone would have had to bring harm to Richard Steenson. Dr
Clarke gave evidence that he had seen Steenson a few short hours before his death. His extremities were cold, he was insensible and his
pulse was weak. The post-mortem examinations were conducted by
Dr Moore, Dr Mulholland and Dr Clarke.

Dr Moore reported the findings. He first looked for any marks on
the body and only found a slight abrasion on the lip. As the dissection began, he removed the scalp from the bone. 'We saw nothing unnatural. We then removed the upper part of the skull to examine the
brain and its membranes. On removing the upper portion of the skull
about two or three ounces of dark liquid blood escaped. The blood vessels on the surface of the brain were gorged and congested with dark
blood. The substance of the larger brain appeared healthy. In the substance of the smaller brain was a smaller quantity of extravasated
blood,' stated Dr Moore.[34] 'I believe the deceased died of extravasation and congestion of the brain. We examined the stomach, liver and
spleen without detection of anything unnatural or unhealthy.' Since
there was no evidence presented that there was any cracking or damage to the skull, it did not appear that Steenson was hit on the head.
He appeared to have died as the result of an aneurysm.

Although testimony of heavy drinking and possible violence the
night before Steenson's death was presented, as well as suspects held
in custody by local police, the investigation was ended by the verdict
of the inquest. The coincidental circumstances were left just as that
– the verdict of death was extravasation and congestion of the brain
and that the deceased had not received violence or injury of any kind.[35]
The evidence produced from the post-mortem had ultimately determined the outcome.

The inquests in which a post-mortem examination was ordered
were deaths in which one or more persons might be liable. These included high profile murder cases, horse and cart accidents occurring
on the road and on fair-days, sudden death involving suspicious circumstances, women dying as a result of childbirth and infant death.
42% of the post-mortem examinations in the coroner's casebook were

performed on infants. Most were babies that could not be identified and it was the duty of the coroner to determine a cause of death as well as to arrange a coffin and grave-digger to bury the unknown child. In high profile murder inquests such as the double homicide of the Shaw Brothers, two post-mortem examinations were done on each body. The cause of death was obvious since both brothers had been shot about the face, head and chest, but the case caused great distress in the district and it was of the utmost importance that it be most thoroughly investigated. The two medical opinions shed more light on the circumstances surrounding the murders, such as the likelihood of there being more than one shooter and the range and distance of the killers to their victims; and it offered more evidence of the motives behind the shootings – based upon the nature of the wounds on the bodies.

Today, doctors who perform autopsies in Ireland are pathologists who specialise in dissecting and analysing the state of the corpse. They take into consideration all physical factors that may have contributed to the death and, through the years these techniques have evolved. One aspect of nineteenth-century post-mortem examinations is that they were random. They were not carried out in many cases where it appears further examination would have yielded more information about the cause of death. It is important to remember that forensic medicine was in its early stages of development, and ordering a post-mortem at all inquests would not have yielded any new findings because that evidence was not being understood in the same way as it is today. Modern DNA is a good reminder of how we as a society have evolved in the art of determining causes of death scientifically. Areas such as toxicology, forensic psychology and criminal investigation including examination of fingerprints have encouraged more specific outcomes of how death occurred as well as creating a profile of murderers.

JEALOUSY, GREED AND ARSENIC
Add a Little Spice to Life

Homicidal poisoning was not an unusual phenomenon in the nineteenth century. Many different plants, herbs and flowers were used to kill unsuspecting victims and metallic poisons such as strychnine or arsenic were easily purchased. These substances were available in most households where they were used to remove rodents and other pests.

When poisoning was suspected, doctors performing post-mortem examinations began by looking at the stomach, oesophagus, intestines and other internal organs for inflammation or blood in areas that might indicate poison as the catalyst for the death. If the physical evidence was unusual or suspicious, organs and fluids were sent off for testing to chemists in the hope of uncovering some such substance. As previously mentioned, Professor John Hodges, lecturer in Medical Jurisprudence at Queen's University Belfast was dedicated to the science of chemistry and completed all chemical analysis sent to him by Waddell.

The onset of signs and symptoms in a person who has been poisoned by arsenic or any metallic or non-metallic irritant, varies depending upon the dosage administered. With arsenic, when a large dosage has been given or acute poisoning has occurred, symptoms usually appear within half an hour to an hour. If a victim is poisoned over time, symptoms of chronic poisoning will appear such as gradual loss of weight, hair loss, loss of appetite; the tongue may be reddened or covered with a thick white coating, but the symptoms prior to death will be the same. Severe pains in the abdominal area or burning in the oesophagus is associated with continuous and painful vomiting and diarrhoea.[36] Another symptom that can arise is constipation. The vomited matter at first consists of normal stomach contents, but later becomes just bile. In some cases, it may be of a 'coffee-grounds' appearance due to altered blood. The victim would suffer from 'an insatiable thirst' and drinking water or any other fluid would only make vomiting more intense. The face of a person poisoned by arsenic is anxious, pinched and the skin cold and clammy. Death occurs by convulsions, coma or cardiac failure. When a post-mortem examination was conducted as transcribed in Waddell's casebook, an inflamed oesophagus, stomach and intestines would be a warning sign of poisoning. An inquest where any of these symptoms were described would be considered suspicious and require further inquiry.

Poisons were not often detected by the intended victims. Arsenic is virtually impossible to detect by appearance, taste or smell when dissolved in very hot or boiling water, such as tea, hot milk or cocoa, gruel or porridge. It is only when it cools that arsenic will become sedimented and the milk and gruel curdled. Therefore persons unknowingly ingesting arsenic would have eaten or drunk quickly with little or no interruption and have had no reason to question what was placed in front of them. One must then ask: Who would likely be a suspect in poisoning cases?

Poisoning usually takes place when someone knows another person very well – it is usually a very close friend or family member who is the murderer. The reason for this is simple – they have access to the food, they are trusted and their motives have gone undetected. They are too close to be suspected. Poisoning was believed to be a characteristic of the female murderer as she would have access to the food, and, as the cook or housekeeper, she would not be held under suspicion by her intended victim. Men with motive to kill might receive help from wives, mothers, sisters or female servants to administer the deadly dosage.

Hot Burning in her Stomach and 'Insatiable Thirst'
The Death of Elisabeth Crawley,
Carrickmacross, Magheross Parish, October 1867
In October of 1867, Elisabeth Crawley was a healthy young woman twenty-nine years of age, married and pregnant with her unborn child due in six weeks time. Although this should have been a harmonious time in her life, it wasn't. It appeared that she and her husband did not have a happy marriage. Her closest friends knew that she was in the habit of drinking heavily, she regularly slept in one of the outhouses[37] and her husband on many occasions had threatened to send her back to her father's home. It was said that her husband, Mr Crawley, was a kind man when she kept from drink. On the other hand, there is no information available as to his disposition when she became intoxicated.

On the evening of 11 October, Elisabeth had been drinking and had gone into one of the outhouses to sleep. Whether deliberately or mistakenly, she left one of her children unattended and an accident occurred. The young child got too close to the hearth fire, was engulfed in flames and died soon after from the severe burns received.

Four days after the fatal event, Elisabeth entered the dwelling house where her husband resided. She was very sick and vomiting continuously. Although the family at first considered that she was ill as a result of alcohol, they soon discovered she was sober. Her husband sent for Dr Taggert and Dr Duffy who promptly attended to her. Elisabeth complained of inward pain and some whey was made to settle her stomach. She immediately vomited up the food. The vomiting continued relentlessly. The suffering woman repeatedly called out for cold water to 'cool the burning pain inside her'.

Ann McDonnell, a qualified professional birthing attendant with a diploma in midwifery from the Rotunda of Dublin was called to see

Elisabeth. When the midwife arrived she found her vomiting, complaining of a great burning in her stomach and calling constantly for
cold water. She gave Elisabeth some of the medicine that was ordered by her attending doctor over the next few days. In evaluating her
patient, McDonnell stated that vomiting was not 'an attendant circumstance on being in the family way'.

It soon became clear that Elisabeth was not going to recover. Expecting death to be likely, Dr Duffy and the coroner carefully collected a portion of the vomited matter to be tested for possible poisons.
Elisabeth Crawley died on 19 October 1867. A post-mortem examination was conducted immediately. Her lungs, heart and liver were healthy,
but it was the region of the gullet, stomach and duodenum, the upper
part of the intestines where the problems were found. The stomach
was partially inflamed and distinctly at the opening part of the gullet.
The bowels had been restricted, and from the autopsy they found that
the upper parts of the intestines were slightly congested.

A chemical analysis of the stomach and other matter was sent to
Dr John Hodges of Belfast. He returned his report stating he could not
discover any poison or traces of it. The verdict was death from natural causes but under such suspicious circumstances so as to cause the
jury to require an analysis of the stomach.[38]

Was Elisabeth Crawley murdered? It appeared that Elisabeth had
unknowingly ingested something that burned and inflamed the inside
of her throat, stomach and intestine. It is unusual that there was no
mention of her unborn child or regard to the foetus; however it might
illustrate that medical professionals and the coroner were convinced
that her pregnancy was not a contributing factor in her death. So
how could the tests that Dr Hodges ran detect no traces of poison? By
1830, chemical analysis could detect most mineral compounds, but
not organic poison.[39] If a herb, flower or plant was used, it is possible
he was unable to find it within the tissues and samples provided.

An example of poisoning by an organic substance exists in the
inquest of Rose O'Neill of Latlorcan in 1862. Rose probably took something such as Savin, made from the shrub *Juniperus Sabina*, which grows
everywhere in the world and is the most common poisonous plant
used to bring about abortions. At high doses, it causes convulsions, haemorrhages, vomiting and convulsive coma, which were her symptoms
prior to death. Although a post-mortem was performed on Rose
O'Neill's body and samples were sent to Dr Hodges, these also were
returned with a negative result.[40]

Another possible reason for not finding any toxic substances in the body of Elisabeth Crawley is that not enough of the poison was in the samples tested. Although arsenic is an element, which means that it cannot be broken down further, and is known to be able to be detected years after a person has died, it is found in such body parts as hair, fingernails and urine. In none of the cases of tissues samples taken were these sent for testing. The Reinch's test used by Dr Hodges is known to fail to take up all the arsenic which may be present in the suspected material.[41]

In trying to determine the matters of the case, one must ask: who would want Elisabeth Crawley dead? Clearly her husband did not appear happy with her drinking problem. It was documented that they were unhappy and he may have blamed her for the death of the child who had been burned a few days prior to her death. Contrary to the possible motives, he did contact two doctors and the midwife from the Rotunda to aid in her possible recovery. However, the testimony of one witness raises suspicion. Mary McEneny was questioned by the coroner and explained that she was present when Elisabeth returned home on 11 October and remained there until the death of the child the next day. She also insisted she was only occasionally in the house on 15 October and had been present when Elisabeth appeared that day with a 'tossed appearance'. She confirmed she was indeed present on the day that Elizabeth became ill. One detail was curious. She told the coroner that she had seen Elisabeth drink and gave her alcohol unknown to her husband. Did Elisabeth's drinks contain more than just alcohol?

EXHUMING BODIES
Waking the Dead for Evidence

The cases which call for exhumation are always unpleasant, and in most cases, disgusting, proceeding where a suspicion of poisoning or violence has arisen some little time after burial of the supposed victim ... no post-mortem should ever be conducted on an empty stomach.

H. Aubrey Husband,
The Students Handbook of Forensic Medicine and Medical Police

When Waddell decided that there was just cause to remove a body from the ground, he conducted a comprehensive investigation. Before examining those inquests where a body was exhumed, it is important to attempt to understand how the coroner determined one case might yield this necessity, while others did not. Some examples of the coroner deciding against exhumation include situations where the deceased was involved in excessive drinking and disorderly behaviour prior to death, previous long-term illnesses and children who had died from burns received in apparent household accidents. It is very clearly stated in many inquests of a suspicious nature that the deceased were 'in good standing with their family' and therefore, the body was not exhumed. One such inquiry was the death of an old man, John McCabe of Shelvins. He had died suddenly, shortly after being engaged in drawing turf, and the coroner was late in being notified – approximately a week after the burial. When Waddell investigated he discovered that McCabe lived 'in good turns' with his family and that he could attach no suspicion to any person. This detail, along with the evidence produced, resulted in a dismissal of exhumation or inquest.[42] Other inquiries more clearly support this consideration. More than once Waddell made a statement similar to the following: 'No suspicion of ill treatment, neglect or foul play can be attached to his wife or any other party, and the deceased being ten or twelve days interred, I did not consider it right or necessary to exhume the body for the purpose of holding an inquest.'[43]

Bearing in mind the feelings of the family was another consideration when deciding to unearth a recently departed relation. Waddell was under pressure to make sure the inquiry into death was in the best interests of the deceased as well as that of the law and justice, while at the same time being respectful of the bereaved relatives. There had been a delay in his notification regarding the death of a young girl, Margaret Curley of Rossnaglogh. By the time Waddell reached the family, the child had already been buried. Margaret died as a result of burns received when she went too close to the fire while stirring the breakfast. She'd been left alone with two of her brothers and sisters while her mother went to mass. Her father had gone directly to Dr Moore of Rockcorry for medicine and treatment, but having lingered painfully for several days, she died. Having spoken to the father and Dr Moore, Waddell was satisfied that there was no reason to exhume the body. There was no suspicion and having interviewed the distraught and grieving family members, he was satisfied.[44]

The word of the local clergy was considered reasonable doubt for further inquiry. While the coroner was inquiring about a man named Dunlop, the Revd William Cooke, minister of the Presbyterian church at Drumkeen, told Waddell that although Dunlop had died very suddenly the man had been 'very poorly the previous week and although not visited by a doctor, he considered his death arose from heart disease'. This testimony was enough for the coroner to end his inquiry into the man's death. Waddell noted that he did not think it necessary or right to exhume the body as it would have been 'most painful to the feelings of the family and an expense to the county not required'.[45]

Suspicious deaths requiring a body to be exhumed could prove expensive. Additional expenses would include grave-diggers' fees for disinterment and re-burial, one or more post-mortem examinations, sending tissues to Dr Hodges of Belfast for analysis and likely additional travelling expenses for the coroner. Such expenses were necessary to obtain a more accurate cause of death. One inquest as seen in Waddell's expense report was listed as follows: Dr Hodges (£5.5.0), Dr Reid (£2.2.0), Dr Moore (£2.2.0) and Dr Rush (£1.1.0); Poor Witnesses (£1.1.0); Raising and Re-interring the deceased (£0.5.0); Accommodation for jury, 3 days (£0.10.6) and Coroner's Fee and Travelling Expenses (£2.2.0). Deciding to dig up the deceased was a carefully made decision. It usually required a large amount of testimony and evidence pointing towards a murder suspect and it would be reasonable to assume that Waddell was expected to produce results in order to justify these expenditures.

Serial Murder in Aghabog? – Digging up the Evidence
Investigating the Deaths of Livingston, McCarter and the Wrights
January and February 1863
The following four inquests, each requiring the body to be exhumed, illustrate one of the largest investigations in Waddell's career. Considering only *nine* exhumations were conducted out of the hundreds of inquests throughout the casebook, it is a startling occurrence.[46] In January and February of 1863, the coroner ordered the exhumation of four bodies – one right after another – from the nearly adjoining townlands of Rakeevan and Drumbrean in the parish of Aghabog. Most unusual was that the deaths were thought to be related and that one or more persons were responsible for the deaths. The case was riddled with rumour and suspicion. Waddell proceeded forward either having been convinced of an outcome of foul play, or in an attempt to quiet and extinguish the fear in the neighbourhood. One other possibility exists – his suspicions were unfounded, he was wrong and a very expensive series of inquests were carried out and paid for by the taxpayers of Co. Monaghan.

On 1 January 1863, William Livingston died suddenly at the home of his sister, Tabitha McCarter, in the townland of Rakeevan. He had just moved in with Tabitha and her adult children, William and Ann McCarter, just three days earlier and his death came as a surprise to all, even taking his advanced age of eighty-six into consideration. The family was still grieving as Tabitha's husband, John McCarter, had just died less than three months earlier. Now her brother had died suddenly and an inquest was held the next day. Waddell arrived to interview the relatives.

Tabitha McCarter told the coroner that her brother had just come to live with her a few days earlier and had been the caretaker at Drumbrean for Mr Brady of Clones. On Monday, 29 December 1862, Livingston took dinner and some light stirabout for supper. After the meal he complained of not feeling well. Over the next two days he was not eating at all, only some new milk, warmed with pepper on it. Tabitha claimed that her brother had showed no signs of sickness, certainly no vomiting, other than being tired. By the early hours of Thursday morning, William was up in the middle of the night calling for a drink to his niece Ann who retrieved one for him. He'd risen to go to the pot (toilet) and went to bed again. At 6a.m. while he was sleeping with his nephew, Livingston died. William told the coroner he had his arms about his uncle when he departed life. The verdict was death from natural causes.[47]

Within three weeks, Tabitha, William and Ann McCarter were arrested for suspicion of murder and held on police custody. Waddell ordered the body of William Livingston to be exhumed from its resting place at Drumkeen Graveyard. The corpse of the old man was taken out of the ground and both Dr Reid and Dr Moore of Rockcorry conducted post-mortem examinations.

It was clear to both physicians performing the autopsy that something artificial had brought about the old man's death. The bowels presented an unhealthy and inflammatory appearance with a considerable amount of blood in the cavity of the abdomen; the intestines presented a turgid appearance. Dr Reid told the coroner that the stomach portion of intestines, liver and kidneys were preserved for analysis and were being sent to Belfast to be tested by Dr Hodges. Although Dr Reid was unable to state the cause of death, he considered it was *not* from natural causes. Dr Moore concurred stating, 'I consider the death of the deceased would be accounted for by the highly inflammatory state of the bowels. The absence of decomposition that is very remarkable considers [sic] a very suspicious circumstance.' Decomposition does not take place quickly when a person has been poisoned with arsenic.

As Waddell and the police continued to gather evidence in the case, three new witnesses came forward. Their evidence contradicted that of Tabitha, William and Ann McCarter and clearly something wasn't adding up. Ann Boyle worked at Tabitha McCarter's house in Rakeevan scutching flax and was present when the deceased, William Livingston, was there. She told the coroner's jury that Livingston had been complaining of not feeling well and stayed to his bed most of the time. Her evidence about one evening that Livingstone was ill did not match up with Tabitha McCarter's. Boyle stated that she had seen William vomiting on several occasions, whereas his sister stated he had not been sick once.

The scutcher also added, 'The deceased took his breakfast of stirabout in Mrs McCarter's with me, but *'twas after he came back from Drumbrean* in the course of the day that he said he was ill,' she said. 'The deceased purged both Tuesday and Wednesday night. On Thursday morning early, he arose to go to the pot but for what purpose, I cannot say. This was about 5a.m. and after that he lay down and I heard him snoring in his sleep.'

The second witness, Biddy Keelan, was also a scutcher for Mrs McCarter working at the house from the time the old man arrived at the McCarter home in Rakeevan until the morning of his death. She did not see the deceased but she could hear him coughing and vomiting throughout the night.

'On Thursday morning, about 5a.m., I heard him call for a drink which Ann McCarter arose to give to him. After this I fell asleep and as I awoke around 7a.m., I heard someone exclaiming that the deceased was dead and William McCarter jumped out on the floor from the bed,' said Keelan.

The third witness to give evidence was James Foster, husband of Sophia McCarter. Sophia was a daughter of Tabitha and the late John McCarter, and sister to William and Ann. Her husband was summoned to provide a deposition that would not prove favourable for her family. Foster told the jury that just seven months earlier in July 1862 he was asked by William McCarter to buy him 2d. worth of sleeping drops from the apothecary in Newbliss. In return, William McCarter would mow his meadow for him. Foster agreed and went to Matthew Hall, the apothecary in Newbliss.

The sleeping drops referred to were laudanum, a variant of opium. Laudanum was regularly taken for various illnesses. As a narcotic, it was highly addictive, however it was 'watered down' in small doses and a lethal dose would have produced much different symptoms from those described. It is for this purpose that the chemical analysis requested by Waddell from Professor Hodges was in search of opium as he considered it might have been the cause of the death. Determining whether it was deliberately given or accidentally taken would be decided in a criminal trial. The depositions now given by Foster would show a possible motive for murder.

James Foster told the coroner and jury that he'd gone to purchase the laudanum from Mathew Hall of Newbliss. He received only half the amount he requested and the apothecary explained that 1d. worth or 60 drops (25 to 30 drops in a dose) would be sufficient to help someone sleep and do them no harm. The most controversial testimony was what Foster had told the apothecary that day. Foster had told Hall that McCarter wanted the drops to put Livingston to *sleep*; that Livingston was a 'watch' for a sister of McCarter's who had married against the mind of her family. He added that the McCarter family wished to carry away some of the sister's property.

'I told Hall this because William McCarter had told this to me,' he said. 'I got the laudanum from Hall and gave it to William McCarter.'

William McCarter being the principal farmer of the land since his father's death just three months earlier may have been threatened by his uncle coming into the house as a 'spy' for one of his siblings.

Dr Hodges' report was returned and read at the next continuation of the inquest held on 11 February 1863. It appeared as follows:

The Report of Professor Hodges of Belfast on the Analysis:
The case of the late William Livingston, Co. Monaghan

Sir,
On Wednesday 21st I received from Sergeant Paul Hunter of Newbliss, Co. Monaghan:

1. A bottle closed with bladder tied
2. A delft pot tied on with bladder and sealed.

These were stated to contain a stomach and portion of the viscera of the late William Livingston which a letter from W. Charles Waddell, Esq., coroner directed to be submitted to chemical examination, a second letter from the coroner dated 24th suggested opium as the probable cause of death.

Having devoted some days to the examination of the various re-agents apparatus and to be employed in the analyses, I opened the vessels and found in the bottle a stomach received by ligatures and containing about 4oz of a dark orange fluid of the consistence of thick gruel and a portion of intestines also secured by ligatures.

The pot contained a liver and a kidney.

The stomach on being examined was found of a bright red colour both on the external and internal coals. The inner lining exhibited a high degree of inflammatory action and yellow lines were observed in several parts such as are characteristic of the presence of sulphurate of Arsenic which is sometimes produced after death by the action of sulphurated hydrogen gas evolved by putrifaction on Arsenic; believing therefore that the condition of the stomach indicated the probable presence of Arsenic, I directed my attention to its discovery.

The contents of the stomach, about 1oz of the liquid being employed, 5oz of the liver and about 1oz of the substance of the stomach were submitted to separate examinations. In each case, new vessels and acids were used. From all the substances examined, I was able to obtain by the process of Reinsch, abundant deposits of metallic arsenic. The identity of metal being subsequently verified by the production from it of crystallised arsenius acid which when dissolved in distilled water and tested by the addition to separate portions of sulphurate hydrogen and hydrochloric acid, ammoniacal nitrate of silver and ammoniacal sulphate of copper gave the characteristic reactions. My opinion therefore is that the portions of the body of the late William Livingston placed in my hands contain a considerable amount of *Arsenic*.

I am Sir,
Your Obedient Servant,
John F. Hodges, MD
Professor Medical Jurisprudence,
Belfast 29 January 1863.

Livingston had been poisoned by an acute dose of arsenic. When a large amount of arsenic is ingested, the symptoms can appear within an hour. The deceased had displayed all the symptoms of poisoning – chronic vomiting, weakness and a burning pain in the stomach increasing his desire for water. All this information had been previously kept quiet by the McCarter family. The inquest of William Livingston ended with a verdict of death from arsenic given to the deceased by some person or persons unknown.[48]

It was at this point that Waddell made another decision. Actually, he made three. He ordered the exhumations of three more bodies after the results of the tests proved that Livingston had been poisoned. They were John McCarter, late of Rakeevan, husband of Tabitha McCarter and father of William and Ann and two others, the late Thomas Wright and his wife, Sarah Wright, both of Drumbrean. The family were not only under suspicion for the murder of Livingston, but were now considered to have murdered their own husband and father and two other persons who also appear to have been relatives. Reports stated that 'a very heinous case of wholesale poisoning' was being investigated and that three other persons who died under the same circumstances were now being exhumed by the coroner.[49] One can only wonder: Was the decision to exhume John McCarter, Thomas Wright and Sarah Wright based upon the information or pressure he received from local police? Or was it his own investigation into the deaths, interviews with witnesses, neighbours and family members that made him follow a 'hunch' or his own intuition that one or more persons in the McCarter family were capable of killing not once – but four times?

Just two days after arsenic was discovered to have killed Livingston, the body of John McCarter was removed from the Drumkeen graveyard.

The Inquest of John McCarter,
Rakeevan, Aghabog Parish, February 1863

John McCarter's body was raised from the ground at the Drumkeen graveyard. He died in October 1862 and it appeared from his post-mortem examination that there were some unusual findings. Dr Moore found 'an injected state of blood vessels in the intestines and stomach' but what he found unusual was a quantity of blood serum (about five or six ounces) lodged in the cavity of the abdomen. Dr Moore said, 'The stomach did not present an appearance of inflammation, but blood serum in the cavity of the abdomen is not a natural thing to meet in the body of a deceased person.' Several samples were sent to Dr Hodges of Belfast to be tested. Regardless of this outcome, Waddell went forward in his quest to uncover the truth about the deaths of Thomas and Sarah Wright.

Looking for Evidence of Murder
The Wrights of Aghabog Parish

One week after the exhumation of John McCarter, the two bodies of an elderly couple who died two years apart, Thomas and Sarah Wright were exhumed at the Aghabog Church of Ireland, located just down the road from the Drumkeen Presbyterian church where Livingston and McCarter were buried. Sarah's body was exhumed just a few days before her husband. As they removed the body from the grave, the coroner, Dr Reid, Dr Robinson, the Revd Ellis Turely, JP and the Revd Alexander Goudy Ross, curate of Aghabog parish, watched the coffin rise. It was clear that they had the right body. Mr James Crawford stated that he had been the grave-digger who interred her coffin into the ground and had nailed in the breastplate that now read 'Sarah

Wright, aged 77 years. Deceased 20 March 1862'. They found the corpse in an advanced stage of decomposition and, on opening the abdomen, found one pint of blood serum. The necessary samples were taken and sent to Professor Hodges.

At the inquest that followed, one key witness was subpoenaed to offer testimony as to the circumstances surrounding the death of the old woman. Mary Gordan told the coroner that she had lived with Sarah Wright for two years. The old woman had been ill for just three weeks before her death and was attended by a woman named Letitia throughout that illness. Letitia prepared all Sarah's food and drinks and gave them to her.

'I was not allowed to be in the room alone with my mistress who often wished to see me. She was also not allowed to see her minister, Revd Mr William Cooke,' Gordan said. The Revd William Cooke had even called to the house to see Sarah just a few days before her death and was not permitted inside by Letitia.

Gordan went on, 'There had been a plate in the buttery with poison on it prepared for putting into stacks for mice and a few days before Mrs Wright's death, I saw the same plate in Letitia's hand quite clean. Previous to her death, Sarah was subject to both purging and vomiting and to such a degree 'twas hard to keep the bed clean around her.'

Thomas Wright's body was not easy to find. It took several attempts digging up three different holes and checking coffins to finally unearth that which was inscribed 'Thomas Wright. Died 15 December 1860. Aged 87 years'. James Clarke, the grave-digger remembered the breastplate clearly as it was he that had nailed it on the coffin on the night the body was interred. The wooden box was opened and the post-mortem carried out at the gravesite while the decomposed body of Thomas Wright remained in the coffin. Dr Andrew Robinson of Newbliss and Dr Moore of Rockcorry found the body in a very advanced stage of decomposition. They removed the liver, spleen and other portions of the abdomen which they placed in jars to be examined by Dr Hodges of Belfast.

The inquests of John McCarter, Sarah Wright and Thomas Wright were continuously adjourned and a date was set for 25 March 1863 when the results of the chemical analysis would be read out for all three cases at the same time. When the results were returned, it became clear that proving murder would be impossible. *No traces of metallic poison could be found in any of the samples of the suspected murder victims.* All three inquests resulted in verdicts of death from natural causes.[50]

Tabitha, Ann and William McCarter were released from police custody as no further mention of charges appeared in the newspaper or in any archival records. It appears that although arsenic was found to have contributed to the death of William Livingston, it could not be proved by what means or by whom the poison was administered. The fact that the family was not convicted for the murder of Livingston is further assumed by death and marriage records. In the years that followed Ann McCarter died at home in 1870 of glanders[51] at the age of forty and her mother, Tabitha died of old age on the farm in Rakeevan in 1876 at the age of eighty-five.[52] William McCarter not only inherited his father's land in Rakeevan, but land in several other townlands in 1863, the same year of the discovery of the murder of his uncle. He was married on 9 November 1866 to Maria McQuag of Aghnacue, a young woman from the townland adjoining his own.[53] William and Jane Gordan served as witnesses to the marriage held at the Aghabog Church of Ireland. William and Maria went on to have more than nine children, including one daughter named *Letitia*. Was this child named after a relative? And were these Gordans relations of Mary Gordan, the caretaker of Sarah Wright who believed that the woman named Letitia murdered her mistress? Coincidences and conjecture surrounding the death of any individual are not conclusive facts in determining a cause of death. A cause of death had been found for each person exhumed. The coroner could use only the facts from medical professionals to uncover the truth in any investigation.

But what went wrong? Did Waddell get carried away with circumstantial evidence provided by suspicious witnesses, pressure from local authorities; or attempt to prove this inevitable outcome only to quell the public's thirst for knowledge? Clearly he had uncovered the McCarter family to be less than honest about the symptoms experienced by Livingston and later, as the tests proved conclusively, that he had indeed ingested arsenic. But what information had he received after Livingston's inquest that prompted him to exhume three more bodies in connection with that case? Trying to reconstruct the information Waddell was privy to during the latter part of the investigation is difficult, if not impossible, after one hundred and forty years. The information is patchy, incidental and relationships between the parties involved can only be inferred from parish and civil records. One advantage that Waddell had over the investigator of today was that he knew the relationships between the parties, the familial bonds, and in speaking with those closest to these families had clearly developed his own theories and ideas – enough to order the exhumation of four persons within four weeks of one another.

When searching through the pieces of random, sometimes suspicious and inconclusive evidence one might just consider the following: Waddell was a thorough and careful coroner. He appeared always to err on the side of caution. In many examples of his own investigations and decision-making regarding whether or not to hold an inquest or exhume bodies that were already buried, he was careful to consider all options and possibilities. It seems highly unlikely that Waddell, in his thirty-year career as the coroner, had a momentary lapse of reason, became a zealot in his quest for the truth. He was steady, reliable and above all, a gentleman. The traces of evidence that remain to substantiate the information to which Waddell was privy are random and highly speculative, if not a creation of a researcher's mind almost two centuries later.

The one person who was poisoned was William Livingston and the question remained: Was he murdered? This would be left up to the criminal courts to prove based upon the evidence gathered at the inquests and throughout the investigation. It appears it was one or more members of the McCarter household. Not only was William McCarter found to have been trying to buy a prescription to give to his uncle to 'make him sleep' but also his mother and sister were found to be lying as to the extent of Livingston's sickness prior to his death. It appears each member of the family was attempting to cover up the facts. Tabitha McCarter, Livingston's own sister, had lied about his vomiting and serious symptoms in the days and hours up to his death. His niece Ann McCarter mentioned providing him with a drink of water, but failed to mention that he had an 'insatiable thirst' indicating that something more than an average sickness was to blame in his death. Possibly all three were threatened that Livingston was there as a 'spy' for a member of their immediate family, whom they had fallen out with, showing motive that one or more in the household were threatened by his presence. After all, it had been arranged for him to come and live with the family supporting the adage 'keep your friends close and your enemies closer'. He lived in the household for only three days. If he was murdered, this was something premeditated before he even came to stay.

Of the four persons whose bodies were exhumed and dissected for testing, only one was proved to have been poisoned. Due to the early testing techniques involved in uncovering poisons within the human body, it is possible that the arsenic found in William Livingston's body was due to the fact he had only recently died and the samples more readily contained the traces of the murderous substance. It is also possible that the three deaths where poison was not found were not only by natural causes but unrelated. Yet, giving the police and Waddell the benefit of the doubt, why suddenly four exhumations within a month, in the same area, with families belonging to the same small parish and community? Much of the evidence involving theories of murder and motive went undocumented in all four cases and it was left to the criminal court and judicial process to determine the fate of those suspected. Was Waddell deluded by the careful planning of one person or persons that sought to murder but went undiscovered?

The name Letitia (also spelled Leticia), although somewhat common in Presbyterian and Anglican records from the nineteenth century, is a curious choice, given the events prior to the birth of William McCarter's daughter. Is it possible he named her after a member of his family? The woman considered the suspect in the death of Sarah Wright was named Letitia. Her surname was a difficult name to transcribe. It appears that her last name might be McArdle, McArther,[54] McCarele or McCarter – in which event may prove that she was a member of the McCarter family of Rakeevan.

What was the McCarter family's connection to the Wrights? The name Thomas Wright appears in land records of 1860 in the townland of Drumbrean in relation to two adjoining plots of land. In one instance, a Thomas Wright sells his tenant right to Henry Hair, brother-in-law of the Revd William Cooke of the Drumkeen Presbyterian church. In the other instance, a Thomas Wright of Drumbrean appears to be renting land to a man named James Foster. As a matter of note, Sophia McCarter, daughter and sister of the accused McCarter family, was married to James Foster. Was this the same James Foster who was called to testify against the McCarter family? If these two were the same man, something close to the truth might imply that land or property was the motive to kill Thomas Wright. There is another possible connection of familial relation to consider. Just five years after the investigation into the deaths and murders of Livingston, McCarter and the Wrights, one unusual case appeared in the coroner's casebook. William Foster, a farmer from the townland of Drumbrean in the parish of Aghabog – who inherited his land from James Foster mentioned above – died under suspicious circumstances. One might consider his connection to the cases of Livingston, McCarter and the Wrights.

Arson on the Farm: Death by Grief or Arsenic?
The Death of William Foster, Drumbrean, November 1868
William Foster's health had greatly deteriorated over the past year. In 1866, he'd inherited land, more than twenty-two acres, from James Foster. Less than two years later all his hard work had been destroyed. His crop had been maliciously burned and he had been grief-stricken since. William told a member of his household, Margaret Manley, 'My heart was broke that Robert Wright was the man that done it [burned the crops] and might the Lord revere him for it.' He was renting the land from Thomas Wright and it appears that possibly the rest of the Wright family did not want him there.

On Thursday, 12 November 1868, William travelled to Newbliss to the Flax Market in good form. On returning home, he shared some bread and tea with his mother and Catherine McCann, possibly a servant in the household. That same night, William began vomiting. First up came the tea and bread, but, having regurgitated all the contents of his stomach, all that was left was yellow bile which he was now coughing up regularly. In the middle of the night, Manley was aroused out of bed on account of William being unwell. He told her he had an 'insatiable thirst'. The combination of his symptoms of vomiting and thirst was suspicious as they are consistent with arsenic poisoning.

Sam Foster, William's brother, found him looking very ill and sent for the doctor, but he did not arrive in time. Sam felt William's pulse but it was already gone and his feet were cold.

Dr Moore performed a post-mortem examination on William Foster. He determined that death arose from the inflammation of the stomach and bowels but from what cause, he could not say. The verdict of death was inflammation of the stomach and bowels.[55]

No tissue samples were sent to be analysed and there is no documentation available that suggests any further investigation into the death was made. Did William Foster die from 'natural causes' or is there someone who might have wanted him dead?

The troubles with his farm clearly affected his health and perhaps contributed to his death within a year after the event. Foster stating that his heart was broken 'that Robert Wright had done it' indicates a close relationship, possibly a kinship with Robert Wright. However, his sudden sickness raises some suspicion. Was William Foster poisoned? Did someone in the household want him gone so as to attempt to take over the farm? It was not a small holding, but instead was in excess of twenty-two acres. The land records show that after William Foster's death, the land at Drumbrean was transferred temporarily to a *Letitia* Foster and later the same year to the Revd William Cooke.

There are many unanswered questions that will likely never be conclusively proved and the theories appear unsubstantiated. Yet one might get a feeling for the position of the coroner, William Charles Waddell, when taking on such an investigation, took on the uncomfortable job of investigating a murder in a devoutly religious, private and tightly-knit community. Waddell was certainly a man of conviction and willing to step up to the tasks and duties expected of him in his role as a coroner. However, had the Aghabog exhumations of 1863 made him shy away from ordering chemical tests on the body of William Foster? As a matter of note, Waddell conducted only two more exhumations over the next thirteen years.

POLITICS AND POLICY
Little Pay and Less Respect

The Coroner's Bill
To the Editor of *The Northern Standard*
Sir – Would it not be an advantage to abolish the office of coroner instead of to increase the county rates by adding to the fees of these respected gentlemen? No doubt the office is ancient, but the altered circumstances of the present time would seem to obviate the necessity of continuing it as a separate office. In cases where inquiry as to a death might be necessary, provision could be made for the nearest magistrate to hold it.
Your obedient servant, a taxpayer,
9 March 1875.[56]

The coroner is an agent for the people, but not everyone agreed on the need for the office of the coroner in the nineteenth century. Some began to question why they as taxpayers were funding coroners to investigate death when the police and magistrates were perfectly capable of carrying out these duties. Since the coroner's inquest considered the liability of a suspect involved in death and then the process continued into criminal or civil court, it appeared to be somewhat of a duplication of efforts. On the other hand, if all public investigations into death were carried out by police who could be responsible for the prosecution of suspects at a later point in time, would it be possible for them to be objective? Or avoid corruption? Ultimately the public would not be able to trust such results. It would cast suspicion and doubts on the survivors of the deceased if police decided further inquiry was required. However, taxpayers (or ratepayers) were frustrated with any rise in costs (as seen in the above letter) and the salary of coroners around the country was being reviewed. It is likely that the 'altered circumstances' that the author in the above letter refers to is modern society and the fact that the coroner's office was beginning to look antiquated.

When Waddell took on the role of coroner, the minimal require-ments to hold the office were to be a resident of the district and to have the necessary 'property qualifications'. The Coroner's Act of 1846 established that the qualifications of coroner meant having *an estate of inheritance of the clear annual value of fifty pounds sterling ... or of an estate of freehold for his own life with a clear yearly value of one hundred pounds sterling ... situated within the district of which he is elected or chos-en to serve the office of coroner.* Such a large landholder would have the money necessary to pay fees to doctors, witnesses, travel expenses and any other items that were essential to perform the duties of the job until he was reimbursed at the next grand jury assizes. Additionally, the position required a man to be available twenty-four hours a day, to work on a part-time basis and to be living in the district. Moreover, it must be a man who could be relied upon. The coroner was paid a fixed fee per inquest, one pound one shilling (£1.1.0) and was reim-bursed approximately every three months for the expenses incurred. A coroner was paid from presentments made by the grand jury and levied from local taxpayers. If the grand jury did not agree with the expenses, or felt that the coroner had not used reasonable judgment in spending the money, they might contest payment. In July 1867, Mr Hugh Swanzy, the coroner of South Monaghan, appealed to the members of the grand jury that he and Waddell should receive the money for their expenses either upfront or within a more reasonable amount of time. Sir George Forster saw no objection to the proposal if they could get agreement from the rest of the members. But no change was made and the men were still required to pay for their own expen-ses and wait until the assizes for reimbursement.[57] In fact, even in the last years of his career as coroner, Waddell was not being fully reim-bursed for his work. In March 1876, Waddell, at the age of seventy-seven, having had experience of conducting inquests in well over 1,300 cases, was reprimanded for the costs of his inquests. He sub-mitted his expenses for holding inquests which totalled £70 17s 4d. Waddell was told by the committee that they recommended that he should only be paid the sum of £65. The law regarding payment of any coroner (with the exception of the Dublin City coroner) meant that at no one pay period between grand jury assizes was any coroner to be reimbursed a sum of more than £65. In addition to this, the grand jury cautioned him in 'employing medical men on inquests when the cause of death was apparent'.[58]

This lack of respect for his experience must have incensed Waddell for several reasons. Would he not know at this point in his long career the difference between death that appeared 'apparent' and one that looked 'suspicious' or was 'unknown'? Doctors who appeared at inquests were required to do so by law when requested to attend. They were paid a fixed fee of £1.1.0 for performing a post-mortem and £1.1.0 for testifying. Most doctors did not want to attend the inquests as it was not worth their time and effort. If the case was lengthy with several adjournments or taking one full workday, they were still paid the same flat fee. If the doctors were resisting, the coroner would have to persuade or encourage the doctor to participate and in the end pay for it out of his own pocket. Waddell had turned in expenses over the twenty years documented in the casebook that were much higher than £75 pounds. No documentation could be found to support that the difference was eventually paid by the Crown.

This system of expenses and fees withheld from coroners is an important concept in the outcome of many inquests and verdicts of death. When an inquest was held, often coroners steered the juries towards expedient or meaningless verdicts, partly through their own ignorance and partly to justify the decision against holding a post-mortem.[59] If a post-mortem was held without revealing new knowledge, could the coroners be held responsible for the fee themselves? The costs of inquests came from the county rates and coroners were always conscious that they might be disallowed. Justices maintained that inquests should only be held in cases of violent death, and breathed fire at those coroners who sought to extend them to cases of 'sudden' and 'unexplained' deaths.[60] It is for this reason that the inquests conducted by Waddell in these uncertain cases should be admired in that he was persistent and thorough in his investigation for the truth; and yet, at the same time, they should be carefully considered with an inquisitive and suspicious eye.

Conflicts of Interest
Witnesses, Doctors, Juries, Time and Money

Doctors were legally required to perform an autopsy and appear at the inquest to reveal the evidence if selected by the coroner to do so.

Although doctors take an oath to study medicine for the greater good of humanity, it is not unreasonable to assume that the time and effort necessary to attend inquests may have encouraged many physicians to expedite not only their often brief review of the body, but additionally the conclusions they drew from them. Asylums and public infirmaries had their own medical officers who most often were the primary witnesses providing testimony into the death of inmates. However, these medical men were not entitled to payment for their evidence at an inquest. This may have been an attempt to keep them *honest* as well as to keep the costs of the Crown to a minimum.

Doctors weren't the only participants that wanted an expedient end to an inquiry into a death. Juries were often steered into convenient verdicts by coroners, so that a post-mortem examination would be rendered useless as the verdict of death was obvious. This was a frequent occurrence in cases of infant deaths. Juries were notorious for returning neutral verdicts in cases of children found floating in water or who died from exposure, as it was well-known that it would be near impossible to find the mother who had killed her child. For example, one infant body found floating in the Ulster Canal in Monaghan town was examined by Dr A. K. Young. His testimony at the inquest revealed that he had viewed only the external marks on the body and stated that 'it was a full grown infant with no marks of violence, it had been born alive but the umbilical cord appeared to have been severed violently very close to the womb of the mother as if it had fallen from her while standing.'[61] Although the child had been placed in the water and drowned, knowing that it would prove an impossible task to find the mother, the coroner and jury returned a verdict that ensured the investigation into death ended there.

Inquests were also expedited in many instances when carried out at the Monaghan District Lunatic Asylum. Waddell was called on to conduct inquests of patients where the death was sudden and especially in cases of suicide. Although these inquests appear to have been conducted in the usual format, as the years went on Waddell wrote down only one line to record the verdict of death of asylum inmates. There could be several reasons for this occurrence. First, because the asylum would be considered to be a 'destination of no return', many persons admitted only left the walls to be buried due to disease; the public may have viewed this with fear and distrust. Additionally, because it was a public institution and the rates for its upkeep were paid by the taxpaying public, an investigation into many deaths only necessitated the arrival and judgement of the coroner. If only the coroner attended, his fee was the only expense to the Crown. His key witness or informant in these cases would have been the asylum doctor, matron or attendants.

Another reason why there may have been a rush to judgement in making a decision on a verdict of death was the time and effort required by the jury. There are many clear examples of the jury becoming frustrated with the time spent on inquests. One example of the jury members' reluctance to participate comes from a transcribed conversation taking place between two jury members before an inquest. At the inquest of Ann McDonald, an inmate of the Monaghan Poorhouse who fell into the hot water boilers while attending to her duties on the morning of 17 May 1872, two jurors were recorded as complaining at the start of the inquest:

> A Juror: Begor it's time I was out of this. I have my own business to attend to.
> Another Juror: Faith then, you'll have to stop here until we find a verdict.
> First Juror: I was on my way to the market when the sergeant stopped me.[62]

It is most likely that the verdict reached stating that Ann McDonald died as a result of an accidental fall resulting in the scalding and inflammation of the bowels was correct.[63] However, if jurors were openly discussing the inconvenience of the inquest, it is fair to consider that they may have had the same attitude towards an inquest of a more serious nature? Would they have had the same attitude towards an elderly person dying suddenly, an 'obvious' farming accident, a child burn-victim, or infanticide; especially when they felt there was little chance of proving a party responsible for the death and even less chance of prosecution? Although it may appear unfair to criticise such a short exchange between two jurors disappointed and angry about the lack of notice about the inquest, it does accurately measure the propensity for failure to reach a proper verdict if some members are interested in having the proceeding over as quickly as possible.

Jurors could also be fined for not attending an inquest as it was their public duty to participate. There are several examples throughout the casebook of jurors being fined for not attending an inquest. One note refers to James McAtee and James Martin who did not answer their names even though there was a hefty £5 fine for non-attendance.[64]

The Case of the Menacing Jurors – the Coroner is Threatened

> Infrequently one is in danger of serious violence. Once, when about to re-
> ceive personal violence, I escaped by describing the pleasing effect that hang-
> ing would produce if the threats made were carried out. The effect was en-
> tirely satisfactory; the gentleman of brawn and liquor became very pale and
> very thirsty, and left me to finish my work.
>
> William S. Wadsworth, MD,
discussing the role of the coroner in his publication
'Post-Mortem Examinations'

One example of anger directed towards the coroner was dramatically
highlighted in his notes when conducting the inquest of Mrs Letitia
Andrews. In the margin of his casebook, he noted this event as 'A
Discreditable Occurrence.'

The inquest was underway. All members of the jury viewed the
body, identified it and upon reaching the dinner hour, he adjourned
the rest of the proceeding until the following Saturday. Upon hearing this decision, the jury became 'very noisy and insisted I should
finish the case'. Waddell told them he could not do this for two reasons: first, that it would take a long day yet to close the inquest; and
second, he had another inquest to proceed with until 5p.m. Waddell
wrote, 'They would hear no reason that I must finish then and, if I
would not, they would attend no more adjournments.'

Dramatically, as he walked from his seat to the door to leave, the
jury moved in his way and stood in a threatening manner in front of
him. They would not allow him to pass out of the room. Waddell stepped on a chair and used it to step up on to the table, and walked across
the table towards the door at the end of the room and left. Having
exited, he informed the police sergeant that in reply to their threat
of no further attendance, he would now fine them £5 each.

Waddell found out later that after he left the room amidst a great
hubbub, the jury put their foreman in the chair in his place in an attempt to act independently to reach a verdict. The other officials in
the room were unco-operative with the angry jurors. Four of the legal
gentlemen arose and left the room. The head constable would not call
any further witnesses as the last witness had concluded his evidence
and the foreman would have got himself into trouble if he presumed
to administer the oath to this witness. In conclusion, Waddell wrote,
'Shortly after this disgraceful scene was brought to a close, the jury
left the inquest for their own houses. When I met them two days after
according to the adjournment, I took no notice of their conduct.'[65]

COMPENSATION FOR EXPENSES OR DONATIONS?

Some witnesses were paid expenses to testify at an inquest. A provision was made in the Coroner's Act of 1846 that stated 'poor witnesses' would receive payment of one shilling for their attendance at
an inquest given that their testimony was necessary in determining
the cause of death. At first glance, it appears that the condition of a
poor witness was not that they were necessarily destitute, but instead
that this provision had been created to compensate those who would
incur an expense as a result of their attending the inquest. When Thomas
Salmon, a cart driver for a man named Joe Campbell of Aughnacloy
was killed,[66] Campbell was subpoenaed as a witness at the inquest held
in Monaghan. Aughnacloy is twelve miles from Monaghan town and
it was considered reasonable that he be compensated for his required
attendance. Campbell was recorded by Waddell as having received one
shilling. Railway fatalities also resulted in several witnesses receiving
payment for their testimony at an inquest since they might occur at
any particular location along a very long track. Those who would need
to leave work for a day or incur unreasonable expenses for their travel
were compensated. Travel accommodations were recorded as being a
primary reason for payment.

One situation that raises an eyebrow is when key witnesses in a
suspected murder are paid for their testimony at an inquest. Such was
the case at the inquest of William Livingston. As Livingston was found
to have been poisoned and clearly by one of the members of his family,
it is questionable that James Foster was paid for his testimony. Foster
was the brother-in-law of one of the accused and his deposition provided evidence that indeed his brother-in-law, William McCarter, had
offered him his services if he would buy some laudanum, to 'help his
uncle sleep'. Was he paid for his testimony or was it a possible expense he incurred from travelling from his townland of Drumbrean
to Newbliss Court house where the inquest was held? Surely travelling less than a few miles down the road could not have been that
large an expense. Is this justice for the dead or does it compromise
the integrity of the truth?

Waddell paid some poor witnesses for testimony, but it is likely
it was to help to compensate them for their tragic loss. For example,
in the case of the death of Elizabeth McMahon, a young child of three
years of age was burned having been left alone by her older brother.[67]
Her father, a neighbour and brother were paid for their testimony at
the inquest that was held in their townland. It cannot be determined

how he justified the expenditure to the county; however it appears that Waddell was deeply sympathetic to the destitution of such families and the loss they had experienced.

There were many other tragic cases of death and many witnesses were not paid for their testimony and one might conclude it was impossible for the county to pay each and every poor bereaved family. However, Waddell was allowed to approve of payment for coffins and burials, including grave-diggers' fees for unidentified bodies, especially those of infants. When conducting an inquest that led him to the haunts of poverty and wretchedness, it was said that Waddell often paid for coffins and burials out of his own pocket in order to help the suffering relatives as it pained his heart.[68] Waddell's compassion is also illustrated by the next case.

Starvation and Death: The Death of Margaret Maghath, Maghernaharne, Ematris Parish, December 1861
Dr Moore of Rockcorry deposed that on Saturday, 14 December 1861, just two weeks before Christmas, he received a dispensary ticket to attend to the family of Michael Maghath. He found Michael along with his wife and child, Margaret, all very ill. He determined the child was suffering from a disease called Pemphigus and prescribed a can of nutrient that was necessary for her recovery. Pemphigus is a disease characterised by large blisters on skin and mucous membranes, often itching or burning. However, the destitute circumstances of the family prevented them from buying this necessity to save their daughter's life.

Two days later, Dr Moore discovered that the child was not any better and delivered the grim news to her parents that he did not expect her to recover. Four days later, Margaret Maghath was dead. Dr Moore told Waddell that the child died 'having been super induced by want of sufficient and proper nourishment'. He examined the body to confirm his diagnosis. The verdict was death from disease caused by want of proper and sufficient nourishment resulting from the very straightened circumstances of her parents.[69]

Waddell saw to it that the parents would at least be able to bury their daughter. He approved that a fee of two shillings and six pence be provided for the burial of the child. Unfortunately, Waddell's personal donations to such families were not recorded within the coroner's casebook.

HIGHLIGHTS
Tension and Tough Cases

There were several cases which showed that the coroner's job was not always an easy one in regard to procedure during an inquest, especially when suspects in murder were in attendance. The coroner's authority was often confused with the process of holding suspects and pressing criminal charges against them in murder cases. Some solicitors used this hazy area in process and understanding as an advantage to their clients' defence. As the following inquest will show, it was imperative in later years to change the law to distinguish where the coroner's authority ended and the criminal and judicial process began.

Eruption in the Courtroom: What is the Coroner's Authority?
The Unsolved Death of Phillip Treanor, Monaghan, December 1869
The coroner was called when Phillip Treanor's body was found lying on the banks of the river outside Monaghan town. His nose had been broken, there were fractures on the skull and from the marks on his hands and arms it appeared as if he'd been trying to defend himself. The circumstances of the death suggested foul play. It appeared that having suffering a beating, he was thrown off the bridge into the Blackwater River, although the possibility existed that he fell. Several men were taken into police custody under suspicion of beating and forcibly drowning the deceased.

The inquest was a highly publicised event and took place over four days at the County Courthouse. In the densely crowded courtroom, prosecutors for the Crown and defence solicitors were passionate in their questioning of witnesses, trying to determine if the men held in custody were responsible for the death of Phillip Treanor. The solicitor for the defence, Mr John Rea, was a well-known Belfast solicitor who was considered to be one of the best criminal lawyers in Ireland. He was the terror of the petty sessions and other magistrates in the north of Ireland as he was reputed for his courtroom theatrics such as rising to address the bench, opening his portmanteau thus revealing his many papers and law books and preparations already made for his own sojourn in prison for expected contempt of court.[70] He described himself as the 'Orange Fenian attorney of the North'.

Living up to his reputation, Mr Rea attempted to run the inquest himself and conduct it as if it were a criminal trial. Mr Treston, a magistrate for the Crown, also attempted to ask questions of witnesses, himself of the belief that the group of men in custody were guilty of the murder of Phillip Treanor. Uncovering the details of the night in question proved difficult and the facts were murky.

A few nights earlier, Treanor had been out with several men drinking heavily at the barracks pub. They had been asked to leave by publican Mary Smith and although they left the building, Treanor and company remained outside continuing to knock on the door requesting more whiskey. As they lingered, another group of men arrived and all appeared to gather for a short time outside the pub. There was drunken talk of a scuffle between the two parties, but soon after, all dispersed and headed home. It was just a short way down the road that Treanor and his party were accosted and beaten with fists and sticks. All the victims fled the scene in different directions and lost each other in the darkness. It was a particularly dark night, a cloudy, moonless sky with no lamp nearby to easily identify the attackers. However, one man in Treanor's party, James McKenna, claimed to recognise one of the men who beat him. McKenna, an animated witness, told the coroner's court that the man who attacked him had a small face with a thin red beard and whiskers. He pointed to one of the accused men sitting in the dock, Richard Garland.

Mr Rea attempted to discredit McKenna's identification of Garland explaining that there were many red-headed men in Monaghan and in fact, three other men in the dock with red hair. How was he sure it was this man? Did he really get a good look at him?

Even McKenna admitted there was no moonlight or lamp nearby on the night of the attack and that it was foggy. He added, 'I was not foggy with drink, but there was a thick fog at the time.'

'Oh, I see. Your brains were not foggy with alcohol, but there was atmospheric fog,' Rea pointed out cynically. The courtroom erupted into laughter.

McKenna retorted, 'I heard some talk about Orangemen that were taken into custody, but I did not know whether they were orange or blue men.' Again there was laughter in the courtroom but McKenna clarified, 'I swear to nothing but what I saw.'

Many witnesses in the neighbourhood testified to hearing noises, voices and carts travelling in the dark of night, but no one was able to identify any of the men who sat accused of beating and throwing Treanor off the bridge. In fact, it wasn't known for sure if the deceased man was thrown into the water. Was it possible that his physical injuries, the broken nose and fractured skull occurred from a severe fall? A. K. Young who performed the post-mortem examination was of the opinion that Treanor was beaten up and then thrown into the water which hastened his death. He said that he'd seen men with much more severe head injuries recover and that it was Treanor being submerged in the water that was likely to have finished him off.

After four days of interviewing witnesses, the coroner instructed the jury to determine the verdict of death. The verdict by the jury of sixteen men determined that the deceased came to his death by injuries received from some persons yet unknown. Mr Rea immediately asked the coroner to discharge the five prisoners: brothers Richard and James Garland, their cousin Francis Garland, and two other friends, James Jackson and James McAvin. Waddell asked the head constable if he had any other charges against the prisoners, to which he answered, 'No.' Waddell then announced the prisoners were discharged. As the crowd cheered loudly and the prisoners began leaving the dock, they were surrounded by a body of police and again taken into custody.

Mr Rea was outraged and spoke directly to Waddell. 'I wish to inform you of contempt of your court that has just been committed by the head constable of police and I think it is desirous that you should take cognisance of it. These men were discharged by your order and as they were leaving the court, the head constable thought it fit to re-arrest them upon a charge from which they have just been discharged. I contend he has no right whatever to do that, unless he had a magistrate's warrant. If Mr Treston thinks fit to have the prisoners re-arrested, let him take informations against them in the court at once. I know very well what he is sitting there for,' he said.

Waddell immediately asked why the prisoners were arrested.

They had been arrested on a charge of murder.

Mr Rea continued to argue and question what was the point of the coroner's court if his clients could be re-arrested after they were not named or found to be culpable of the death of Phillip Treanor? He was most appalled by the fact that the police had arrested the men without a warrant. Mr Rea begged the coroner to exert his authority, but Waddell could only state that he had discharged his duty and that he was done. The coroner's court was over. Mr Rea would now have to make his appeal to the Queen's Bench.

To the delight of the crowd in the courtroom, Mr Rea went on to give a speech to all who would listen about the injustices done by the police and the how the police had ruled the county for too long. The crowd applauded and began to get unruly. Mr Rea then instructed the prisoners to 'go home' at which point, they rose from their seats only to be stopped again by the police.

'You shouldn't tell them to do that,' said Waddell. He felt that this was a very irregular proceeding and stated that he was of the opinion that no authority but the Queen's Bench could interfere.

Suddenly several judges appeared in the courtroom to hear an explanation for the re-arrest of the prisoners as well as gathering information to be used in the upcoming trial should there be enough evidence to prosecute. After a short amount of time it was determined that there was not sufficient evidence for holding the prisoners.

Mr Rea shouted to the prisoners, 'Go home immediately and if any man attempts to interfere with you, knock him down!' There was great cheering in the courtroom as the free men left the room. There was no further attempt made by police to arrest them. Waddell was later considered by those in the court to have withstood and subdued Mr Rea valiantly.

WADDELL V. SWANZY

With two different coroners' districts in Co. Monaghan, Waddell and Swanzy were called by the police to cover each other's cases occasionally. One might get the impression that Waddell and Swanzy may have had differences from time to time based on some of the notes recorded by Waddell. As Dr Brian Farrell, the Dublin city coroner has pointed out, 'There are times when coroners disagree. This often happens when the jurisdiction where a body is found is in question and an issue may arise between two coroners. One way to describe such disagreement might be reflected by the phrase, "It's my body".' There are indications in the text of Waddell's casebook implying that there may have been some tension between Waddell and Swanzy on a few occasions. For example, Thomas Johnston was killed and terribly mutilated by the machinery at his father's mill in July 1857. Waddell stated, 'I attended at the hour appointed, 9a.m., but on reaching the house did not consider it necessary to prosecute the inquiry any further.' He added, 'On reaching the deceased's house, I saw Mr Swanzy leaving it. He had returned home sooner than expected, though aware that owing to his absence, the case had been reported to me. I left home at an early hour and had without the knowledge of the police or any of them being present, hurried over to the inquest, which annoyed them very much as 'twas in consequence of the report and request of the police I had attended.' Another such example of a cross-over between the two men's services was an entry on 27

May 1867 documenting the inquiry into the death of John Timlin. Waddell's entry stated, 'The sudden death of John Timlin of Corsilloga (Aughnamullen) near Rockcorry was reported to me. I attended there early the next day, inquired into the case, but from what I learned did not consider it right to proceed with the matter; more particularly, as on reaching the police barracks, I learned the case belonged to Mr Swanzy's district, but of his attendance the police were very doubtful.' It is unclear why Swanzy's attendance was doubtful; however, it is a point that he felt warranted documentation. The effort required travelling and the time spent on the inquest when both men arrived was unnecessary and might have caused friction from time to time.

Regardless of Waddell's documentation of overlap in coverage of the county regarding the dead, the relationship between the two Co. Monaghan coroners appears to have been harmonious. Hugh Swanzy was a solicitor.[71] As the son of Henry Swanzy and Rose Rosborough, a prominent and well-known family, he was educated in Newry and served as a solicitor in the county for many years. Is it possible that the gentleman and the solicitor, although both from prominent families, did not always see eye to eye? Or were they a good team covering the investigation of death in the county? Several forensic and medical jurisprudence texts from the nineteenth century pass the opinion that medical men working as coroners bring great knowledge in determining a cause of death and yet, attorneys and solicitors are expert in following the procedures of a court of law. It is worth pointing out that when the two men questioned the grand jury about their compensation and expenses for their jobs, it was indeed Swanzy who did the talking. Although well-educated and experienced in speaking to authorities, it appears that Waddell left the negotiating and politics to Swanzy.

THE GRAVE IS CLOSED OVER ALL THAT WAS MORTAL OF WILLIAM C. WADDELL

William Charles Waddell served faithfully as the North Monaghan county coroner for thirty-two years investigating, organising and determining a cause of death for more than 1,300 persons. His judgement and decision-making may be questioned but his record-keeping and attention to his duties cannot. Over twenty years in volume two of his casebook he appears to have carefully recorded those dying under suspicious, sudden or unusual circumstances. In the spring of 1878, Waddell became ill. He had caught a cold that eventually affected his lungs. He died on 4 May 1878 at the age of seventy-nine and is buried at the Cahans Presbyterian church at Lisnaveane in the parish of Tullycorbet. His gravestone reads as follows:

> In memory of William Charles Waddell who departed this life 4th May 1878 aged 79 years; also of Maria Orr Waddell, his wife, who departed this life, 4th May 1886, aged 82 years. 'He giveth his beloved sleep'.

In the chapters that follow, it becomes increasingly difficult to comprehend why seemingly obvious deaths were under the scrutiny of the state. Only now, looking back at the some of the issues facing our nineteenth-century ancestors such as infanticide, domestic abuse, mental illness, dysfunctional family dynamics and larger societal constraints that contributed to homicide, may we begin to use our modern understanding of the complex web of human behaviour to truly understand our own culture born out of the problems extending not very far back in our history. These stories are painful, detailed, gruesome and sad and deserve to be remembered; for those who have suffered in these pages were the silent martyrs who created the need for change in our contemporary society. *These are all true stories of death*, and here for the first time these forgotten souls, many buried in unmarked graves around the county, are remembered.

CHAPTER TWO

INFANTICIDE
CHILD MURDER IN MONAGHAN

I saw where in the shroud did lurk,
A curious frame of nature's work;
A flowerette crush'd in the bud
A nameless piece of Babyhood,
Was in her cradle-coffin lying;
Extinct, with scarce the sense of dying;
So soon to exchange the imprisoning womb,
For darker closets of the tomb.

– Charles Lamb, 'On an infant dying as soon as born'

Upon close examination of the infant deaths recorded by the coroner in Co. Monaghan, it is apparent that most of these newborns were murdered. They were the 'illegitimate' children of unmarried mothers – women who were either abandoned by the father, fearful of becoming social outcasts or simply found themselves in trouble with no one to count on. Infanticide and 'baby-dropping' (the dumping of anonymous babies in exposed places) were commonplace in nineteenth-century Ireland and the tiny bodies of infants were bundled, tied, and drowned, strangled with cords or bare hands, suffocated with bed covers, violently beaten or left to the elements of the countryside, hidden from sight or found by animals and unsuspecting passers-by.

Some babies, as well as their mothers, died as a result of the trauma of childbirth, even with the help of midwives and physicians. In some cases, misdiagnosis and dated procedures often encouraged death rather than a passage for life as doctors lacked the pre-natal technology to save the mother's or baby's life. Mothers died from haemorrhaging and infants of premature and stillborn birth. Midwifery in the nineteenth century was under the scrutiny of the medical profession, as obstetrics was being more carefully studied and there was a growing interest in overcoming the large number of deaths. The midwife's knowledge, judgement and years of experience were often discounted even when using the same techniques as a physician, simply because they were not proper scholars of medicine. Skilled in the art of delivery, these women were also accomplished in techniques of terminating life that were often undetectable upon investigation. An unmarried mother could request the use of these talents to end the life of her baby immediately after the birth. Contrary to premeditated fatalities, a midwife might find herself in jail if death occurred while delivering a legitimate child to a married woman. The law investigated her delivery techniques and attempted to point out the errors made by the medically untrained 'witch'.

THE SCOURGE OF ILLEGITIMACY

As one would expect, infant murder was much more likely to occur in conjunction with illegitimacy, poverty and brutality.[1] Women and children were part of a value-system that attached a label, either 'legitimate' or 'illegitimate', to every newborn infant, as well as a distribution of resources that placed the illegitimate child and its mother, but not its father, in serious danger of destitution.[2] These women were the object of public scorn, viewed as sexually loose women, looked down upon by the Church and their children considered outcasts. If they did not have the support of their family, some found ways to provide for their children by begging, gaining admission into the workhouse, and in some severe cases resorted to prostitution. Of course, all these options could be averted by simply hiding the pregnancy and ending the child's life soon after birth. Given the options, it is not surprising that many women giving birth to illegitimate children were driven to commit infanticide.

One personal account of illegitimacy from an anonymous man, born in 1906, depicts how these children were treated in the early twentieth century. One can assume it to be a similar experience to those children born forty years earlier.

> I was reared in a workhouse, in fact I was born in a workhouse. I was illegitimate ... I was supposed to be very good looking as a grown up boy and if I dated a girl or a girl dated me the next thing she'd drop me all because I was illegitimate. That was a horrible crime in the Victorian age. Oh Lord God of Almighty, you were like the untouchables in India, the right type of company wouldn't go with you. You were an outcast and you had to go for the lowest of the lowest, somebody in the same category as yourself.
>
> If any woman years ago got into trouble with a man and made her in the family way, the quicker she was got away to America overnight the bet-

ter. They'd be ashamed that it happened. They were taken undercover at night, put on a boat and over to America. They were never let back again. For adultery you were chased. The parish would chase ye. The priest and all, ye couldn't live it down.[3]

Married women too had reasons for disposing of their infants, yet this occurred less frequently. Another child on an already financially-burdened family, domestic disharmony or post-natal depression are some possible reasons for disposing of a legitimate infant, but because a married woman was in a respectable position (i.e. having a husband), it was not as likely. In one case, a woman named Mary McMahon was charged with the murder of her child after it was found floating in the Ulster Canal.[4] The evidence showed the child alive and well at 6a.m., but by 7.30a.m. it was found floating in the water. The argument presented at her trial was: 'There was no motive for the crime; for this was the case of a married woman, and not that of some unhappy being who, in her anxiety to hide her shame, might be tempted to destroy her offspring.'[5] She was acquitted by the jury. This case emphasises that in the eyes of society and the justice system, unmarried women had motive to commit infanticide and married women did not.

ABORTION

If a woman by her magic destroys the child she has conceived of somebody, she shall do penance for half a year with an allowance of bread and water, and abstain for two years from wine and meat.
                                   – Penitential of Finnian (7th century)

In the nineteenth century, infanticide and abortion really were alternative ways of disposing of unwanted (usually illegitimate) children.[6] Abortion could be procured sometimes through 'the most drastic purgatives and emmenagogues, of which aloes and gamboges are the chief ingredients ... certain herbs and plants, particularly rue and savine pulled in a particular manner are believed by the country people to have a like end.'[7] Other products used to induce abortion were 'innocent' items on sale, like cantharides and diachylon (lead) plasters, or purgatives like juniper oil. Some newspaper advertisements boasted propriety remedies for menstrual disorders, 'female ailments', but everyone knew they were thinly (but legally) disguised abortifacients.[8]

The Master Gets Rid of Evidence
The Death of Rose O'Neill, Latlorkin, Monaghan Parish, April 1862
Rose O'Neill had lived for ten years as a servant with the family of

Mr John Crow of the *Eight Tates*.[9] She fell ill and her sisters Alice, Biddy and Ann went to visit her. Alice arrived first and found Rose speechless. She was not replying to any questions, but instead had a 'wild look'. Rose had always been a strong healthy girl, not subject to fits, but had more than one when Alice was present. During these fits, Rose's arms were working violently with fists firmly clenched and she had to be held down.

Ann also saw her going through these fits, each one lasting about ten minutes. Ann stated, 'Up until the time of her decease, all that time (from early in the day until early evening), she never once appeared to recognise me.' Ann knew that Rose was known to take medicine when nothing ailed her, and knew that she had taken medicine to procure an abortion six years earlier. The sisters believed Rose to be taking medicines and herbs to destroy the foetus inside her. Savin, made from the shrub *Juniperus Sabina*, is a very common poisonous plant used to bring about abortions. At high doses, it causes convulsions, haemorrhages, vomiting and convulsive coma.

The master of a house employing domestic servants was obliged to supply food and lodgings but not medical attention or medicine for his servants.[10] Ann told the coroner that there were some powders in Rose's room which her master, John Crow, desired to be thrown in to the fire. Why did he destroy evidence that might have been able to answer the cause of her death? Was John Crow the father of the child? Or was he just a caring man concerned that she was taking a substance that would kill her?

Her body was exhumed and the authorities ordered a post-mortem examination which revealed that Rose's brain, heart, lungs and abdomen were healthy and she was indeed four months pregnant. No cause of death could be determined and the jury requested the stomach of the deceased and its contents be sent for analysis. Dr Hodges of Belfast was sent the contents and returned the following letter:

> On the 23rd April, I commenced the examination of the portions of the viscera and contents of the stomach of the late Rose O'Neill as directed by William Charles Waddell, Esq., coroner of Co. Monaghan. The examination was completed this day. No trace of the presence of mineral or vegetable poison was discovered in any of the substances received by me.
> John F. Hodges, MD, F.C.S.
> Professor of Medical Jurisprudence, Queen's University, Belfast[11]

With no other witnesses being produced, the jury returned the following verdict: Death on 15 April 1862 under circumstances of strong suspicion but the cause leading to death unknown. William Wilde once stated about abortion, 'Can we wonder at the ignorant Irish girl wishing to conceal her shame by the destruction of her offspring, in a country acknowledged to be one of the most moral in Europe, and where caste is more certainly lost by the circumstance of pregnancy before or without marriage, when, in other lands boasted to be the most civilised, induced abortion, even among married females, in the upper ranks of life, is spoken of in society without reserve?'[12]

METHODS OF THE CHILD MURDERESS

There were several ways in which infanticide was committed. Most infants were suffocated, strangled, drowned, or struck with a violent blow to the head to stop their breathing. Others were left to the elements – referred to as exposure. These are cases where the evidence is clear and straightforward, even if the suspected mother could not be identified or convicted. For example, Dr Robert Moore while performing a post-mortem examination on a dead infant stated, 'There were no marks of injury and the umbilical cord was well and carefully tied and from its whole appearance, consider the deceased had lived 8 to 10 days subsequent to its birth. On an internal examination, I saw from the state of the lungs that the deceased had lived and from the milk in its stomach that it had been suckled within perhaps half an hour of its death. The right side of the heart was distended with blood and the lungs also presented a congested appearance from which consider the child was suffocated and which appearances would be caused by immersion into water ... The verdict was deceased came to its death by suffocation and most probably from drowning.'[13] The mother was never found and therefore not prosecuted. Another infant was found by James McBerney in Monaghan town at Scroggy's Bridge.[14] When it was examined by Dr Young, it was found to have a 'mark of violence on the windpipe'.[15] More gruesome yet was the post-mortem examination by Dr Manwhinny of a child found by Mary Gould in the townland of Greagh Hill. The doctor testified, 'The corpse has a mark around its neck; the eyes were dark and protruding as also the lips and mouth. The heart and lungs were full of blood and congested.'[16] He was clear that the death was the result of strangulation.

Although the evidence in cases of violent death is apparent, it is when a neutral verdict resulted, such as 'unknown', 'natural causes', 'accidental suffocation' or 'stillborn', that a view into the methods of infanticide can be seen, as well as the difficulty in proving it. These unmarried mothers, desperate to rid themselves of their illegitimate offspring devised a plan of how to dispose of their child or gained advice from midwives on the techniques least likely to attract suspicion. Injuries to the head or neck could always be blamed by the midwife on the extra pressure exerted during a difficult delivery; strangulation by the umbilical cord was used, as death could be blamed on accidental entwining of the neck during birth; a midwife might sit her client over a bucket of water and if the baby drowned before it cried and took breath, the lungs would show no sign of inflation and suggest stillbirth; suffocation could be attributed to the bed covers smothering the child or overlying the mother on top of the child.[17] In these cases, the lack of proof corresponds with a neutral or unsolved verdict and no charges were filed against the mother or any other parties.

Death from 'Natural Causes'?
The Death of the Infant Child of Ann Soraghan,
Feragh, Monaghan Parish, July 1872
On 28 July 1872, Constable McDonald received information that a child had been found in Sparks Lake (the Convent Lake) in Monaghan town. He was aware that Ann Soraghan had just given birth to a child. Thinking the dead baby might be hers, he went in search of her and found Ann in the service of Sam Skeath. When confronted, Anne admitted that she had been confined earlier that week with a male child in the house of James Henderson of Leagh and she would show him where the child was buried.

The coroner began an investigation, organised a jury and asked Dr Reid to perform a post-mortem examination. He found the child to be full-term, but because the body was already in an advanced state of decomposition could not find any marks of foul play. He found the internal organs to be healthy and considered that the baby lived for some hours; the umbilical cord had not been properly severed.

John Henderson and his wife were also questioned. John stated that Ann Soraghan appeared at his home on 19 July and complained of being sick. Once in the house, his wife told him that Ann was not just sick, but would soon give birth to a child and asked him to retrieve the midwife, Mrs Duffy. John and his male servant went to the house of Mrs Duffy, but she refused to attend. By the time they returned, his wife told him that she heard the cries of the child from the other room. It had been born, but thirty minutes after the birth

Ann left the house with the child. The next day, Mrs Henderson went to the home of Ann Soraghan to check on her and her newborn child. When she arrived at the house, the child was in the cradle but the mother told her it was dead. She left immediately and never got a look at the child.

It was never explained how the child ended up in the lake, but it may have been placed there by its mother as a method of burial. Without any physical evidence that Ann had extinguished the life of her child, the jury found that the death resulted from 'natural causes'.[18]

SECRETS AND LIES
Concealing the Pregnancy and Birth

Concealing a pregnancy was difficult but not impossible. It was done for many reasons – out of the shame brought upon the woman, her family and the unborn child, the inability to obtain employment – and it showed premeditation towards ending the child's life. Some unmarried women, having concealed their pregnancy, appear to have chosen to leave their home near the time of their confinement, seeking out a place to deliver the child in the presence of strangers, and having disposed of the child, they moved on. The workhouse was sometimes used for this purpose. A woman would travel to an area where she would not be recognised, deliver her child at the local workhouse, leave with the baby and the body of the infant would be found dead later on. Often the workhouse was the first place where the police would begin their investigation into such an infant death.[19] When the body of an infant was discovered, a common question to persons of the surrounding area was: had they any idea of who its parent might be or if there were any young unmarried women who had lately had a child.[20] When such a corpse was found in the field of John Kelly of Corclare in the parish of Errigal Truagh under some dry grass, it was reported that 'there was a young woman in the neighbourhood for a couple of days considered to be in the family way'.[21] One young girl was spotted in the townland of Derrynahesco, parish of Tedavnet, placing a bundle in a hole at the end of a bridge. The witness watching the girl stated that she thought it was 'a bag of feathers', until she went out to have a look and discovered the body of the infant. Upon examination, she stated she would not be able to identify the girl if she saw her again.[22] For many women, travelling away from their homes to have their child and dispose of it was an effort worth making, allowing them the possibility of returning to a normal life back at home having taken care of their 'problem', their reputations and lives intact.

A pregnant servant's condition was more likely to go unnoticed by her employers than in a more modest establishment, and she had a better opportunity of secretly delivering and then 'dumping' the body.[23] The stories of pregnant servant girls concealing their condition and giving birth secretly in their bedrooms to babies that were either wilfully killed in a mother's panic or died as an inevitable consequence of a botched self-delivery, were a hardy perennial.[24] In 1864 at the house of Mary Ann and George Fleming, Mary Ann Hoey working as a servant in the house concealed her pregnancy right up to the time of delivery. She lied to Mrs Fleming when asked if she was pregnant, possibly because she wanted to keep her job. Another likely reason was that she planned to destroy the child quickly after its birth. The child was found by Mrs Fleming, dead, rolled up in a towel, with a black cloth about its head, stuffed between the bolster and the bed tick. Dr Young in performing the post-mortem examination could not determine whether the child was born alive or dead and the verdict was 'death from natural causes'.[25] No charges were brought against Mary Ann Hoey. There was a theory that 'baby-dropping in the wealthier districts of London could be traced back to nearby houses, as servants would not venture far from their places of employment at night for fear of being spotted'.[26] If this idea holds true to the countryside of Co. Monaghan, could two of the infant corpses found by the gamekeeper for Lord Cremorne at the Dartrey Demense be traced back to the big house?[27] There were several unmarried women mentioned in the coroner's casebook as having given birth to illegitimate children while employed as domestic servants at 'big houses' in the county.[28]

Concealment of the birth of a child was a crime punishable by law. However, the legal definition for 'concealment of birth' meant that the child was *found dead and a suspect named*. Trying a suspect for 'exposure' meant that the child was *found alive*. The case of Sarah Goodfellow in 1873 appears to be the only woman investigated by W. C. Waddell who was convicted for the crime of concealing the birth of a child.

Hidden Under The Floor:
The Death of the Infant Child of Sarah Goodfellow,
Kilmore East, Ematris Parish, May 1873
On 30 April 1873, Constable James Finegan received information that Sarah Goodfellow had lately delivered a child and he went to

her residence. When he arrived, he made a search inside the house, and, on the dirt floor, saw where some earth had been disturbed. He began to dig and at a depth of two feet he found a flag and beneath it the body of a young child. He took charge of the body and while on his way back to the barracks, he came upon Sarah Goodfellow. He arrested her and charged her with having given birth to a child, concealing her situation and destroying the child.

Dr Moore did the post-mortem examination and found that the child was full-term and had been alive. He found around its neck a 'mark of ligature' with the effusion of blood beneath the mark. The head and brains were gorged with blood and the blood vessels ruptured in many places causing effusion of blood beneath the skin and brain. He concluded that the child came to its death by strangulation and that its death followed immediately after its birth. Dr Moore was also called upon to go to the house of Robert Goodfellow, Sarah's father, to examine her; she appeared to have given birth to a child within the past several days.

The verdict determined the child came to its death within about a week previous to 1 May 1873 from strangulation, but how or by whose means, the jury had no evidence to show.[29] Sarah Goodfellow was held as a prisoner and committed for trial on a charge of wilful murder to be held at the Monaghan assizes in July. A woman named Mary Garrity, presumably the midwife, was also in custody charged with aiding and abetting the crime and was remanded for a week.[30] A few months later in July, Sarah Goodfellow appeared in court, described as a 'respectably dressed, good-looking young woman' who pleaded guilty to concealing the birth of her child. The magistrate hearing the case said 'he had read the informations and there was nothing in them to lead him to believe that anything further had been done to the child beyond concealing its birth.' He therefore took a lenient view of the case and Sarah Goodfellow was convicted of concealing the birth of her child. She was sentenced to prison for three months from her date of committal.[31] Why did the magistrate ignore the physical evidence in this case? It appears that pleading guilty to concealment was enough to satisfy the court and a charge of wilful murder was dropped.

Mental weakness was another defence for women who chose to conceal their pregnancy. Essy Kells of Derrins in Currin parish was described by her sister Mary West as having 'a very weak mind'. Essy worked scutching flax and lived with her sister and husband. One morning she revealed to her sister and a Mrs Lancashire that she had given birth to a child and told them the identity of the father. The child was dead. Essy had gone unattended throughout the delivery of the child and the family were totally ignorant of the situation. There were no marks of violence on the body and it was determined that the afterbirth was still attached to the child because it was either stillborn or that it died of neglect due to the 'imbecility of the mother'.[32]

The killing of newborns immediately following their birth was in some cases carried out with the help of midwives and family members. Mary Kelly of Cormeen had delivered a child that was allegedly born dead. Mary Reilly, the midwife, took the child to wash and dress it, but the Kelly sisters insisted that before the child had been prepared it was already dead. Mary's sister Margaret said, 'I kept the body safe for four days and four nights (in her bed) that it might be seen in case any reports on the subject should be raised (at a later date).' Someone had tipped off the police that Mary Kelly had delivered a child and Constable Finegan went to investigate. At first Margaret denied that her sister had delivered a child, but finally showed him where the child had been put. She had placed it in water, presumably a lake or canal. A drag was used to retrieve the body and a post-mortem examination was performed. The child showed no marks of external violence and the lungs were well inflated to show the child had breathed. The heart was healthy, but the right side was filled with dark blood. All the other organs were healthy. There was also no food in its stomach. The verdict stated only that the deceased was born alive but how or by what means it came to its death the jury had not been shown. No charges were pressed against the women.[33] In another case, an unmarried young girl, Eliza Croarken, was in labour, but those around her believed she was having an attack of convulsions and not expected to live. The girl's grandfather, Mr Schoales, and witness Mary O'Neill stated they had no idea the girl was pregnant until they found the infant lying in the bed – dead. They considered it had not been born alive as there was always a person in the room. The child was delivered underneath the bedding and likely suffocated as a result of the ignorance of the caretakers and the mother's mental state. The verdict was death from accidental suffocation in consequence of the state of unconsciousness of the mother.[34] Did they know about the impending birth but were helping to end its life? It would be difficult to prove they were not telling the truth in a court of law. No charges were filed.

One noteworthy case was that of nineteen-year-old Elizabeth Smith, alias Lee, who was indicted in September 1882 in Clones for 'feloniously, wilfully and of malice aforethought, killing and murdering her illegitimate son, Thomas Smith'.[35] The evidence presented at trial told the story. Elizabeth was admitted as an inmate to the Union Workhouse at Clones on 20 August and gave birth to a male child the next morning. She left the workhouse two weeks later with the child in her arms and on 18 September the dead body of an infant child was found in a drain in the townland of Altartate Glebe, lying on its side and partly under the water. It was identified by a tuck on its clothing and mark on its neck as being the child of Elizabeth Smith. Dr Richard Henry of Clones was of the opinion the child was suffocated before being put in the water and the defence argued that it might have been accidentally smothered against its mother's breast. After two hours of deliberation, the jury returned a verdict of guilty and strongly recommended mercy in sentencing the accused. A shocking sentence was then handed down by the judge. Elizabeth Smith was sentenced to be hanged at Monaghan County Jail on 13 January 1883. The judge added that he hoped the recommendation would be mercifully considered by the Executive. An immediate appeal was made to the Lord Lieutenant. Elizabeth Smith had no prior record and her sentence was commuted to life imprisonment. Elizabeth served just five years of a penal sentence at Mountjoy and Grangegorman Prisons. She was released on 15 December 1887.[36]

With the exception of the sentencing of Elizabeth Smith, it appears that the judicial system in Co. Monaghan was lenient in its treatment of unmarried women concealing their pregnancy. The attitudes towards sexual misbehaviour in Ulster were described as 'lax' in comparison to the rest of the country at the time and this was confirmed when the official statistics on the incidence of illegitimacy became available for the first time with civil registration of births in 1864. Illegitimate births in the north-east registration division of the country amounted to 6.2% of the total number of registered births, roughly the same as the ratio recorded in England and Wales at this period and almost twice that recorded in Ireland as a whole.[37] A possible explanation is the prosperity of industry in Ulster at this time. As work became available in the mills, more young men and women were able to work outside the home to make an income, often for the first time. As they became more financially independent of their parents, so did the desire to become socially independent. The result of this newfound freedom appears to have led to disaster for some women who found themselves pregnant – without a husband.

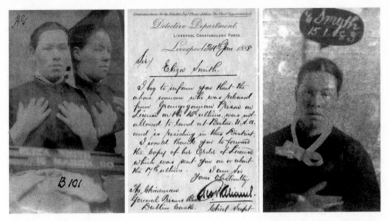

Left: *Prison photo of convicted murderer Elizabeth Smith (alias Lee), taken when she (age 19) was first committed to Mountjoy Prison on 15 January 1883. [Elizabeth Smith, GPB, PEN 1890, National Archives, Dublin] Elizabeth was released on licence (parole) on 15 December 1887.* **Right**: *Picture taken upon her re-arrest in March 1890. She had not informed authorities of her change of residence and so served two months in Liverpool Prison. She was released on 20 May 1890.* **Centre**: *Letter from Liverpool Constabulary explaining the location of Elizabeth Smith. The letter dated 24 January 1888, informs the General Prisons Board, Dublin Castle, that Elizabeth was not allowed to land at Boston, USA and had returned. She would continue to live in Liverpool.*

The judicial system was often lenient towards illegitimacy, but this did not reflect the social and religious attitudes. The woman who gave birth to a child outside lawful marriage was seen as an offender against the principles of sexual morality as put forward by Church authorities. The statutes and regulations laid down for the government of different dioceses made clear that such women were in fact regarded as offenders to be punished. For example, a common penalty for unmarried women with illegitimate babies was to withhold either temporarily or altogether the ceremony of Churching,[38] the repurification of a woman after childbirth; or baptism of the child.[39] These unfortunate women and children were often refused religious privileges and considered outcasts within their own faith.

BURYING THE BODY OF EVIDENCE

The bodies found in Co. Monaghan were discovered in open fields, underneath bushes, buried in the churchyard, but very frequently in water – along the edges of lakes and streams, buried under heavy stones or floating in a bundle along the Ulster canal.

The bodies of the infants were often found covered with heavy stones along the water's edge or in a bundle or sack, the stones used to weigh down the body. In August 1872, fifteen-year-old Eugene Brady and John Early were sent out to the Convent Lake by Hugh Fitzpatrick to set up a net to go fishing.[40] He found a bundle next to the water near the convent where the cows went to drink and thought it to be a drowned pup. John Early took out his knife and opened the bag. He saw three stones, pushed the stones off and saw the child. Fitzpatrick immediately contacted the police.[41] Other children were found in a similar fashion in the Convent Lake over the years. Another example of such an infant 'burial' was discovered by Robert Kearney while in Cloncaw, Donagh parish, on the way to visit his daughter. When coming towards a pool of water, his dog got hold of something and began to beat around after it as if it were a rat. It was the head of a child. When the body was taken out of the water, it appeared to have had a heavy stone placed on it.[42]

In many other parts of the country the remains of babies buried in water, marked by a few stones along the edge of the shore, are thought to be the graves of babies from the famine, unbaptised infants or both. It is evident that illegitimate children in Co. Monaghan were found in water, but it cannot be determined if this was necessarily a burial tradition or just one method of deposing of the bodies. It was believed in the nineteenth century in some Christian churches that unbaptised infants were not supposed to come within the pale of perfect redemption, but passed into a state of almost non-existence. Such children were therefore never buried in consecrated ground, but in graveyards set apart for that purpose.[43]

There are thought to be many different burial grounds around the county for children who weren't baptised. One such location is in Mullaghbawn, another at the railway near the graveyard at St Mary's Church in Carrickmacross and another along the hedge of the Old Monaghan Graveyard outside Monaghan town to mention just a few.[44] There are stories in local oral tradition of various makeshift graveyards for unbaptised children in fields around the county. The likely reason for such burial practices was the regulations handed down by the Roman Catholic Church. The burial of children who had not been baptised was prohibited in consecrated ground (that is, with other family members) and abnormal interment practices, and particular beliefs concerning the destiny of such souls in the otherworld became common. Similarly, with regard to abandoned and murdered children or miscarried and aborted foetuses, different death customs have prevailed

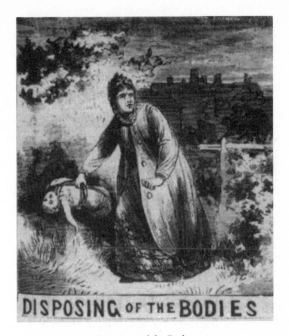

DISPOSING OF THE BODIES

Disposing of the Bodies
Illustrated London News, 1870

and it was believed that such souls lacked status in the afterlife.[45] Is it possible that the frequent occurrence of illegitimate and murdered children being buried in water in Co. Monaghan was an attempt to ensure the safety of the souls of these children? The manner in which unbaptised babies were buried and the location of the burial places signifies their liminal status in both human and supernatural terms according to Irish tradition.[46]

One story handed down in Co. Monaghan is that of *An Féar Gortach* (Hungry Grass). It is a general belief in Irish tradition that a person might suddenly walk on a certain piece of ground and be overcome with consuming hunger which would result in his or her dying of starvation unless he or she could eat something immediately. This was said to occur where famine victims had died, wherever a dead body had touched the ground for instance, or where food had been eaten and no crumbs left behind. In other instances, however, *an féar gortach* is believed to occur where an unbaptised child had been buried.[47]

However, some women did secretly bury their children in the churchyard. In September 1859, Edward Hughes was performing his duties in the chapel churchyard in Monaghan when his attention was drawn to the exposed body of an infant child in the retired part of the graveyard.[48] Another child was found in the chapel graveyard in Monaghan by two Roman Catholic clergymen. They told the police of an uninterred child being found inside a small box beside a hollow, slightly scraped in the ground. They had the box carried into town and discovered the remains of a premature child of five months who had died approximately three weeks before.[49] One woman was actually seen bringing a bundle into the Monaghan chapel, leaving it to be discovered. The sickly delicate young woman was observed by Ann Woods, the cleaning woman for the chapel, as she stooped down on her hands and knees next to the confessional with a small bundle of white cloth. Ann later told the coroner, 'On learning that she was not going to confess, I desired her to remove farther off and not to remain within hearing. After some time, I saw her come down from the gallery where the deceased was afterwards found. The woman was quite a stranger to me and I would not know her if I saw her again.'[50] And what became of the corpses of the children that were found and autopsied? Waddell's expenses show that coffins were purchased for these infants and they were buried, although it was not determined where.

Some infants were exposed to the elements, where their decomposing bodies were found by animals and torn apart. Robert Blakely was out walking around his farm in Clones when he observed some crows clustered together. He stated, 'Having my gun in my hand, I went towards them (the crows) to see what they were at, when I saw the body of the deceased. They were pecking at it.'[51] In the townland of Clonamully, Tedavnet parish, James Robinson was busy driving his pig off the road when 'she suddenly started off and ran to the body of an infant'. When he tried to get the child's body away from the pig, she seized it and ran off with it but, by that time, one of the legs was torn off.[52]

THE INFANT INQUEST

There was pressure on the coroner to carefully choose the inquests he performed as the county ratepayers paid his salary and costs. In the case of infant death, it became a tricky and frustrating situation. Because it was near impossible to prove the murder of an infant and attitudes of jury members of the time were forgiving towards unmarried mothers desperate to extinguish 'their bastardy', there was often a

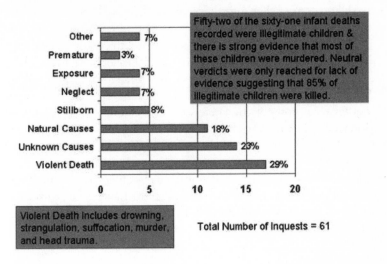

Verdicts of Infant Inquests

Fifty-two of the sixty-one infant deaths recorded were illegitimate children & there is strong evidence that most of these children were murdered. Neutral verdicts were only reached for lack of evidence suggesting that 85% of illegitimate children were killed.

- Other — 7%
- Premature — 3%
- Exposure — 7%
- Neglect — 7%
- Stillborn — 8%
- Natural Causes — 18%
- Unknown Causes — 23%
- Violent Death — 29%

Violent Death includes drowning, strangulation, suffocation, murder, and head trauma.

Total Number of Inquests = 61

Verdicts of Inquests: Infant deaths recorded by W. C. Waddell (1856–1876)

'why bother?' attitude towards inquests and post-mortems in the case of infants, induced by the workings of the judicial system.[53] Doctors were reluctant to provide their time at inquests for very little money and police had no evidence other than an unidentifiable body to begin an investigation. If an autopsy was held and the coroner's jury found sufficient evidence to prosecute a suspect, almost always the mother, the chances of a verdict of murder at the assizes were slim to none. It can be assumed that many suspicious deaths of infants went uninvestigated as the lack of resources and evidence would not warrant any further inquiry.

Sixty-one infant inquests were recorded by W. C. Waddell from 1856 to 1876.[54] Fifty-two of those recorded were illegitimate babies born to unmarried mothers. In the cases of children being found, without knowing the identity of the mother, they were presumed to be illegitimate. The verdicts in such cases range from stillborn death to death by violence. In the chart above, 79% of the infant deaths recorded were verdicts of non-violent death. However all murdered and deserted children were believed to be illegitimate[55] and the disproportionately high number of 'illegitimates' in infant inquests suggests that there was something wrong with the many neutral verdicts, since illegitimates were the most at risk from infanticide.

The number of illegitimate infant deaths and murders recorded, more than likely underestimates the actual number. Logically we must consider the cases that went unreported, the burials of live-borns as stillborns, deaths which the coroner did not deem worthy of recording and investigating for lack of evidence and the many cases where the body of the infant was simply not found. Lionel Rose, in his book, *The Massacre of the Innocents: Infanticide in Britain 1800-1939*, found that it was reasonable to assume that for every one infant reported, another went unreported. There were two coroners working in Co. Monaghan. The findings here reflect only the cases investigated by W. C. Waddell, not those of Hugh Swanzy, Esq. To estimate a figure closer to the actual number of infanticide cases, the figures would again double if taking into account the cases of Swanzy. Rather than 52 illegitimate infant deaths investigated, the figure is more likely to be 208 – this figure still possibly being an underestimation of the actual number.

WHEN THE SUSPECT IS THE FATHER

In thirty-seven inquests, it was proved a baby died as a result of violence such as drowning, physical trauma to the body (usually the head), deliberate neglect, strangulation, suffocation or exposure. Only one of those inquests, the case of Mary Maguire, resulted in a murder trial against a man – the father was suspected of killing the child. As with all cases of infanticide in nineteenth-century Ireland, the issue of paternity was thought to be a motive for the crime.

Murder on Suspicion of Illegitimate Birth?
The Murder of the Infant Mary Maguire, Clones, August 1875
The tiny body of four-month-old Mary Maguire was laid to rest on the first day of September 1875 in the Abbey Graveyard in Clones. She had been bathed and wrapped in a shroud. Within twenty-four hours, the police had received information that the child came to its death by violence. They took swift action by placing a guard at the grave, arrested the child's father, Peter Maguire, and arranged to have the body raised for an inquest and an investigation into the circumstances under which the child died.[56]
    Just one day earlier, Anne Kelly, who lived next door to the Maguire family on Pound Hill, had a visit from her neighbour, Margaret Maguire. Margaret had given birth to a baby girl just four months

earlier and the child had been ill of late. Anne had gone with Margaret to take baby Mary to Dr Hoskins to get some medicine. Dr Hoskins had prescribed some powders, but told Margaret that because the child appeared emaciated he was afraid she would not live.

Anne rented a room to Mary McCabe and the two lived in the house next to the Maguires. Mary was new to Pound Hill and had just moved in three weeks earlier. She didn't know much about the Maguires, but told Anne that while she was away that she heard the couple arguing. Margaret had come over following the shouting, asked to borrow a shawl and left the house.

Margaret and Peter Maguire, both just twenty years old had been married on 1 May 1875, about the same time as the child's birth, and a story was circulating that Peter did not regard the child in a friendly manner. His character was questionable from the start of their relationship. On their marriage licence, under the title of occupation, he is described as a 'gentleman with no profession except knocking about'.[57] Rumours were spreading that Peter may have had doubts about the paternity of the child.[58] However, Anne had seen him nurse and kiss the child on several occasions and at those times, he appeared quite fond of his daughter.

Being concerned about the shouting in the house and Margaret's quick departure, Anne waited about thirty minutes and went over to the Maguires' house to visit and see if there was any serious problem. As Anne entered their home, she saw that Margaret had returned. She was sitting with her baby on her knee and her husband Peter was next to her. He had a hold of the baby's wrists. The infant appeared to be very ill and was vomiting. Anne noticed that the baby's head was enlarged and one of its eyes was swollen. The eyelid was a bluish colour. Anne asked if she might take the child in her arms to observe it more closely and Margaret handed the baby over to her.

Margaret then looked at Peter and asked, 'What ails the child?'

'Nothing ails it. 'Tis just crying,' he replied.

With her hand open, Margaret then took her arm back and swinging forward, hit Peter in the side of the head. She began to wail. 'Oh my baby, O my baby, my baby, O my poor wee Mary.'

The mother appeared to be greatly disturbed – clearly distraught about her child's condition.

At this point, Anne was feeling desperate. With the baby in her arms, she dropped to her knees and asked Peter, 'What have you done to the child?'

'I've done nothing to it,' he said.

Anne then decided there was nothing more she could do. She decided to return home and leave them to sort out the situation.

An hour and a half later, she and Mary McCabe returned to the Maguires' house and discovered the baby was dead.

Margaret McAvina, the wet nurse, Margaret and Peter were there. The wet nurse mentioned that she had called earlier in the day to nurse the child who was in good health at that time. She appeared shocked the child was dead. Now the friends and neighbours could only look on in dismay at the mother sitting beside the cradle containing the body of her dead child. Peter was standing next to his wife.

The mother, mourning the loss of her child, turned to Anne and asked, 'Will you wash the child?'

Anne quickly answered, 'I've had four children of my own that died. I never washed any of them, but I'll do it.'

As Anne removed the child's clothing, she noticed black pitch plasters on its chest and back. She guessed that Margaret must have put them on in an attempt to heal the child since she knew Dr Hoskins had never prescribed plasters. Most upsetting was the state of the baby's head; it was swollen and there was a slight discolouration on its cheek. Placing her hand on its head, she noticed that it was very soft to the touch.

After she finished preparing the tiny body for the wake, Peter reached into his pocket, pulled out a shilling and gave it to his wife to buy Anne a glass of whiskey for her trouble. Anne immediately refused to take any money or whiskey, at which time Margaret said to her husband, 'It would be fitter for you to spend the money in buying a shroud for the body than in paying for whiskey.' He did not answer.

The wake began a short time after. Anne observed Margaret drinking. She was in great distress, very nervous and 'faintish'. She heard Margaret say at one point throughout the evening that she would have been better had she not been married at all, then she would not have had to have gone through this. Peter heard her, but said nothing.

Anne then began speaking with a friend, Michael Trudden. She drew his attention to the state of the child's head. He observed that the head appeared to be a little swollen above one of the ears, but could not say whether he thought it was discoloured or not.

John O'Neill was at the wake. Margaret began throwing comments towards her husband. John claimed to hear Margaret say, 'I hope that those who were to stand sponsors [for baptism] for the child and did not do so, will meet a sudden death.' It was to John she referred when she made the statement. She then said to her husband, 'I had to work at Mr Dudgeon's and the hot suck (hot goat or cow milk given to the child as a substitute for mother's milk) is what killed the child.' Margaret continued giving out to her husband, 'If you had lifted the child out of the cradle when she was smothering, she would not be dead.' Peter made no reply. John took credit for Peter's silence, as he claimed he would not let him respond to Margaret's comments and additionally that he didn't feel that the wake was any place for the couple to get into an argument. By 11p.m., Margaret was raving, 'Oh my poor wee Mary, my poor wee Mary' and Peter then helped her up the stairs to go to bed.

The inquest was held on 4 September 1875. The examination of the body revealed the most substantial evidence in the case. Dr Henry and Dr O'Reilly performed the post-mortem examination. The eyes were closed, the body plump and well-nourished. They found the two black pitch plasters on the child's chest and back and a slight mark on top of the head. There was also a black mark behind the left ear.

On cutting the scalp open from ear to ear, Dr Henry found that it was not only puffy, but that a quantity of fluid escaped and on removing the scalp found that there was a quantity of clotted blood. He told the coroner's jury, 'We found the left parietal [skull] bone and left temporal [cheek] bone fractured and resting on the brain. We also found the covering of the brain torn on the same side and the frontal [forehead] bone broken on the right side, the fracture extending to the ear. On removing the skull we found dark bloody spots on the upper part of the brain ... In regard to the chest (covered with the plaster), when it was opened, we found nothing abnormal and nothing to account for death,' he said.

The conclusion was that death was caused by extensive fractures of the bones in the head and extravasations of blood on the brain. Dr Henry concluded, 'It is our opinion that the child's death was the result of violence. I do not think it could possibly live more than an hour and a half or two hours after receiving these injuries. It could have died in fifteen minutes. The child was healthy as far as we could see. After such a trauma to the head, the child would be likely to vomit. An ordinary blow would not inflict those injuries. I do not think that one blow could cause them. The injuries could not have resulted from a fall out of the arms of a person nursing a child.'

Mr Knight, the defence attorney cross-examining Dr Henry, had two points of contention. First, that Margaret Maguire had put the black pitch plasters on the child's chest and back – possibly the child died of pleurisy. If the child had pleurisy, it would have had fluid on the chest and possibly in other internal organs.

Dr Henry replied, 'Although I opened the chest, I did not find fluid. Because there was not a distension of the abdomen, I did not proceed any further.'

Mr Knight was attempting to show the jury that there could be other potential factors leading to the child's death that had not been thoroughly examined. Dr Henry made the comment, 'No human being could live under such injuries as those inflicted on the child.'

The second point of argument made by Mr Knight was that the child might have accidentally received the fatal injuries to her head by a fall. To this Dr Henry responded, 'If the mother fell with the child in her arms in a certain position *it is possible, but hardly probable*, that the injuries I have described could have been inflicted.' He continued, 'An ordinary blow would not inflict the injuries unless one side of the head was resting on a hard resisting substance. In such a case both sides might be fractured by the one blow.'

At the end of the inquest, many questions were still unanswered. How did the child receive these injuries? Did some person hit the child as it lay with its head against a solid surface, fracturing the skull and cheekbone on the left, while the right-side facing the hard surface was fractured and contused by the sheer force of the blow? Did someone stand on the child's head? Did the child fall from a height, such as from the arms of one of its parents? If so, was it done intentionally or was it a terrible accident?

By the time the inquest concluded, the coroner felt that there was not sufficient evidence to charge Peter Maguire with the death of the baby. The jury's verdict was as follows: 'We find that the deceased child came to its death on 31 August by extensive injuries received on her head; but how or by what means these injuries were inflicted there is no evidence to show.'

The coroner then stated, 'As far as I am concerned, the prisoner is discharged.'

Although the coroner concluded there was not enough evidence against the suspect as a result of the inquest, the Crown court in co-operation with the police could hold their own investigation and bring charges against a suspect at the assizes. As Peter Maguire sat in the courtroom, he was released from custody by the coroner but immediately arrested again by the police.

By the time of the first hearing on 1 October, both Peter and Margaret Maguire had been arrested for 'having willingly and maliciously

killed their infant child, Mary Maguire, aged four months.'[59] Peter
was in custody having been remanded on a magistrate's warrant since
the time of the inquest. Margaret was stated to be unwell and had been
discharged to her home by Mr Wall, JP, after her arrest. Dr O'Reilly
certified that her health would be endangered if she were confined in
a bridewell.

At the start of the proceedings, there was a dispute between the
lawyers and judges about the absence of Margaret Maguire. Dr Henry
was sent to check on her and see if she was well enough to attend the
trial. Margaret was at home in an 'excited state' and very weak. She
had suffered a haemorrhage and was confined to bed. Dr Henry was
to determine if she was well enough to leave her home to attend the
trial. A car was sent to bring her to court. Margaret arrived and the
trial commenced.

Mr Knight and Mr Armstrong defended the Maguires. Mr Knight
began by reviewing Dr Henry's post-mortem examination evidence.
Again, as he had done at the inquest, he began to question Dr Henry
as to possible accidental causes for the wounds to the child's head.

'If the mother fell from a height with the child in her arms the
injuries might have been accidentally inflicted, but in such case the
person who had the child in her arms might be killed too,' said Dr
Henry. 'I said in reply to Mr Dudgeon (one of the prosecutors) at the
coroner's inquest that the injuries might have been caused accidentally. It is *possible* the injuries I saw were the result of an accident.'

Mr Dungeon, the prosecutor, cross-examined Dr Henry and asked, 'What kind of accident would cause it [the trauma to the child's
head]?'

Dr Henry answered, 'Falling from a great height.'

'What height?' he asked.

Mr Armstrong, the defence attorney, objected to the question
but the court allowed it. Although Dr Henry's response was not recorded, it can be assumed that the point attempting to be made is
that although possible, it was highly unlikely the child could have
received such injuries by falling from or while in the arms of its
mother (or father).

Anne Kelly, Margaret McAvina, Martha Reilly[60] and Mary Mc-
Cabe were questioned. Each told their account of the events on 31
August. There was one witness for the prosecution, Eliza Howe, who
recollected seeing Peter Maguire go into his house on that afternoon.
After a considerable amount of time, she had heard Margaret Ma-
guire crying and saying, 'My baby is going to die and I wouldn't have

that for all that ever appertained to me!' Eliza heard Peter respond, but she did not know what he said. This occurred before Anne Kelly went into the Maguire's. She also stated that 'the child had been ill for some time before.'

The case for the prosecution was weak as pointed out by Mr Arm-strong in his closing arguments. He contended that the evidence for the prosecution had entirely failed to cast even a suspicion of guilt on Peter or Margaret Maguire. He dwelt on the absence of all motive for the crime, showing that, according to the evidence of the witnesses produced by the police, both parents had manifested the greatest af-fection for their first and only child. The evidence of Dr Henry which had stated that the injuries might have been caused accidentally was also strongly in favour of the persons accused. No jury would find a verdict of guilty on the evidence adduced, and therefore, he would ask the magistrates to refuse the informations.[61]

The case of Margaret Maguire was refused [not enough evidence to proceed further] and the magistrates returned Peter Maguire for trial at the Monaghan spring assizes on the charge of murder. Peter Maguire remained in custody until March when the spring assizes took place. He again appeared in court. The evidence was again reviewed and a verdict of 'no bill' was brought forth. He was discharged.[62]

There is no further information to suggest anyone was ever charged in the murder of the infant Mary Maguire. In evaluating the evidence it appears that all the witnesses questioned had seen the child in the months prior to the day of her death and knew her to be suffering from an illness, but did not report any wounds or marks about the child's head at that time. The most compelling evidence appears to be that of Margaret McAvina. She had shown up early in the after-noon to nurse the child. It did not appear to have any injuries. When she arrived at the house later that day, the child was dead and there was trauma about the head. Unfortunately, there was no testimony provided by either Peter or Margaret Maguire. The prosecution clearly could not prove motive on the part of Margaret or Peter Maguire although the injuries to the child's head were significant.

Did Peter Maguire suspect that the child was not his own? Why did John O'Neill not stand as a sponsor at the child's baptism? It is interesting that the only other man involved in this tragic story was one who would not participate in the religious celebration of the child's birth. What did he object to? A possible theory exists: Peter Maguire suspecting the child was not his own, having married this woman, unhappy with his situation and feeling angry, resentful and deceived, lost patience with an already sickly and crying child, struck or stepped on the child crushing its skull in the mother's absence. Given the attitudes towards illegitimate children in the nineteenth century, a man marrying into such a situation could be motivated towards such a crime. The case was left unsolved.

ABANDONMENT BY THE FATHER
Legal Recourse

Women facing a pregnancy alone without the support of the father were publicly shamed and their earning power was greatly reduced, giving them a dependant that they could not support. There was no law in place to make a father provide support for the illegitimate child and no means to prove paternity. In these cases, there were only a few legal processes in place to attempt to protect the woman and the offspring. They were: 1. Damages awarded in cases of seduction; 2. Enforcement of promises made to the girl by the said man to help with the child's maintenance; and 3. Damages awarded against the man for impairing the girl's earning potential by making her pregnant.[63] In 1875, Catherine Murtagh of Ballybay was charged by James Mc-Geough of Drumgor for exposing and deserting her infant child. She had been working as a servant in the house of the complainant's father, who had seduced her, and in the course of time she had given birth to a male child. He refused to give her any support and she took him to court. Murtagh obtained a decree of £21 against him. To evade payment of the money, the father signed over his farm and effects to his son [the complainant] and the result was that Murtagh and her child received nothing. Being destitute, she went with the child to the complainant's house, met with his wife, gave her the child, and then went away. She was charged with child desertion for having left the child behind her. Mr McWilliam, representing Catherine Murtagh, spoke to the magistrates passionately about the harsh conduct of James McGeough and his father and asked that the court give his client the full amount the court allowed. The court dismissed the case with 15 shilling costs.[64]

In another similar abandonment case in 1858, Sarah McGrayons was put in Monaghan Jail for leaving her child in the shop of a man named Kierney in Ballybay, charging him with being the father. When her child was brought to the jail, it appeared very delicate and sickly and it died there in the arms of its mother.[65]

Women with illegitimate children who lived at the workhouse often pleaded with the Monaghan Union board members to get monies from the fathers, as was recorded in the minutes of the meetings that were published in *The Northern Standard*, 3 October 1863.

> The Master laid before the board the names of several women who had illegitimate children with them in the house, supported by the union.
>
> Mr Lloyd expressed a desire to make the fathers of these children pay the cost of their support, if possible.
>
> After an investigation of the circumstances connected with each case, the board deferred proceedings against all the fathers with one exception. Mr J. C. Wright said that in this case the father had been processed and the Barrister dismissed the case in consequence of the mother having settled the matter with the father and received a sum of money from him.
>
> Mr E. W. Lucas and Mr Lloyd were of the opinion that settlement could only be held good against the mother as long as she was out of the house, but that having brought the children into the house to be supported by the union, the father became liable for the support of the children while in the house. It was decided that the case should be laid before the solicitor of the union to be proceeded with in the manner he thought best. Mr Hamilton thought that if the case was again dismissed by the Chairman of the County, an appeal should be lodged and the issue tried in a superior court. After admitting three paupers the board rose.

> *The Northern Standard*, 5 March 1864
> Co. Monaghan Spring Assizes: Putative Father Case
> The Guardians of Monaghan Union vs. Patrick Mohan
> This was an appeal from the decision of the Chairman at Quarter Sessions. The mother of the children, at present an inmate in the Union workhouse, deposed that the respondent Mohan was the father of two children, who were supported by the Guardians of the Union. An agreement on her part to forego all claims on Mohan, on payment of a sum of £4 was put in as corroborative evidence against Mohan. Mohan alleged that the agreement was not made by him, but by his brother, and was executed under constraint as he was about to get married. He also deposed that he had no connection with the woman. The judge held the agreement corroborative evidence which with the evidence of the Relieving Officer of the Union, he considered sufficiently corroborative to authorise him to reverse the decision made below, and to decree that the respondent should pay for the support of his illegitimate children.

Of the many cases in which infants were found dead in the countryside of Co. Monaghan, one can only imagine the stories of trouble and abandonment for the mothers who decided to keep their illegitimate children. Every child had a father and every case of illegitimacy bore its own sad story. What were the repercussions for men who admitted paternity to illegitimate children without the covenant of marriage? As most illegitimate children were born to the poor and farming classes, an unplanned marriage or the pregnancy of an unmarried daughter could prove disastrous for a delicately balanced family. Preserving the family holding relied upon the orderly transfer from one generation to the next and depended upon a system of marriage in order to avoid upset to the pattern of succession. Therefore, to destroy a girl's character was to destroy the intricate mutual obligations and expectancies of the rural family.[66] 'Bastards' broke the bonds of familial inheritance which linked members of rural Irish families and damaged their reputation in the community. This does not excuse the men who abandoned pregnant women; however, it does offer an explanation. They were often motivated by the fear of losing status and a holding that the family had worked for generations.

BEGGARS, PROSTITUTES AND THE WORKHOUSE

Illegitimate children created a whole new set of problems for the women who gave birth to them and, more often than not, threw them into destitution. There were not many employment opportunities for unmarried mothers. Some were forced to beg for money and food, others became prostitutes and many used the workhouse for shelter, subsistence and childcare. Poverty was not seen as a social cause, but was an outward manifestation of the failure of individuals to secure work and support themselves as a result of their own particular vices such as idleness, sloth or laziness. However, when individuals were destitute through illness or misfortune, they were perceived in a new light as the 'deserving poor'. It was for this category of people that the workhouse was intended.

The workhouse was not an institution of absolute confinement, but instead one that was used by women especially when they were vulnerable, burdened with the lethargy of pregnancy and the weakness of childbirth and nursing, and the fathers of their children were not obliged to pay anything towards their maintenance.[67] It was especially useful as a makeshift home from time to time to leave their children and ensure their health and safety. Frequently a woman would gain entry into the workhouse with her child, and then abandon it there as she knew it would be taken care of properly for a short time. During this time she would attempt to earn money either by begging or working in the fields at harvest time, or by other means. It was desirable to have the child in the workhouse during times of great economic hardship because of her inability to mind the child and work at the same time. This was not without repercussions; it was still required that the mother pay for the care of her child while in the establishment.[68]

In the case of Betty Doyle, she was eager to have her child placed in the workhouse by a friend in order to use the time to go out begging for money. She was found out and charged by the Guardians of the Poor of Monaghan Union for having deserted her child. The story was reported in *The Northern Standard*, Friday, 8 October 1875 as follows:

Child Desertion

The Guardians of the Poor of Monaghan Union charged a woman named Betty Doyle described as a tramp, with having on 25 August last, deserted her male child, aged twelve months, and left it chargeable on the rates.

Mr Douglass, relieving officer, appeared on behalf of the Guardians.

Alice MacGonnell said the defendant lodged with her for some time last summer. She last saw her two months ago. Defendant said at that time she would pay anybody well who would get her child into the workhouse, and if she (witness) would do it, the defendant would not forget her.

She [Betty Doyle] told witness that her name was Betty McGeough. She did not know whether the defendant was married or not. She said the child was her own.

Mary Duffy said the defendant came to her house one very wet evening and she gave her lodging for the night. She left the next morning, leaving the child behind her. Witness took the child to the workhouse and a few days after it was admitted.

Defendant said she left the child with the last witness and told her to take good care of it.

Mr Murray – Are you willing to take the child out of the workhouse now?
Defendant – Yes.
Mr Murray – Are you able to pay for its support there for the past six weeks?
Defendant – No. I have no money.
Mr Young – How do you get your livelihood?
Defendant – I look for it.
Mr Young – You are a sturdy beggar. Are you married?
Defendant – No.

The magistrates discharged the defendant on her promising to take the child out of the workhouse.

Women who were incarcerated either in the local jail or in prison also used the workhouse as a 'surrogate mother' in a time of need. Sarah McCarville, alias Sarah Brown, single mother of two, was in trouble with the law for various crimes from 1870 onwards, most of which involved robbery; in fact she was arrested and put in jail over

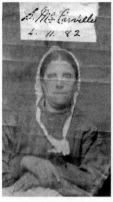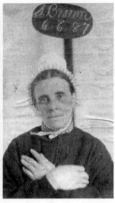

Sarah McCarville (alias Brown) [Sarah McCarville, GPB, PEN 1886/129 & Sarah Browne; GPB, PEN 1890/48] The picture on the left is Sarah upon her committal to Mountjoy on 4 November 1882. The picture to the right is her upon her release from prison 6 June 1887 under the name Sarah Brown. Sarah was arrested over 41 times and was incarcerated for much of her life over a span of 20 years.

40 times. Having been sentenced finally to penal servitude for seven years at Mountjoy, she corresponded frequently with the master of the workhouse to apply for admittance of her son who was frail and weak.[69] Although her behaviour in and outside of prison was questionable – she frequently threatened the life of other prisoners and was violent towards prison guards – she did continue to ensure the care of her children. There were many others like her.

Prostitutes were another group of women who had 'survival' instinct. In the nineteenth century they were an *invisible* group judged as social outcasts, viewed by philanthropists as 'fallen women' and accepted as an inevitable feature of society. In the case histories of prostitutes, often published in the annual reports of rescue agencies, they were portrayed as women whose lives were destroyed by sexual experience (having been seduced) and usually came from the lower classes.[70] There were prostitutes in Co. Monaghan, although references to them appear only randomly when they came into contact with the law or, in the case of Catherine Byrne of Carrickmacross, when found dead. In March 1876, the body of Catherine Byrne was found drowned in the canal. She is described as 'a native of Carrickmacross, where her father and mother live, and early in life acquired habits of intemperance which led to a course of infamy. She became a prostitute years ago, and went under the nickname of "the Gawk".'[71]

A most common feature of prostitutes was that they were single mothers with fatherless children, who for reasons other than their occupation were in frequent trouble with the law. Many were arrested for stealing, presumably for money or items that could be sold to support them and their children. Elisabeth Finnegan, a twenty-six-

year-old single mother and prostitute from Clones, was convicted on
5 July 1883 at the Co. Monaghan assizes for stealing £110. She was
sentenced to five years penal servitude at Mountjoy where she corresponded regularly with the master of the Monaghan workhouse to
ensure the care of her child while she served her sentence.[72] Another
woman referred to in the coroner's inquests was Mary McGarvey, a
witness in the trial of Terence McGuigan in Castleblayney. She was
an admitted prostitute who had served four years at Mountjoy prison
for robbery.[73] In testimony given, it was revealed that she had been
sitting in the pub crying that 'she had left her orphan children at
Castlebellingham'.[74] It may appear that by getting into trouble with
the law and spending long durations incarcerated these women were
ignorant, callous or uncaring towards their children, but the risks they
were willing to take to care for them depicts the true nature of the
relationship between mother and child.

DEATH IN CHILDBIRTH AND THE PRACTICE OF MIDWIFERY

Most women had birth attendants or midwives, traditional handy-
women who guided them through the experience of childbirth. In
many cases, the midwife was the only person present in the room
with the woman delivering her child and was a greatly trusted and
relied upon member of the female population in their time of need.
In the nineteenth century, a new focus on gynaecological science and
surgery was being used to reinforce all existing assumptions about
women and femininity: that women were passive and pure by nature
and their primary biological purpose was to bear children. Further-
more, the medical profession began investigating and criticising the
practices of midwives, characterising them as lurid, boozy and ignorant women – a witch in her lair – who would dispose of unwanted
babies for a price. There were midwives who would perform abortions
and fake stillbirth deaths for a fee; however, many were in the business of delivering healthy mothers and children successfully through
the birth process. In fact, the average general practitioner felt some
threat to his livelihood from the midwives, whose trade was crowded[75] and in the late 1860s there was discussion that legislation should
be passed to make midwives register to prove they were qualified for
their practice. It would make them less of an economic threat, subordinate to the doctors, but it would also get rid of those in the profession who were unskilled and committing criminal abuses.

Of the fourteen cases when a mother died as a direct result of complications during childbirth, only two were unmarried. These were 'legitimate' cases where married, *respectable* women had died and therefore it was necessary to initiate an investigation into the circumstances and cause of death. One salient feature of these inquests is the attitude of physicians who offered criticism of the attendance, behaviour and skill of the midwives. Most often doctors chastised and condemned the midwives' lack of improper training when a death took place without their requesting 'expert' help from a physician. For example, Susan McCleary died after childbirth when her midwife, Betty Caulfield, was unable to extract the afterbirth. Susan died from internal haemorrhaging and the midwife, presumably thinking she could handle the situation herself, did not call for the doctor. The doctor was called to testify at the inquest and told the jury, 'Had a properly qualified practitioner attended the deceased, the probability is that she would have come safely through her confinement. Afterbirth is a fact attendant on all confinements and that this was properly dealt with, we have no evidence whatever.'[76] The removal of afterbirth was a frequent problem for midwives and physicians, yet it is only criticised in the absence of a *qualified* practitioner.

On the other hand, if the midwife did send word to the physician during a difficult time in the delivery, there might be a different attitude taken towards her actions. For example, Rose Martin, a nineteen-year-old pregnant girl, very near the time of giving birth, walked nine miles from her home in the townland of Magherashaghry in the parish of Currin to the Cootehill Market in her bare feet on a very cold day in December 1860. Upon her return, she complained of not feeling well – her labour had started. The midwife, Margaret Reilly, was called and the child was safely delivered. Margaret was described as 'a middle-aged woman much employed and considered to be fortunate on such occasions'. Unfortunately, a problem arose; Margaret was not able to remove the afterbirth from the mother's body and immediately sent for Dr Taylor of Drum. Sadly, Rose died before the doctor reached the house. At the inquest, the midwife was praised by Dr Taylor in his deposition to the coroner's jury that 'the treatment she [deceased] received was careful and considerate and such as is usual in similar circumstances.' However, he added, 'Had a qualified practitioner been present 'tis possible her life might have been preserved, but the long walk taken on 30th was quite sufficient to have an injurious effect on so slight a person as the deceased.'[77] The words 'qualified practitioner' clearly show the opinion of the time that only male physicians (women were not allowed to attend medical school to become doctors) were capable of properly attending to and diagnosing women in labour – even though most midwives had attended in hundreds of cases. It is also important to note that the walk that Rose Martin took on the day she went into labour would have absolutely nothing to do with the afterbirth becoming lodged in her abdomen. Dr Taylor himself might not have been successful in removing it and saving the woman's life.

Another example of a midwife considered responsible for the death of a mother was the case of Mrs Robert Clarke who died in childbirth. Mrs Clarke was buried soon after her death and, shortly thereafter, a rumour began to circulate that there was neglect on the part of the family and gross and culpable mismanagement on the part of the midwife who attended her. The midwife was described as a person without either the necessary experience or information for such a duty and who immediately after the death of the young woman left the country. Inquiries were made and in a statement to the Stranooden police, Robert Clarke, the deceased's husband, stated that 'he did not wish nor did any of his family that the body of the deceased should be raised for the purpose of an inquest being held and that he did not think there had been any wilful neglect or mismanagement on the part of any one. He also reported that the midwife had left the country and gone to America.'[78] Was she so afraid of prosecution that she fled the country? Was she inexperienced?

Witch-Trial or Poor Medical Practices by a Midwife?
The Death of Mrs Margaret Johnston,
Clones, Clones Parish, October 1860
After nine long months, Margaret Johnston began having labour pains on a Sunday for her first child with her husband, Thomas. They were greatly anticipating the birth like most new parents and Margaret had planned to have a midwife attend the birth to ensure a successful delivery. The midwife, Ellen Brady, had a 'great name' in her field of employment and her services were in wide request.[79]

By Tuesday, the pains were strong enough to have their servant, Bridget Sherry, collect the midwife. When Ellen Brady arrived at the Johnston's house, Margaret was trying to comfort herself by lying in bed for a while, then having a cup of tea by the fire, back to her bed, then back to the fire. The expecting mother was restless. Ellen, with the help of Bridget Sherry, carried Margaret's bed to the kitchen fireside as was the custom as it was the spot where the birth usually took place. Unfortunately, nothing seemed to be working. Margaret was complaining and switching positions to either lying in her bed, or crouching by the fire on her knees. Before early morning the bed was removed back to her room; the child was still not ready to come.

By Wednesday afternoon, the midwife made a decision to aid the progress of the labour and help deliver the baby by performing an 'operation'. She instructed Bridget to help her. This operation lasted for three hours from 4p.m. to 7p.m. that evening. Mary Tibby, Margaret's sister-in-law, stopped by on Wednesday evening having heard that Margaret had still not given birth to the child. She walked in on the operation being performed by the midwife and servant. Margaret appeared to be in great pain with a great deal of blood pouring out from between her legs. She was moaning and yelling that the midwife was hurting her and begged her to be easy. Mary went out and told her brother to call for Dr Moorehead. Ellen Brady was very unhappy when she discovered that the doctor was coming. The expectant mother and the midwife, both exhausted, fell asleep until an hour later when the doctor arrived.

Dr Moorehead came in to find Margaret Johnston, still very pregnant, lying on a mattress beside her bed. Her pulse was very low and upon examining her found that she suffered from 'very injurious treatment'. The operation performed by Ellen Brady was that of *Dilatation* – artificial manipulation to promote dilation of the cervix to bring about delivery of the child. Much injury had been done to the private parts (genitals) and there were lacerations on the neck of the uterus from which blood was flowing freely, even though labour had made little progress. These cuts were likely made in order to reach inside the patient to cut the cervix in an attempt to remove the baby from her body. Dr Moorehead gave the patient a *draught* to suspend the haemorrhage and after some time, the haemorrhage did cease. He desired her to be kept quiet, get light nourishing of food and drink and not allowed to go into labour. He left shortly after these instructions late on Wednesday night.

In the early hours of Thursday morning, Margaret, still in much pain, called Mary Tibby over and told her that 'the child was dead and swelled and would take her life', even though Dr Moorehead had said that the child was still living. Dr Moorehead had also delivered more bad news during his visit. He told Mary Tibby and Thomas Johnston that 'there was no chance of Margaret living. The injuries she suffered from were sufficient to cause death'. Now they could only pray and hope for a miracle.

The miracle never came. Margaret delivered a stillborn child two days later on Friday night, 28 September 1860. Mary Tibby said she could not stay in the room with her anymore as there was 'a bad smell coming from her'. Dr Moorehead stated that *gangrene* had set in which produces a stench resembling rotting apples. Margaret lingered for eight more days until her death on 4 October 1860.

An inquest was held and charges were brought against the midwife, Ellen Brady for 'unskilful treatment as a midwife'. She appeared at the Monaghan spring assizes in March 1861. Before calling the case to the attention of the court, Justice Edmund Hayes made the following statement to the jury:[80]

There is, however, in what is called the bail calendar, one offence on which I think it right to detain you for a moment. That is, a person has been committed for causing death by unskilful treatment as a midwife. That gentlemen, is not an offence of everyday occurrence and probably that circumstance demands some observation upon it. It will be your duty, gentlemen, in examining the witnesses against this woman, who stands charged with the offence, to have your attention directed to this principal point – whether under all the circumstances of the case, this woman has been guilty of gross rashness or gross negligence in discharge of the office which she may have undertaken to perform. That gentlemen is a question, which on the hearing of the evidence for the prosecution you are to ask yourself. The law will not allow any person even under the guise of rendering assistance to another in the time of need, to trifle with human life, or to undertake the performance of duty which they know or feel themselves incapacitated to perform, more especially, if more able assistance is available at the time. The one would amount to rashness, in interfering with things that did not belong to their capacity to perform, then they should bring to the performance all due diligence. If a person fails in that respect, and if there be gross negligence and death has ensued, it will be your duty to find the bill. On the other hand, if you come to the conclusion that this person possibly accustomed to matters of this kind, yet not used to dealing with cases of sudden emergency, such as frequently arises, death may have unfortunately happened on account of the skill brought to bear on this case, which had proved useful in other cases, not being sufficient to deal with this one. – If on the whole, you think this woman brought reasonable skill and reasonable diligence to the discharge of her duty, then, gentlemen it would be your duty to ignore the bill. If there should be a doubt in the case, probably you will come to the conclusion that it is better in a case of this kind that further postponement should not take place – new facts not being likely to come out, that the charge should not be kept hanging over her; but that she should be found not guilty.'[81]

Bridget Sherry, Mary Tibby and Dr John Moorehead were questioned before the jury. Both Bridget and Mary were asked if the midwife was drinking at any time throughout the process of the delivery. Bridget stated that she did not see the midwife take any drink the night of the operation. Mary stated that she did see the prisoner (Ellen Brady) take a little whiskey, but she was in no way affected by it. An attempt was being made by the prosecution to stereotype the midwife as a 'drinking slattern'.

Dr Moorehead took the stand and under cross-examination stated, 'Dilatation was formerly practised but is now abandoned. I am of the opinion that if a male practitioner used dilatation, it would be criminal.'

He continued, 'I never knew of it being practiced by a doctor, but heard of midwives doing it. The suffering of the patient (Margaret Johnston) from the injuries would be vastly greater than those arising from natural child birth. When I first saw Mrs Johnston she was suffering more pain than she would under the pains of labour.'

Midwife Ellen Brady was found guilty and sentenced to four months imprisonment.[82] Was this verdict justified? Although dilatation was no longer used by midwives or physicians, Ellen Brady, with all her years of experience, may have been successful in the past using this technique. Under the circumstances, Margaret Johnston was three days in labour, and being concerned with the safety and welfare of the child and mother, there is no reason to believe she made the decision to perform such a procedure other than to expedite the birth in an attempt to save lives. In any event, considering the instructions given to the jury, they came to the conclusion that she did not have reasonable skill, took on the responsibility of performing an operation she was not qualified for and therefore came to a guilty verdict.

Tragedies in Childbirth: Some Individual Accounts
Sir William Wilde once wrote that 'it was a popular belief among some of the lower orders that a woman dying during pregnancy was saved hereafter in virtue of the sinless offspring which she carried'.[83] These cases of women dying in childbirth are tragic – leaving a husband, the newborn infant and other children without a wife and mother. Most of these women haemorrhaged during or after delivery and could not be saved by midwives or physicians. The inquest of Ellen Murphy on 8 September 1875 illustrates the circumstances in such a case. The inquest reads as follows:

8.1144, Murphy, Ellen
8 September 1875
An inquest was held on the body of Ellen Murphy on 8 September 1875 in

the townland of Cornapaste in the parish of Currin. Mary Murphy deposed on the evening of the 5th, 'I was at the house of the deceased being sent for – she had been well and safely delivered of her 7th [seventh] child about 9p.m. I went in to see her and remained about an hour during which she had been ill and departed life. A midwife had been engaged to attend the deceased but had not arrived and deceased had taken ill unexpectedly.' Bridget McDonald deposed was with the deceased prior to the child being born. 'Soon after, I came in and the deceased became faint and weak; there was no external haemorrhage.' Dr Richard Sherry deposed that from the adduced evidence he considers the deceased died from internal haemorrhage. The verdict was death on 5 September 1875 from internal haemorrhage after confinement of a female child.[84]

The Northern Standard published a few lines describing the feeling in the locality of Laurel Hill where Ellen Murphy lived:

> A woman very much respected in the neighbourhood took suddenly ill and was confined; no person being with her at the time, she died two hours afterwards ... much sorrow is felt for this woman's family in the locality. She was the mother of seven children.[85]

There is one case of all the infant deaths and murders listed that is in a category all its own. It is a strange and disturbing tale resulting from misdiagnosis and ignorance on the part of all concerned.

Puerperal Fever: The Death of Biddy McManus and her Infant,
January 1857, Clones, Parish of Clones
Biddy McManus was admitted as a patient to the Clones Fever Hospital by Dr Knight on Sunday evening, 4 January 1857 with a fever and an inflamed leg.[86] She was put into a bed; some powders were prescribed as well as warm fumigation. On Monday morning, she requested Mary Ann McDonald, attendant, to send a priest to visit her. The priest attended to her and left.

Later that night, Mary Ann was sitting up and heard noises in the ward. She discovered it was Biddy McManus and went in to check on her. Biddy said she must have been 'raving in her sleep'. Elisa Bowen, matron of the hospital, went in about twenty minutes later to check on her. When Mrs Bowen came out of the room, she told Mary Ann McDonald, 'I saw a child's leg sticking out of the bed covers.'

Mary Ann went in to investigate and saw the same thing – an infant's tiny leg was sticking out from underneath the bed covers. She observed a clean cut on the knee of the child, but it was not bleeding.

Mary Ann asked Biddy, 'What is that?'

Biddy responded, 'Some dirt.'

Mary Anne requested, 'Can I see the child?'

Biddy would not let her see the child and immediately gathered the bed clothes around it. She also saw a small white-handled pen-knife lying on the bolster at Biddy's head.[87] When Mrs Bowen came back in to the room, Mary Ann took the pen knife, showed it to Mrs Bowen and closed the blades. There were spots of blood on the knife along with clotted hair.

Both Mary Ann and Mrs Bowen were concerned that the child might be killed by the mother and decided to stay in the room with Biddy McManus for the night until the arrival of Dr Knight in the morning. At one point in the middle of the night, Mrs Bowen left the room to check on another patient. After she had gone, Biddy spoke to Mary Ann pleading with her that she 'had given birth to a child and wished that Mary Ann would take it and hide it, and say nothing about it.'

Dr Knight arrived the next morning and the women relayed the details of the events the previous night as well as the present condition of Biddy McManus. Dr Knight did not see anything unusual about her appearance the days before and did not know she was pregnant. He then went in and asked her if she had given birth to a child. At first she denied it and started moving about as if to examine her own bed. She then admitted having had a child but that she had 'gone out and placed it beside the canal and supposed the dogs had eaten it.' He knew this could not be true and Dr Knight was determined to remove her to another bed in an attempt to locate the child. In the process Biddy attempted to cover herself with a blanket, but it was discovered that the baby was at her back, below her shoulders. It was taken from between her shift and skin, tied up in a red handkerchief. The infant was quite dead and the upper part of the head was cut and carved, so much so that the brain was almost gone.[88]

Biddy, when asked who the father of her child was, said, 'His name was Maguire, but he has gone to America.' The child was born at seven months and Dr Knight considered it was born alive.

Dr Knight did not consider Elisa Bowen or Mary Ann McDonald guilty of neglect in their attendance on the woman and stated that he had 'every reason to believe that his directions were attended to and the medicine for the deceased duly given'. However, why did these women wait until morning to try to remove the child from her? They had already removed the penknife that could have been used as a weapon against them, so what were they waiting for? They must have already known the child was dead since they stayed in the room the entire night, and there was no report of hearing any sounds coming from the child. One possible explanation involves the politics of hospitals and similar organisations. No member of staff would treat a patient or make a decision before consulting the doctor. It was protocol for most medical institutions that only the doctor was able to make decisions and determine treatment, and those duties were then carried out by the staff. It must have been a desperate situation as the women didn't once attempt to move Biddy throughout the night. Yet, why didn't they call Dr Knight? She was still suffering from what they believed to be typhus, had an inflamed leg, had also given birth to a child – and killed it. What kind of treatment was Biddy receiving?

By Wednesday morning, 7 January 1875, just four days after her admission to the hospital, Biddy McManus was dead. One interesting piece of information stated by Dr Knight in the coroner's report reads as follows, 'From the reports in town on Wednesday morning of her death and the cause of it, I proceeded to the hospital and found her dead, but on carefully examining the body found no marks of injury, while the body presented a natural appearance considering all the facts of the case.'

Puerperal fever or childbed fever is an abnormal condition that results from infection of the placental site following delivery or abortion and is characterised in mild form by fever but in serious cases the infection may spread through the uterine wall or pass into the bloodstream.[89] The symptoms of puerperal fever can range over fever, delirium, convulsions, ranting and slurred speech, rage towards the child and/or the father, severe depression, etc. In the nineteenth century, puerperal fever was not believed to be an actual infection or physical problem, but instead defined as 'puerperal insanity' and psychiatric explanation defined it as 'that after childbirth a woman's mind was abnormally weak, her constitution depleted and her control over her behaviour diminished.'[90] Puerperal fever very often resulted in the death of the infant and the mother as was the case with Biddy McManus and her child. The most terrible act of the puerperal maniac was child murder. It was during the nineteenth century that the infanticidal woman first became the subject of psychiatric as well as legal discourse. Her crime was the worst that could be imagined by a society that exalted maternity.

The symptoms of typhus and typhoid fevers were similar enough to puerperal fever that the two were often easily confused, and puerperal fever even viewed as a variant of typhus, a disease caused by several microrganisms and transmitted by lice and fleas. High fever, depression, delirium, headache, a peculiar eruption of reddish spots on the body, the tongue dry displaying brown crust – are all signs of typhus fever. In addition to being diagnosed with typhus, Biddy had an inflamed leg which is often associated with puerperal fever as infections can result and manifest themselves in the skin. Hard red patches appear, the leg swells; sometimes this is called 'white leg'. It is extremely painful due to the presence of a thrombophlebitis, the inflammation of a vein owing to a clot of blood that remains attached to its place of origin, and in the case of puerperal fever, can be traced back to a bacterial infection of the uterus.[91] Although puerperal fever most often occurs after the baby has been delivered, if there was infection in the body prior to the delivery or if the baby was stillborn, the signs of the fever could immediately appear.

It is possible that Dr Knight was unfamiliar with puerperal fever? Even after he found out that Biddy had given birth to a child, killed it, then died the next day, his testimony supported the verdict at the inquest which was 'death from complications of typhus fever'. Or did he ignore puerperal fever as a possible cause of death as Biddy had already been admitted for typhus? Of course the possibility exists she did have typhus and was concealing her pregnancy, but the derangement that followed combined with the infection in her leg (the site of the infection was believed to have originated in her uterus) supports the existence of puerperal fever.

The psychiatric definition of puerperal fever ignored the social problems of unmarried, abused and destitute mothers and the shocks, adjustments and psychological traumas of the maternal role. Biddy had been concealing her pregnancy which indicates a potential for premeditation to destroy it. Also the information that the father of the child had gone to America would certainly only enhance the severe depression and delirium associated with puerperal fever and prove deadly to the infant and the mother.

This is the only clear case in which puerperal fever appears to have contributed to the death of an infant in the coroner's casebook – but how many others were there? We have no way of knowing except to identify that in such a case as that of Biddy McManus, where very clear signs of puerperal fever were apparent, it still went unrecognised or unacknowledged. How many of the women who murdered their newborn infants were suffering from 'childbed fever' in Co. Monaghan?

Illegitimacy, perpetuated by social, political and religious fears and beliefs, contributed to hundreds of infant deaths in Co. Monaghan in the nineteenth century. It should be considered that, although some women committed infanticide and willingly ended the lives of their children, their action should not be defined without understanding that they too were victims of the society they lived in. A child born out of wedlock often excluded them from their religion, limited their employment and earning power and often sent them, literally, to the poorhouse. They were shunned within their communities, viewed as a plague on traditional life and their children were seen as a threat to land inheritance. Regardless of the choice each woman made, they should all be seen as survivors – strong women in the history of the county who made hard decisions under extremely difficult conditions.

CHAPTER THREE

MANSIONS OF DESPAIR
SUICIDE AND THE ASYLUM

Kilmainham Jail: Prisoner No. 520. Hugh Stewart; born in Truagh, Co. Monaghan; Age 36; Height 5'6"; Brown hair, grey eyes, fresh complexion; Can read and write; Presbyterian faith; Convicted for talking to a spirit in his head, refuses to eat or dress himself and knocked his head against a wall; Classified as a dangerous lunatic; Committed 14 August 1865 by G. Wyse, Esq., from A Division; Discharged 9 November 1865.
– Kilmainham Jail Registers, National Archives, Dublin.

Many of the persons recorded as *lunatics* or *insane* in the coroner's casebook were physically healthy individuals who had displayed signs of depression, anger or violence and were sent to jails, prisons or asylums where they contracted diseases and died; others committed suicide. Vaguely defined mental disorders were suggested as reasons why they might have become mentally and physically weak. However, this chapter is not an attempt to correct misdiagnosis, instead, it is an opportunity to expose both a society that was intolerant of behaviour perceived as 'abnormal' and the changes that occurred within rural families and communities which translated to an increase in 'insanity' in the post-famine population at large.

Monaghan was not different from other counties in Ireland dealing with the constant loss of children to emigration, especially those not favoured with inheritance or dowry. A sense of loss and isolation followed the massive rural population decline.

Tensions between inheriting son and ageing parents who still controlled the farm or between young and old in the transfer of land contributed to changes in marriage patterns and birth rates. Additionally, the male dominance in this rural society put women at a disadvantage, even at the cost of their life expectancy.[1] The result of these changes was an increase in persons being branded as 'lunatics' – a label for various problems ranging from depression to aggressive, violent or even criminal behaviour – which required family members either to manage their care in the home or to commit them to an institution such as the District Lunatic Asylum. Although some did suffer from organic mental illnesses, others only displayed behaviour that was not consistent with expectations and traditional responses to their environment and so were threatened with committal to the asylum. This was especially true of children unwilling to accept their particular position within the family, refusing to listen or accommodate their parents' needs.

Luckily, the information contained within the inquests provides us with an understanding of the behaviour of persons considered insane and the conditions under which death occurred. The picture that emerges tells us that the behaviour of the 'lunatics', 'maniacs' and 'melancholics' disturbed the sane and disrupted the societal status quo of expected and controlled behaviour. It also shows the inability of rural families, communities at large and medical professionals to fully understand these behaviour and the decisions made regarding the treatment of these afflicted 'lunatics'.

THE DISTRICT LUNATIC ASYLUM

The demand for the asylum grew from the needs of the community. Before the opening of the Monaghan District Lunatic Asylum, lunatics were either housed at the jail along with the vagrants, prostitutes and petty criminals or sent from counties Armagh, Fermanagh, Cavan and Monaghan to the Armagh asylum. Exceptions to such committals were women who were instead sent to the workhouse because they displayed controllable or manageable behaviour. When the Monaghan asylum began receiving patients in May 1869 to service the general population of Cavan and Monaghan, it received a transfer of twenty-one male and twenty female patients from the already overcrowded Armagh asylum.[2] The Monaghan asylum located in Roosky, Monaghan town, was converted into what is known today as St Davnet's Psychiatric Hospital.

Although the coroner's inquests record inmates from the asylum, not all inmates who died within its walls were seen and recorded by the coroner. Only by reviewing the death records of asylum inmates, held at the North Eastern Health Board, can we see who comprised the population of asylum inmates as well as the causes of their death.

The majority of patients were single, male and with an average age of 35 years. They were primarily farmers and sons of farmers. The

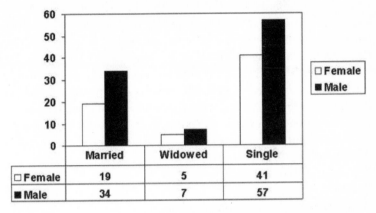

Number of Asylum Inmate Deaths
Recorded at the Registrars Office in Monaghan from 1869-1876

	Married	Widowed	Single
□ Female	19	5	41
■ Male	34	7	57

Unknown marital status = 9 male; 2 female
Total Deaths Recorded = 174

Number of Asylum Inmate Deaths [Sample taken over span of 7 years]

majority of female inmates were also single with an average age of 38 years. Some were the unmarried daughters of farmers, while others were beggars and prostitutes. These demographics are reflective of asylum inmates at other institutions around the country and reveal that Co. Monaghan shared similar social issues. One major cause of this increase in mental illnesses or *perceived* insanity in the rural population was *familism* – a term used to describe the way in which the desires and interests of the individual were subordinated to the welfare of the family in late nineteenth- and early twentieth-century Ireland.[3] Land was no longer divided into separate plots for each child and a spouse, instead it was given to, or inherited in its entirety by, the eldest son. Parents did not always hand over the land in a timely fashion and, without land, a man would have much more difficulty finding a wife. Siblings were left either to work the family farm as servants, or to make the decision to emigrate. For those who worked in industry, the money made would go towards providing for the family. In many cases, marriage would not occur, if at all, until a man was in his thirties or later; with women in their late twenties or early thirties. Women getting married at a later age often meant families were smaller.

Those who did not marry might work a farm they did not own, live as subordinates to their parents well into middle age, and were not able to have a relationship, a sexual relationship, with a member of the opposite sex. These constrictions spread a contagious spirit of despair. Many bachelors were showing signs of what we today would call schizophrenia, believed to have been brought on owing to the postponement of adulthood and later the 'identity crisis' of the Irish bachelor.[4] Hugh Stewart, for example, was sent to Kilmainham aged thirty-four, for talking to a spirit in his head.

One death recorded in the coroner's reports was that of a single young man who killed himself. His father could only account for his death by saying that 'fever' ran in the family. This fever could be interpreted to mean sickness or depression. It is possible there was typhus or typhoid fever in the family, but it is more likely that the father was not willing to share any of the other factors that may have contributed to his son's suicide.

Single Man, 28 Years Old, Son of a Farmer
The Suicide of John Brown,
Glasdrumman, Clontibret Parish, September 1871
The body of a young man was found nude, floating in a pool of water two feet deep (a public sewer) in the townland of Kilnacran, and for a short time, his identity was unknown.[5] By the end of the week, he was identified as John Brown, the twenty-eight-year-old son of farmer Robert Brown of Glasdrumman in the parish of Clontibret.

Robert Brown told the coroner's jury that his son had assisted him in gathering some corn on Tuesday 19 September, and later on in the day he'd left his son alone while he went to Ballybay with his daughter. When he arrived home that evening, John was gone. The father had enquired of the neighbours as to his whereabouts, but could not find him. The next day he had heard of a young man being drowned and not knowing who he was, he went to see him and found it was the body of his own son. He told the coroner's jury, 'I cannot at all account for his being naked when found in the water. Fever had been in my family for months past and I think he was taking it and it affected his mind.'[6]

Women suffered the same illnesses as the men; however, they were considered different from men in relation to the reasons for their insanity. They were still believed to be the 'weaker' sex and by their natural constitution were considered not strong enough to handle being romantically spurned by men. Femininity in itself was considered a natural limitation giving women a predisposition for insanity. The

term 'female malady' is often referred to in the medical research and
literature of the nineteenth century.[7] The very nature of their committals and death were more romanticised versions of mental illness
such as 'melancholy madness' and 'natural weakness'. Aggressive behaviour was considered abnormal to the true nature of a woman's disposition and as a result, these women were often committed to the
asylum to correct this abnormality. Ann Lovett, a seventy-five-year-
old woman and inmate of the Clones workhouse, was found dead in
her bed one February morning in 1871. When her death was investigated, Dr Gillespie, doctor for the workhouse, told the coroner he believed that the woman died due to the rupture of a blood vessel on
her brain because she had got involved in an argument the day previous. Ann Lovett had been scolding another woman and he believed
that her irritable temper had finally got the best of her.[8] Ann was a
spinster and had previously been an inmate at the asylum. As discussed in chapter two, many women who had not followed a traditional
path in life – birth of an illegitimate child, unmarried, unskilled, displayed anger or aggression towards family members or others in the
community – were women most vulnerable to public scrutiny, perceived mental aberration and were either admitted to the workhouse
or committed to the jail or asylum.

Diseases of Institutions: Causes of Death

If inmates were not sick before reaching the jail or asylum, it was
likely they would be after they arrived. The deaths of patients varied
but most died from diseases contracted inside the institutions themselves. Contagious diseases ranged from consumption or phthisis (a
variant of tuberculosis) to bowel diseases such as typhus and diarrhoea, sometimes called 'asylum dysentery'.

Other vague descriptions such as 'general debility', 'nervous ex-
haustion' and 'paralysis' were considered causes of death. In many cases,
these verdicts were a combination of behaviour and symptoms such
as old age, epileptic seizures, lack of nourishment and lack of sleep.
In the case of Mary Hearty (a woman committed as a dangerous lunatic to the County Jail on 18 April 1860), she appeared to be in good
health, but had stopped eating. Because her attacks (presumably epileptic seizures) were so severe and frequent as to be almost without
interruption, she could no longer swallow food and as a result died
from a combination of starvation and convulsions.[9]

Most inquests for both the jail and the asylum were brief and
rarely gave much detail about the nature of the committal, other than

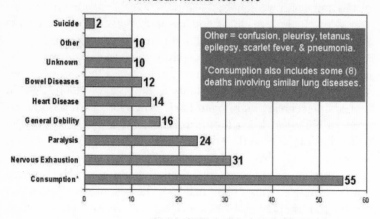

Diseases of Asylum Inmates
From Death Records 1869-1876

Disease	Deaths
Suicide	2
Other	10
Unknown	10
Bowel Diseases	12
Heart Disease	14
General Debility	16
Paralysis	24
Nervous Exhaustion	31
Consumption*	55

Other = confusion, pleurisy, tetanus, epilepsy, scarlet fever, & pneumonia.

*Consumption also includes some (8) deaths involving similar lung diseases.

=Total of 174 deaths recorded in seven years

Diseases of Asylum Inmates. Taken from death records held at the Registar's Office, North-Eastern Health Board, Monaghan.

the dates and the verdict of death. They appeared in the following format:

> An inquest was held on view of the body of Ann Caulfield 9 July 1868 in the town of Monaghan, parish of Monaghan. John Temple deposed that deceased was committed from Monaghan workhouse 14 August 1866 as a dangerous lunatic and continued so till her death on the 8 July. She was a woman of about 70 years old. Surgeon Young attended her. Miss Ann Irwin deposed to deceased being in good health when admitted into the jail. About a month since there was a change for the worse when she drew Dr Young's attention to it. Since then he saw her almost daily and sometimes twice yet she continued to decline up to the time of her death on the 8th. She suffered much from her legs that were covered with sores. Mr Young considered her death the result of debility of constitution. The verdict was death on 8 July 1868 from debility of constitution.

> On this 9th day of February 1876, I attended at the Monaghan County Asylum to enquire into the circumstances of the death of Philip Monaghan, aged 29 years and for 20 months an inmate of asylum and whose decease was caused by consumption.

Committed to the Asylum
The unfortunate people committed and left by family members at the asylum with no chance of release were usually then ignored, disowned and forgotten about by their family. Having a family member

at the asylum would be seen as bringing great shame on the family. Even in the mid twentieth century this was still the case in Co. Monaghan. Tommy Crow, a former asylum attendant at St Davnet's Psychiatric Hospital says that even in the 1950s and 1960s some patients were basically 'disowned by their relatives'.

'They didn't want to know them,' says Mr Crow. 'A lot of them had been sent in and their relatives forgot about them. They were just *forgotten*. We had an awful time trying to get the relatives to accept that these were human beings – their own flesh and blood. It took years to get the relatives to come around.'

In order for patients to be admitted (committed) to the asylum they needed to be evaluated by one or more physicians and diagnosed as curable or incurable. Curable patients were allowed to eventually leave under the care of friends and relatives, but the criteria for discharge depended largely on institutional convenience and the commitment of someone to take responsibility for them. The incurable were either permanent residents based upon their behaviour or kept due to the advanced state of disease, usually resulting in death.

Asylum patients were considered to be persons with 'deranged brains' who could only be evaluated through their conversation and conduct, which was compared with normal behaviour in society and with their behaviour prior to becoming insane. From this perspective, insanity was characterised by social disabilities and there was an emphasis on correcting their behaviour.[10] Although the doctor at the asylum would diagnose patients, it was the nurses and attendants who spent the most time with patients and therefore could best evaluate their progress or lack thereof. An employee manual entitled *Handbook* was given to the asylum staff in regard to how to treat the lunatics. 'Delusions' were not to be ridiculed but ignored and 'misapprehensions which so commonly exist in the minds of the insane' were to be explained 'rationally'.[11] It is clear that the *Handbook* left this up to the attendants' intuition and observation skills. Regardless of patients' mental illness or disability, attendants were expected to correct their behaviour in all areas such as poor manners in eating, cleanliness, anger and outbursts in conversation, and overall 'habits of order'. The morality of the time encouraged teaching inmates to follow the rules of the asylum which included cleanliness, the 'right' habits, order and the expulsion of bad thoughts to creating the 'right' ones.

As welcome as the asylum was to the surrounding community, it wasn't a house of health, cures and discharge – but one of death. Most of these people were simply offered shelter and food, put out of sight from the community and given a place to die. For those who were eventually allowed to leave, it was not unusual for a person to revert back to old behaviour and patterns of thinking after release. Articles in the newspaper reported former asylum inmates, persons once regarded as dangerous lunatics, melancholics or maniacs allegedly cured by their time and treatment in the asylum, having been released only to end their lives by committing suicide:

Determined Suicide

On Sunday morning last a suicide of a most determined character took place in the townland of Brackly, about four miles from Ballybay, when a respectable farmer named William Hagan put an end to his own existence under circumstances of a most appalling nature.

The unfortunate deceased was upwards of sixty years of age and the father of a large family. It appears that about two years ago, he showed some symptoms of mental aberration, and was placed for a short time in the Monaghan asylum. After stopping in the institution for some time, he apparently recovered his reason, and was brought home. Up to the period of the horrible occurrence he conducted himself so as to excite no suspicion of his sanity, nor any apprehension of danger. On Sunday morning last, his son and daughter-in-law who lived in the house with him, heard him moving about his room and in a short time after, the servant maid, having occasion to pass through his room, discovered him lying on the bed in a most shocking condition and quite dead, he having used both a knife and razor not upon his throat, as is usual in such cases, but actually disembowelling himself. An inquest was held on the body by Hugh Swanzy, coroner for the district and a respectable jury, when a verdict was returned that the deceased committed suicide when in a state of unsound mind. Much sympathy is felt for the relatives of the deceased in their affliction.

It is somewhat extraordinary that in a rural district, this is the third suicide which has been committed during the last three months, within a radius of three miles from deceased's late residence. – Cor.[12]

INSANE IN THE MEMBRANE
Defining Insanity

Who was considered insane? No clear cut medical definition has been offered for the lunatic. The terminology used to refer to lunatics is interchangeable. Sometimes the words lunacy, insanity, lunatic, idiot, madman and fool were used generically to refer to all different types of persons and behaviour. There were terms that attempted to define the behaviour of individuals for the purposes of committal to an appropriate institution. For example, a 'criminal lunatic', was a term used to define anyone who committed a crime, namely an insane person who had committed a crime, or had been accused of one. 'Dangerous lunatics' were persons who displayed violent behaviour towards a family member, attempted suicide or had been discovered only 'under circumstances denoting ... a purpose of committing some crime'.[13] Some medical terms, although not politically correct or sensitive in our contemporary social climate, attempted to define the madman. Depression was defined by the term 'melancholic'; those showing signs of delusion or obsession, such as 'religious mania', were 'manic'. The mentally retarded were referred to as 'weak-minded', 'idiots' and 'imbeciles'.

Those who committed suicide were described in the coroner's inquests as living 'under melancholy' or committing the act while 'temporarily insane'. The custom of adding 'while temporarily insane' to the verdict of the inquest of a suicide actually grew from a desire to prevent indignity being shown the deceased (post mortem) and cruel punishment being inflicted upon the innocent relatives by the clergy. 'The balance of his mind was upset' (or other descriptions to that effect) was a common 'let-out' phrase used to allow burial in sanctified ground.[14] Attempted suicide was always taken as irrefutable proof a person's insanity as it was believed that no healthy mind could permit such an act so directly opposed to the natural instinct of self-preservation as self-destruction.[15]

SUICIDES
Why Did They Do It?

Many people then (and perhaps still now), including my late father, would have been offended if the word suicide was used to describe his death. Yet, there is no other way to describe what happened. He voluntarily embarked upon a course of action in the full knowledge that it would bring about his own death. Such is the definition of suicide.

— Michael J. Kelleher, *Suicide and the Irish*

Upon being examined carefully, the evidence recorded in suicide inquests depicting depression, aggression, violence and mental aberration can be linked with familial and societal constraints. Tensions within the family, changes in marriage patterns, emigration, alcoholism and economic pressures were the predominant causes for these behaviours, yet in the nineteenth century, heredity, self-indulgence, moral weakness and even a person's diet was believed to cause insanity.

HEREDITY
You Didn't Get it from 'My' Side of the Family

Insanity, some argued, was an inherited factor acquired from one's ancestors in the same way as wealth or social standing.[16] An inherited trait of insanity combined with physical or moral weakness in a person would be scrutinised and considered the probable cause of the illness. Women were considered the highest risk for moral weaknesses, unable to handle such issues as love affairs, mental anxiety, religious excitement, spousal arguments or grief.

Melancholy Madness
The Death of Jane Divine, Hollywood, Tedavnet Parish, June 1872
In the case of Jane Divine, her inherited trait of 'melancholy madness' combined with her physically weak state is the explanation offered for her suicide. In June of 1872, the twenty-two-year-old servant had been living at the house of James Fiddes, Esq., of Hollywood in the parish of Tedavnet and labouring under what Dr William Woods described as 'Melancholy Madness'.[17] He stated for the coroner's jury that this affliction ran in her family and was increased by her state of bodily health – a well developed attack of English cholera.[18] Her body was seen floating in the lake on the estate by Robert Brown, who along with his brother and James McGuiness took possession of a boat to row out to fetch her poor body from the weeds. It was reported that for several days she had been in a very depressed state of mind and that her 'melancholy madness' drove her to drown herself in the lake.[19]

THE FAMILY AND MADNESS

Lunacy: Alexander Richardson of Drumsaul against Thomas Richardson of Drumsaul. The defendant, a fine-looking young man, about 18 years of age, was sent to Monaghan Asylum as a dangerous lunatic.
– *The Northern Standard*, 31 August 1872

The family was merely a setting for an unaccountable change in a person's life, a change which other family members could only describe as going 'out of his/her mind'.[20] It was within the family and within their own homes, that the behaviour of all who dwelt there could be measured and evaluated. The vast majority of those persons committed to the asylum were sent there by the families. Madness existed only to the extent that some person other than the lunatic defined it as such.[21] The asylum was an option for family members unable or unwilling to continue to care for the 'madman'. In many cases, the insanity of the person was reflective of the problems and issues within the dynamic of the family itself. Anyone who rebelled or showed signs of violence and aggression was considered crazy – especially when expected behaviour dictated their absolute conformity and cooperation with their parents.

Often these 'dangerous lunatics' were expressing violence in conflict-ridden social relations in which the dominance of one over the other was the origin of committal.[22] The reasons brought forth to justify why, in particular, parents were committing their children, reflect the cultural values and expected responses that defined what was considered normal behaviour. In this way, everyday conflicts of 'children' (in their late adolescence and twenties) were translated into forms of madness.

Does Choking his Mother Make him Crazy?
The Case of John McCluskey, Roosky Lane, Monaghan, June 1875
Parents had considerable authority over their grown-up children and the asylum was often used for punishment and discipline when they became rebellious. The example of John McCluskey of Roosky Lane, Monaghan is such a possible case. His mother Bridget stated that her twenty-two-year-old son had come home from Scotland three months previously and six weeks later had begun to exhibit symptoms of madness and became violent with her. On the night of 15 December 1874 he attempted to go out of the house after dark in his nightshirt. When she tried to stop him, he caught hold of her by the throat and tried to choke her. A month later on 9 January 1875 he knocked her down, kicked her and tried to take her life.[23] She appealed to Dr Woods, medical officer of the Monaghan dispensary district and had John examined. Dr Woods determined that he was a person of unsound mind and an order was made for his committal to the asylum as a dangerous lunatic. Although he died as a result of asylum dysentery just six months later, the evidence is inconclusive as to whether he was insane or not.[24] We only have his mother's account of his violent nature towards her since his return from Scotland.

Is it possible that this was a case of family conflict defined as madness – or was he really suffering from a mental illness? As men were usually older than their wives, there were many widows in control of farms having complete authority over the family, especially their sons. Until parents died or handed the land over to their children, they were expected to behave according to their demands, work on the farm as unpaid labourers and were not allowed to marry without their parents' consent. It appears John McCluskey was a migratory worker, which usually meant leaving in May and arriving home in November after six months of hard fieldwork for little pay and poor treatment. Many of the migratory workers, once they had their few pounds saved and felt secure for the winter, had no inclination to do any work on their holdings when they returned.[25] Could the changes that John McCluskey's mother described as symptoms of madness have resulted from his lack of discipline in regard to her authority and his non-co-operation upon his return?

In another case, Rose McKeever was convicted for the repetitive crime of assaulting her relatives and breaking their windows. She was sent to the county jail on several different occasions and because of her outrageous and uncontrollable conduct in jail, the jail matron and staff requested that Dr A. K. Young evaluate her for possible committal to the District Lunatic Asylum. The question to be answered was 'Is she insane?' Below is a copy of his response to the jail authorities.

Medical Report on the Case of Rose McKeever
A Prisoner in the Gaol of Monaghan
Gentlemen,
I have made inquires as to the previous and present state of Rose McKeever now a prisoner in this jail.
I find all her committals have been for assaults and breaking of windows ... That on every occasion of committal, except the first, her conduct has been violent and outrageous in the jail –
That she is, and always has been, except in the first instance, a great worry to the resident officers in the jail – and is a terror to the matron and assistant – and from the continuous and long sustained noises she makes by day and night in her cell, when the fit of ill humour possesses her, she is a disturbance and vexation to all the female side of the prison, as has been stated to me –
That she has committed several acts of outrage whilst in confinement, and is not in the least controlled by punishment, even in the dark cell, where she continues to do as much mischief and make more noise than in other departments –
That at times she will seem to be very amiably submissive, sometimes to one person, sometimes to another – and without any apparent provocation, she will again break out into violence of manner towards those she had lately submitted to –
That on getting out of jail she has walked to the relatives in this neighbourhood of those who live 20 miles off who had her committed, and smashed their windows for revenge –

That the matron of the jail is in fear of her life from her violence and threats towards her –

That even her own clergyman, the RC chaplain, lost control over her and she refused to submit to him –

That her last committal from Petty Sessions of Carrickmacross being for 5 months, viz – two months for one outrage, two months for a second, and one for a third shows she must be esteemed as intolerable nuisance in that neighbourhood –

The opinion forced upon my mind is that some fatal catastrophe will probably result sooner or later from this extraordinary and very ungovernable temper –

From the above circumstances, I have no doubt the woman is not morally sane – but she has not suffered from any mental delusions by which I would feel warranted to certify that she is a lunatic.

I am gentlemen, your obedient servant,
A. K. Young, Medical Superintendent
April 1870, The Terrace, Monaghan

Rose McKeever had exceptional energy for fighting against the staff at the jail, the parish priest and her family. What events occurred in her life making her reject the church and show such violent behaviour towards her family? It is surprising they were unable to have her sent to the asylum since any violence towards relatives, neighbours or self-mutilation was usually the ticket to committal.

In most cases, no record of violent or abnormal behaviour was recorded until a major incident occurred and the authorities became involved. There were many instances in which families admitted there had been problems for months or years, but nothing had been done as the person had not assaulted or threatened to assault someone.[26] In the following case, a young woman was considered to be 'out of her mind' for years, kept in her home and physically restrained to prevent her from committing acts of violence. This method of treatment did not prevent a tragic outcome – murder.

Tied up too Long: Homicide by a Lunatic
The Murder of Mary McCarron, April 1873,
Rakelly, Errigal Truagh Parish
One Wednesday morning in April 1873, Owen McCarron woke early and readied himself to leave his home in Rakelly for the Aughnacloy market. His preparation included saying goodbye to his wife, Mary, and securing his daughter, Catherine – by tying her to a stake in the corner of one of the rooms in the house. Although described by many

Local Inspector's Report on inmate Rose McKeever, 7 April 1870, Monaghan Gaol, 'Inspected this terrible woman Rose McKeever who seems more like a wild beast than a rational human being. She has her cell in an abominable state evidently by urinating on the floor and stamping through it. It has been reported to me that when she demanded a urinal she took it and immediately smashed it against the wall – She showed me dark spots on her person which she asserted was given her by attempts made to handcuff her – but as she is continually abusing herself, I think it is likely she did this herself. She has so terrified the matron (Miss Irwin) that she dare not go near her and her health (ie, Miss Irwins) is giving way in consequence – I have directed the cell to be cleaned out immediately and clored of lime used in the washing of the cell.' – Thomas Young, Local Inspector.

as quiet and harmless, according to those closest to her, she had random violent outbursts. At those times she was a threat to others, that is, members of her family.

Just eight months earlier, Catherine's aunt, Sarah, ordered the young woman out of her home because she was afraid of her. The girl retaliated by smashing one of the windows of Sarah's house with a spade. As a result, Owen began taking the precaution of tying his daughter up with a rope and securing her until his return. The only diagnosis provided for Catherine was that of her father, who told the coroner's jury that his daughter had been out of her mind for the past six years. She was twenty-nine-years of age and considered by her family to be insane and a dangerous lunatic.

On that fateful day when Owen left for the Aughnacloy market, he didn't realise it was the last time he would see his wife, Mary, alive. Just a few hours after his departure, his sister, Sarah, saw Catherine passing by her door with a large, heavy ash stick in her hand. Sarah spoke to Catherine from the front door of her home, but upon her doing so, Catherine shouted back, 'Keep your head in or I'll make you.'

About twenty minutes later, Sarah's sister, Alice, appeared and instructed Sarah, 'Hurry and come over for Mary is lying in the street!'

The women rushed to the spot and found Mary McCarron, Catherine's mother, barely recognisable, bleeding from wounds to her face and head, scarcely alive. Their brother, James, appeared as well as several neighbours. James retrieved some salt and water to try and revive Mary, but it was too late. She was already dead. James was shown a large stick with at least twelve inches of it smeared with blood. There was also a large stone, covered in blood, that lay nearby.

About fifteen minutes later, Catherine McCarron was seen returning to her own house.

The unfortunate daughter, when left alone with her mother, must have succeeded in breaking loose. Catherine then struck her mother with the very stake to which she had been tied, knocked her down, and then battered her skull and face with a large stone, inflicting a number of terrible wounds.

Returning later that afternoon, Owen McCarron entered his home to find his wife lying dead in a pool of her own blood on the floor. Her features were disfigured and unrecognisable and her skull fractured in several places.[27] His daughter, Catherine, was tied and sitting in a corner of the house.

An inquest was held the next day. The family and Dr Richard Henry of the Aughnacloy Dispensary testified to the events of the previous day. Dr Henry, who performed the post-mortem examination, told the coroner's jury, 'The bones on the right side of the skull are smashed in and broken into small pieces. There was a flesh wound on the back of the head, one on the right side of the face, and one on the centre of the forehead all lending to the broken bones. Any one of them would be quite sufficient to cause death. A large stick has now been shown me which would be sufficient to cause the wounds on the back of the head and sufficient to cause death. A stone has now been shown me which would be equal to cause the other wounds and also cause death.'

After hearing all the testimony, the jury returned the following verdict, 'We find that Mary McCarron came to her death on Wednesday 9th day of April 1873 from certain wounds inflicted on her by her daughter, Catherine McCarron.'[28] The accused was then ordered to be sent to jail until the summer assizes.

It appears Catherine sat in jail from April until the summer assizes took place on 12 July 1873. That day she stood before the Crown court in Monaghan charged with the murder of her mother. A jury was empanelled to try to determine whether the prisoner was a person of sound mind and capable of pleading to the indictment. After evidence was given by Dr Robertson, Medical Superintendent of the Monaghan Lunatic Asylum, the jury had no choice but to find Catherine McCarron incapable of standing trial and she was ordered to be detained at the asylum.[29]

It cannot be determined if Catherine was mentally ill with a long history of aggressive and violent behaviour, or a healthy woman, perfectly sensible, just driven to murder by being tied up for hours at a time. Was she a victim of controlling, overbearing parents who perceived her as 'crazy' when she did not obey their orders or disagreed with them as was the case with many other adult children of the time? If she were sane, it would not be unanticipated that by being physically restrained she might become so enraged she might attempt to kill her captors. She had broken the window at her aunt's home, yet there is no record of her physically attacking anyone, including family members. It is unfortunate there was no mention in the inquest or in the details of the trial as to why Catherine McCarron killed her mother, other than insanity. The absence of discussion during the inquest as to her treatment by her father (why he tied her to a stake in the corner of the room) is easily explained. Physical restraint of asylum patients was a common form of treatment in response to aggressive or violent behaviour. Her father declaring his daughter a dangerous lunatic and using physical restraints as a method of treatment to control behaviour was in keeping with treatment in institutions of the insane at that time. In any event, this tragic story illustrates how family members only needed to present a case describing the violent behaviour of the suspected lunatic and thereby justify their treatment within the home.

LOVE AND MARRIAGE AND MONEY

Marriage was another source of conflict within the family in the post-famine years. Prior to the famine, peasant children married whom they pleased, when they pleased, large families were common and the principal farmer, the father, would continually sub-divide the land so that more children could settle and work the land-holding. These sub-divisions proved disastrous over time as many a holding was so reduced and the land so exhausted that in bad seasons, there was an acute shortage of potatoes. In the decades to follow, land was inherited or given as a gift in its entirety and the custom of the eldest child obtaining that right was established. It has been stated that this practice of 'impartible inheritance' (and its associated trappings, such as the 'match') made sacrificial victims of all siblings but one.[30] Other sons and daughters made up the gathering stream of emigration and those risking life in Ireland married more circumspectly.[31] Those who remained often became the aunts and uncles staying on at home, living a life of celibacy. It was this group that were likely candidates in later life for committal to the asylum.

Contrary to the sacrifice of the siblings who would receive nothing in regard to inheritance or land, sacrifice was a part of the compromised situation of eldest child participating in an arranged marriage. They were usually loveless unions, involving class conflicts, creating sibling rivalry, problems between ageing mother and daughter-in-law over control of the son and the home, and they also occurred later in life. The average age of the man was 38 years; the woman, 30 years.[32] The reasons for marrying later varied; however, a primary factor was that the land would be strained to support the second family with the first having yet to disperse (die off). Another factor was that a more 'mature' woman would have labouring skills and a dowry. The marriage was usually arranged by the man or his parents sending someone to the woman's house to make the suggestion of marriage and allow the woman's parents to think on it. If they agreed, they would all meet and the negotiations of dowry would begin. The dowry was paid on the morning of the marriage, before the ceremony took place.[33]

Money Changes Everything
The Death of Nathanial Beatty,
Kilmore West, Ematris Parish, August 1861
Marriages were negotiated and the success and prosperity of such partnerships was based on money, property and children. One can only

consider that any discrepancy in the founding principles of the union would create problems between the parties. In the following case of Nathanial Beatty, it appears that money was the catalyst for problems between him and his new wife.

Nathanial Beatty, a twenty-six-year-old man, had been married for just two months. The union was not one of happiness and it preyed much on his mind.[34] He and the wife were arguing over the matter of fortune and she had left him. He told Marshal Lindsay, a relative and friend, that 'he wished somebody would put a ball through his heart and put him out of his pain'. Before his wife could return and the two might reconcile, Nathanial's body was found in a well by Margaret Killet. She had gone to the well to draw some water when she saw a man's hat and some cloth floating on the surface. As she drew the fabric nearer, she realised it was a man's coat and suddenly a bloated, wide-eyed face rose up from beneath the water. Terrified, she ran away to get help. She returned with John Reilly and asked him to go back, identify the man and retrieve him from the well as she could not bring herself to return to the scene.

Standing near or in front of the well, Nathanial had put a gun to his left breast and squeezed the trigger, sending a bullet through his heart causing death. The verdict was death from a gunshot wound inflicted by him whilst labouring under great mental anxiety and affliction. Although one can never know all the reasons a person decides to take his own life, based upon the method of suicide and placement of the wound, it could be representative of his broken heart. Another factor not considered was love. Emotional bonding might not be reciprocated in an arranged marriage.

Robbery and Desperation
The Suicide of Jane Boylan, Monaghan, Monaghan Parish, August 1858

In non-traditional relationships, such as the case of Jane Boylan, it is apparent that the inability to support oneself financially could create incredible mental strain and anguish, especially for women. She and her husband were estranged from one another and Jane had been living with Mary Connolly for two years. She'd returned from Scotland having seen some friends and family and was in a very disturbed state of mind. As she and Mary discussed her visit, Jane appeared deeply troubled and told Mary that she had robbed her brother of a sovereign while there. She stated that she wished he would come and take her and hang her and other times threatened that she would drown herself in the canal.

Soon after the visit, Mary Connelly went and got Jane's husband. They all took evening tea together and the next morning breakfasted together. At that time he said he would pay for a room for Jane and give her one shilling a week – being as much as he could afford and with which, under Mary's management, she might do very well. After his departure from the house, Jane stayed with Mary for two more days and then left.

Later that same evening she was arrested for being disorderly and drunk by James Burr, a constable. Mary was confined to the jail for twenty-four hours for the incident.

The next day, 17 August, Mary McGlone saw Jane at Scroggs Bridge in Monaghan town.[35] They chatted for a few minutes. Jane appeared greatly disturbed and in low spirits. It was the last time she was seen alive. Jane's body was found in the canal four days later. When her corpse was taken out of the water, they found two stones about 16lbs each, tied in an apron around her body and no marks of violence. The verdict was death from having thrown herself into the canal on the evening of Thursday 19 August 1858 whilst labouring under great mental excitement.[36]

Looking for Love in all the Wrong Places
The Suicide of Archibald Little,
Tavanagh, Errigal Truagh Parish, January 1871
It is difficult to tell if lack of female companionship, bachelorhood, celibacy or a mental illness was to blame for the choices made by Archibald Little, but it would be reasonable to assume that these factors did not contribute to a healthy lifestyle for the single man.

Archy had been missing for two months. His brother, William Little (of Favour Royal) a coachman, identified the body as it lay on the bank of the river where it had been placed by constables O'Brien and Morgan of Aughnacloy station after they found it floating in the Blackwater River. William told the authorities that he'd not known Archy to be a party man or have any enemies, which was important testimony given the state of the body. A cord had been tied around Archy's neck and then fastened above the left knee in a position impossible for a submerged man to become untangled. Had Archy been murdered? Dr John Mulligan of Aughnacloy didn't believe there was any foul play and determined that the body had been submerged in water before death. Additionally, there were no marks of violence on his body but upon making a search in his pockets, they found a pound note, a key and a large pocket knife. At his place of residence in the home of Mr Booth, they found a box in his room which contained £4 of money, a few coppers and a packet of poison. It was then revealed by Constable Martin Bohen that he'd held a warrant for Archy Little on a charge of *bestiality* since 12 December 1870 for an offence committed on 4 December 1870. It now appeared that Archy Little might have had cause to kill himself for fear of prosecution as he'd been missing since the time of the incident. Although bestiality was a crime discussed in Outrage papers with a matter-of-fact detachment, it was punishable by penal servitude.[37] The verdict was suffocation by drowning in the Blackwater River between 15 December 1870 and 20 January 1871.[38] Without any suspects or reasonable cause to believe someone did harm to Archibald Little, it is more likely that Archy, fearful of prosecution, committed suicide.

EMIGRATION
A Society in Mourning

Give us, sir, our farm, our green fields, our house, and every spot and nook that we had before. We love the place, sir, for its own sake; it is the place of our fathers, and our hearts are in it.
     – William Carleton, *Traits and Stories of the Irish Peasantry*

Mass-emigration affected all those who were left behind (after the famine); in fact admissions to lunatic asylums in Ireland increased nearly 500 per cent.[39] Those who emigrated were usually the children who would not benefit from inheritance or dowry, leaving the ageing parents with the eldest child and any other siblings who were too young or too scared to leave. Besides suffering the loss of their friends, brothers, sisters, aunts, uncles and children, there were changes to the fate of each group as a result of these departures. In Co. Monaghan there were now fewer people to work the land and life was dictated by 'familism' (interests of the individual were subordinated to the welfare of the family).[40] Parents, now more cautious, often held back the gift of land as well as the approval of marriage, and many children advancing into their middle years (thirties and early forties), with still no prospect of marriage or of economic independence, and emigration a much more daunting prospect, their discontent could have become unmanageable within the confines of the family.[41] In turn, parents could easily end up alone and die in the workhouse or asylum. Additionally, some could only watch as, year by year, they were unable to manage the land-holding without the additional manpower of those children who were gone. The farm, depending upon the size of the holding, could easily slip away from them.

Land, Livestock and Love Lost in America
The Death of Patrick Prunty, Corcreeghy, Kilmore Parish, August 1863
For some, the emotional and economic loss of children was too great a burden. Evidence of this can be seen in the death of Patrick Prunty. On the morning of 23 August 1863, Catherine Prunty was walking from Sunday mass towards her home at Corcreeghy in the parish of Kilmore when she met one of her children on the road. The child told her that 'grandpapa was hanging in the room' at home. Catherine ran to the house and looking through the window saw the old man, suspended from a beam, hanging from a rope, dead. She and her husband cut the old man down and offered the explanation that 'for some time past [he] was greatly depressed in mind, from various causes – loss of one of his farms, the death of cattle, and for more than a year not hearing from his son in America'. The verdict was death from strangulation by hanging himself whilst in affliction of mind.[42]

The Absence of the Children
The Death of David Hill, Cordoolough, Tullycorbet Parish, February 1865
John Hill, son of David Hill, told the coroner that his father was in a state of great mental depression respecting some of his family who were absent from him and thus accounted for what he had done. Early on the morning of 19 February 1865, his sister had come and told him that their father had attempted to take his life. On going to him, he found that his father had inflicted a wound on his neck. David had used a sharp instrument to puncture and slice the front part of his neck. The doctor was sent for and he attempted to repair the wound. However, over the next several days David was unable to swallow any food. As a result he lingered for several more days and died on 27 February. Michael Lennon, who had long known the deceased, claimed that the old man appeared to live in harmony with his family but, during his last six months, his mind had become weak and childish and he was suffering from anxiety at the absence of members of the family. Michael believed this was why the old man took his own life. The verdict reached at the inquest was that death resulted from an incised wound, inflicted while labouring under temporary insanity.[43]

Without the support of a family or living in a traditional family unit, some poor souls fell by the wayside. They were forced to beg, rely on the kindness of strangers, and live day-to-day without any security for their future. Men without land or a job and women without husbands or children to secure their future would end up at the poorhouse. In the following story, hard economic times and lack of a stable family environment appear to have contributed to the fatal decisions made by the deceased.

Poverty and Hard Times: Sleeping at the Forge
The Suicide of William Mullen, Monaghan, Monaghan Parish, June 1871
William Mullen was a casualty of hard times, subject to repeated blows of economic, social and personal misfortune. He had worked for many years in the brewery in Monaghan town and was quite well known.[44] It is uncertain at which point he stopped working, but it became quite obvious that he was in trouble as he was destitute. William was weak, suffering from ill-health and it appeared that he was not taking proper care of himself.[45]

On the evening of 12 June 1871, John Gavin heard that a man was lying in his yard. He went down with John Herbert and there saw the man lying across a low wall. They raised him up, immediately recognised him as William Mullen and assisted out of the yard. He was very weak and one of Gavin's servants brought him some bread and milk. On discovering he had no money, Gavin gave him a few pence and a man named Herbert brought him to lodgings for the night. After William left, Gavin noticed some blood on the spot where he had been lying down.

About noon the next day, William went to Phil Kernaghan's forge asking if he might rest himself there for the afternoon. He'd had a habit of visiting the forge and lying there for the day to get some rest. Usually, he was allowed to do so. However, this time he was refused. He pleaded to stay through the night as he was planning to gain admission to the poorhouse the next morning. Again he was refused and went away. Around 8p.m. that night, some police came by and took William to the county infirmary. He'd been found in a field having attempted to kill himself. He had inflicted a gash on his throat from which he was bleeding.

William told Constable Tierney that the cut was caused by falling on a bottle in Mrs Vallely's yard, but afterwards acknowledged that he did it to himself with a small pocket knife. The cut was not serious, but weakened his already debilitated constitution. William Mullen died the next day from an 'organic disease accelerated by the loss of blood consequent on his rash act'. He was sixty-five-years old.

INTEMPERANCE AND INSANITY

Chronic heavy drinking without other irrational behaviour was not yet generally seen as having a connection with mental disturbance.[46] One narrow category in which alcohol-related suicide was considered was that of the demented – persons who are deprived of reason. It was believed that chronic alcohol poisoning caused a form of mania known as *delirium tremens*. A heavy drinking session that brought on depression or prolonged drunkenness was believed to lead to complete dementia. One medical professional went as far to say that 'it was a proven fact that a very large proportion of these alcoholic suicides were found on inquiry to have bad family histories.'[47]

A 'Bout' of Excessive Drinking: The Suicide and Death of Michael Duffy, Monaghan, Monaghan Parish, June 1868

Ann Quaid knew that Michael Duffy had been drinking for some days past and that his mind was disturbed from the excessive drinking. He became paranoid telling her that he thought the police were after him. On the evening of 26 June 1868, Michael took a walk with his wife and came back into the house. About 10.15p.m. he was in the kitchen and went to lock the outer door. He gave his hat to Ann to hang up and she left the room to tend to the errand. Immediately afterwards, she heard a splash as if a person were vomiting and then a moan. She lit a candle and went to see what caused such strange and unsettling noises. There in the candlelight she met Michael – with a razor in his hand and blood pouring from his neck on to the ground. She was so shocked that she fell backwards in the dark and began to scream. This caused great consternation and confusion and the neighbours began rushing in after hearing the alarm.

The coroner was called on that evening to see the dying man. He found Michael lying in bed on his back and bleeding profusely from a very large wound on his neck. The man had already lost a great deal of blood and Mr Waddell determined there was nothing that he could do for him. Michael was sent to the county infirmary.

Dr Young at the Monaghan infirmary received Michael Duffy and secured the bleeding vessel in his throat, although he had bled very much. The wound occupied about one-third of the throat between his two ears. The tongue and epilates were separated from the windpipe and the wound extended to the spine. Michael died at midnight. The verdict was death from a severe wound in his throat inflicted by himself while in a state of temporary insanity from a bout of excessive drinking.[48]

RELIGION
Driving People Insane?

A Lunatic
A single woman about 50 years of age, named Ginley, said to be affected
with 'religious mania' was committed to Monaghan District Lunatic Asylum as a dangerous lunatic on the information of her brother and Dr Woods
of Monaghan dispensary district.
– *The Northern Standard*, September 1875

Religion during the nineteenth century was believed to be the origin
of some of the extreme cases of lunacy and abnormal mental behaviour as some persons suffered from a fixed or maniacal fury about religion and were classified as suffering from 'religious mania' or 'religious insanity'.

A revivalist campaign was being carried on in various parts of
Ulster during the mid-to-late part of the century and was appearing
in random parts of the population revealing the extent to which some
minds could be disturbed by frenzied religious activity. The Catholic
Church was fervent in being allowed the same freedom to preach to
their members, while simultaneously Presbyterian preachers, were trying to save Irish Catholics from the errors of popery. Crowds were gathering to listen to preachers; two Presbyterian clergymen who conducted a prayer meeting at Drum, Co. Monaghan, asserted that at
least three hundred of those present had seen God descending from
a black cloud.[49]

The government was in a precarious situation in regard to how
they dealt with religion in jails and asylums. They needed to ensure
that all inmates were accommodated in the practice of their religion
and asylum chaplains were appointed to each institution. Given the
belief that 'religious excitement' could be harmful, there was some concern that the asylum chaplains might have a disturbing influence on
patients.[50]

They're All Out to Get Me: The Suicide and Death of Bernard Daly,
Monaghan, Monaghan Parish, April 1865
It is unknown if there was great religious fever in the air when the
priest celebrated mass one Sunday in April 1865 at the Monaghan
jail, but it is clear that Berny Daly was in attendance – a dangerous
man with paranoid delusions that everyone he met was trying to kill
him. Immediately following mass, he went to his cell, twisted a sheet
like a rope, formed it in a loop around his chin and hung himself. Two

other prisoners broke down the door and found Berny hanging from the wooden rack on the wall – dead.[51]

Religious Fever, the Bible and Butcher Knives
The Suicide and Death of Elizabeth Heasty,
Monaghan, Monaghan Parish, December 1871
Elizabeth Heasty, a thirty-eight-year-old married woman was living with her husband John in Monaghan town.[52] Over a period of seven weeks Elizabeth often complained of pains in her head and heart and it was becoming obvious to those closest to her that she was suffering from some sort of 'religious insanity'. She insisted her husband read to her as much as possible from religious works and would then instruct him to go and read the same to their children. She kept to her bed merely getting up to have it made. When her dinner was brought up to her room by her servant, Jane White, it was returned as she was consistently asleep. On Christmas Eve, John Heasty went up to his wife's room to check on her as, yet again, the dinner had come back untouched. When he opened the door, he saw blood about her neck and shoulders. Elizabeth was dead. When pulling down the bed covers, John found two butcher's knives. The smaller one was sharp and covered with blood; the larger knife appeared not to have been used. Elizabeth had cut a wound four inches long on her neck and carved a large wound into her belly, extending from the breast down to the pelvis – from this wound the bowels protruded.[53] Dr William Temple determined that she must have died within minutes. The inquest was held on Christmas Day 1871.[54]

WOMEN AND MADNESS
A Crime Against God and Man?

Then I peeled off all the paper I could reach standing on the floor. It sticks horribly and the pattern just enjoys it! All those strangled heads and bulbous eyes and waddling fungus growths just shriek with derision! I am getting angry enough to do something desperate. To jump out of the window would be admirable exercise, but the bars are too strong to even try. Besides I wouldn't do it. Of course not. I know well enough that a step like that is improper and might be misconstrued. I don't like to look out of the windows even – there are so many of those creeping women, and they creep so fast. I wonder if they all come out of the wall-paper as I did?
– Charlotte Perkins Gillman, an excerpt from
The Yellow Wallpaper, 1892

In nineteenth-century psychiatry, women were believed to be more vulnerable to insanity than men, to experience it in specifically feminine ways and to be differently affected by it in the conduct of their lives.[55] In defining women as dangerous lunatics, their behaviour was evaluated based upon male-dominated concepts of normality and morality. There was a 'natural' revolution going on – redefining maternity, femininity, Darwinism and the origin of the species. This focus meant that there were many studies determining differences between the sexes – specifically, that men and women were different by nature and therefore expected to accept what they were naturally capable of. It was these natural limitations that confined women to certain moral and social codes that many women found constricting and suffocating.

There was a growing need for understanding lunacy as many women were being admitted to asylums suffering from various problems, very often 'fevers', 'loss of appetite' and 'melancholy'. Academic research and studies show that this was occurring for a variety of reasons, including living in a pre-defined society where women were subjugated to a relatively limited amount of 'space'. They were relegated to work at home and care of the children, or else they were working as domestic servants, factory workers, prostitutes, and, often in the upper-classes, as nurses and teachers. Additionally, women were seeing the advantages their male counterparts had – a wide variety of professions, education and financial independence, to name a few – and they were becoming frustrated and often 'melancholy' as a result of the lack of freedom in their lives.

DOMESTIC SERVICE
A Matter of Life and Death

Domestic service was the major employment for women in Ireland in the nineteenth century. In 1881, forty-eight per cent of employed women were in the domestic class.[56] To be a live-in domestic servant was an acceptable position for daughters as parents liked the idea of room and board as well as wages being offered. There was a risk involved in such work for these women. Domestic servants were vulnerable to exploitation by their employers – owing to their sex, age, isolation from their families and subordinate position. Victorian culture demanded that servants be properly treated, but gross abuses were frighteningly common. Nothing protected the backstairs maid from the unwanted attentions of a scion of the house.[57] The total control of servant by master, which was, in fact, reinforced by legislation, meant that the domestic servant had little discretion over the day-to-day conduct of her life.[58]

A Difference with the Master: The Death of Agnes Martin
Monaghan, Monaghan Parish, September 1872
James Martin deposed to the coroner's jury that his sister's body was found by John Keenan and Sergeant McKey in the canal at Bessmount Bridge in the townland of Drumacruttan. When James arrived to view the body, Mr Humphrey Breakey, the master, was also there and had identified the body as that of Agnes Martin. A cart was then sent by Mr Breakey to remove the body to the Monaghan infirmary. James said, 'I have no idea as to what might have led her to drown herself, save that it might have arisen from a difference between our master, Mr Breakey, yet of whom I have heard her speak of as a very kind Master ...'
Agnes Martin was sixteen years of age.[59]

LEGENDS OF MONAGHAN
Folklore and the Sisters of St Louis

Folklore serves a society or culture by sanctioning and validating religious, social, political and economic institutions and plays an important role as an educative device in its transmission from one generation to another.[60] Some of the stories that are created project the emotional life of the characters into safe, externalised, sanctioned forms of the original story, showing a subconscious objection to laying bare the secrets of the soul. The legend of the sleepwalking nun, Sister Mary Keough, is such a story. It has continued in oral tradition in Monaghan town up until the present time. Her inquest, however, will tell another story, one in which the harsh realities of her suicide were carefully shrouded and covered by a kind people, shocked and shamed, but protective and loving in the careful creation of the story of her death.

The Sisters of Mercy and the Sisters of St Louis were well-respected and credited with teaching self-respect as well as helping to end the feeling of Catholics being second-class citizens in post-penal Ireland.[61] There was much opposition to the orders of nuns establishing themselves in Ireland. For example, Father Alessandro Gavazzi, an Evangelical Protestant preacher, gave a speech in Belfast in 1859 stating, 'Remember that you have concealed, under a cover of gentleness, the worst species of Inquisition ever in your Ireland; I speak of the bad, tyrannical unscriptural system of nunneries and nuns and nunism. O my brethren ... you do not know what nuns are. They are the slaves, the despairing victims, of priestly tyranny ... they live in despair ... under the gentle veil they hide their fear from you; they are in despair ... they are in despair ... they are in despair and generally speaking these poor nuns die before they are forty years of age.' It was therefore of significant importance to the Catholic population that the nuns were held in high-regard and that their behaviour was clearly respected as they adhered to high-moral behaviour within the community. The Sisters of St Louis in Monaghan town were praised and held in high regard for the success they were having with their boarding school for girls.[62] An example of their teaching philosophy is as follows:

> About your work, my dear child, have no fears. The children who have confided in you are young, and you have an opportunity to observe and study them, and to learn for yourself from experience the best way to manage them. You are their visible angel; you will not be without the help of their invisible guardians in forming them to the love and fear of God ... Teach them above all things the fear of offending God and a vivid faith in the truth that God sees everything.
> – Letter from Abbé de Régny received by Sr Claire stating some philosophies of the Sisters of Mercy

One can assume that the suicide of a nun was a rather shocking and traumatic event for the Catholic community in 1875 for the above social and political reasons; not to mention a scandalous and embarrassing one. It also reveals the importance of oral tradition in its need for contradictory accounts of a fatality; a desire to cover up and, at the same time, romanticise the circumstances of such a death.

Walking on Water: The Legend of the Sleepwalking Nun
The Suicide of Sister Mary Keough, January 1875,
Monaghan, Monaghan Parish
The superioress of the Sisters of St Louis in Monaghan, Mary Beale, was concerned about one of the women in her order, Sister Mary Keough. Mary had been with the order for twelve years, since she was eighteen years old,[63] and was usually in good health. For two months past, the Mother Superior and others noticed that Mary had a significant loss of appetite and depression of spirits. She also told the Revd L. J. O'Neill that Mary had been absent from her duties and recreations repeatedly. Mary said she was also suffering from a lingering headache. The Mother Superior told Mary that she insisted on calling Dr Ross for her and the appointment had been scheduled for 6 January.

The morning of her doctor's appointment, Sister Mary Keough was missing.

Later that morning a man named Myles Blake Burke, Esq., Constabulary Company Inspector, received a note from the bishop stating that there was a nun missing and wishing him to go immediately to the convent. Burke and some of his men searched the grounds and came upon a cape, lying at the water's edge of the convent lake. It appeared to have been driven to the edge of the lake by the wind and Burke believed that Sister Mary's body was in the water. Later in the day, with a boat out on the lake, Constable Fletcher hooked the dress of the deceased with a drag. Mary was dead, found in water eight feet deep, about twenty yards from shore. She was not fully dressed when found and appeared to have on her nightdress with something additional thrown over her shoulders.[64] The verdict was that Sister Mary Keough came to her death on 6 January 1875 from drowning while labouring under temporary insanity.[65]

It has been 127 years since the death of Sister Mary Keough, yet the story remains in oral tradition even in the twenty-first century. Some accounts of this story from Monaghan town are told as follows:

> A nun was sleepwalking out of the convent, out towards the lake and an older nun followed her. She had been worried about the younger nun. The older nun then observed her walking out on the water, actually walking on the surface of the water toward the crannóg. And on seeing this she shouted at the young nun, who woke up, and then fell underneath the water where she drowned.[66]

Most accounts of the story are the same as the above. It has even been stated that the 'unofficial' tour for new students at the convent school, even today, includes a short mention of the sleepwalking nun. It is interesting that, in the oral tradition, the unfortunate young woman is not held accountable for her actions, she is in a dream-like state, and only when discovered and interrupted does she fall into the water to her death. Of course, she is also given Christ-like powers in that she can walk on the water. There is no mention of the story of her sickness, only to say that the elder nun was concerned about her. There are still some persons in the area who believe that sleepwalkers not aware of their actions could perform any action while in this unconscious state – including walking on water.

It was reported that Sister Mary Keough drowned herself on the day of her scheduled appointment with the doctor. She had been suffering from a loss of appetite and she was depressed for two months.

Although it cannot be known what events were occurring at the convent two months earlier, one possible suggestion is that migratory workers, both women and men, returned from and went to Scotland in the beginning of November. Was she lamenting over someone who left? Or involved with someone who returned? Is it possible she was pregnant? Was she actually suffering from a mental illness? Was this just a simple case of losing interest in her vows and/or status as a nun, as she had been with the order since she was eighteen years old and was now turning thirty? One idea does emerge: she appears to have lost her faith. If one of the philosophies of the convent was to teach the young girls how to love and fear God and serve as their 'visible angels', what made her make this fateful decision?

The behaviour of the persons defined as 'insane' and 'dangerous lunatics' when closely examined do not always show mental illness, but instead depict persons unhappy with their position within society, and most often, within the family. Asylums and jails were used as a method of disposal for those members of the family that were noncompliant with their station and duties, making them no longer a threat to parental authority. Such institutions were used to attempt to control this aggressive and unacceptable behaviour. Many persons were committed to the asylum and met an untimely death from disease. Others were driven to suicide by poverty, lack of proper diet and shelter and a restriction of their personal freedom by religion and society. It can be surmised that this behaviour, by modern day standards, might not be considered abnormal, but instead illustrates angry, frustrated and depressed individuals desperately searching for a solution in very difficult situations.

CHAPTER FOUR

BEHIND CLOSED DOORS
DANGERS IN THE HOME

We all run and hide to the safety of our homes to secure ourselves from the storms outside. And sometimes it is confused as to which side of the door more dangers lurk.

— M.M.

Deaths that occurred in and around the homestead, behind the closed doors of the families of Co. Monaghan, reflect the hazardous chores and household tasks necessary to maintain the integrity of the landholding and the importance of the unique roles and responsibilities of each member of the family. Fatal accidents occurred often in homes and on farms. Infants, young children and the elderly were most at risk of accidental death. Children under the age of five were frequently left alone with infants and given adult responsibilities for their care. Fatalities resulted from burns by fire and boiling water, suffocation and drowning in nearby streams and lakes, and other structures and instruments unsafe by design. Duties performed by the elderly such as shovelling manure, working in the fields picking potatoes and taking care of grandchildren often proved too much for their ageing bodies. Medicines, cures and superstitions were sometimes useful when accidents did occur, but they were primitive.

The home, intended to be a place of comfort and security, in some cases became a dark prison – a place where violent, unspeakable crimes were committed. Domestic abuse was prevalent, a cruelty whose victims were not protected by laws or shielded by social reform. The Aggravated Assaults on Women and Children Act of 1853 in England, was unfortunately not adopted in Ireland and many women had no legal recourse and often no family support. Some women lost their lives violently at the hands of their husbands. Married women were at great risk of being abused and even murdered – especially those unable to have children. Some men who were unable to show their virility via fertility (children were essential in order to pass on the land) became shamed and enraged. The elderly were also exposed to various forms of torture. Lacking proper shelter and food, sick and unable to provide for themselves, some of the old and infirm were vulnerable to neglect at the hands of uncaring relatives or at the mercy of neighbours, friends and strangers.

One salient feature of life in the home in Co. Monaghan in the post-famine years was the importance placed upon the family working together to maintain the integrity of the homestead. Those family members who stayed, who remained working on the farm and continued to work, endeavoured to carry out their responsibilities in the traditional roles that preserved the qualities of the family. The deaths that resulted from the customary activities and work performed at home on the farm were tragic and heartbreaking, yet they provide an inside look at the nature of the duties of each part of the family, young and old, as well as the expectations placed upon each – the mother and father, brothers and sisters, the elderly and the children.

THE HOME AS A DEATH TRAP

Most homes in Co. Monaghan had one to three rooms, thatched roofs with stone and mud walls and were poorly built. Throughout the century, living conditions were described as small and inadequate, and cabins were over-populated. The following is a description of the typical home of the average farmer or tenant in Currin parish in 1835:

> A glance at the wretched hovels, scantily covered with straw, surrounded and almost entombed in mire, which everywhere present themselves throughout the parish, sufficiently testify that the total absence of all activity in industry is one source of the wretchedness and misery which almost overwhelms the land ... The most substantial of their mud-built houses resist the elements for a few years only, and remain long in dilapidation before they are restored. There are exceptions of stone-built dwellings to this almost universal substitution of mud perceivable in the parish, the more numerous in the western section.[1]

There is a similar description of homes in the parish of Ematris:

> The mud houses, divided into 3 apartments, seldom exceed 1-storey high, furnished occasionally with small glass windows but often without them, an earthen floor with no ceiling, and universally thatched with straw, one extremity appropriated as a bedroom for the family, the opposite for the cattle, and the centre a kitchen and dining-room for the whole household.[2]

It was the tenant who made repairs and performed the necessary maintenance on the home, although the law (before 1870) presumed that
all permanent improvements such as drains, buildings, roads and fences,
if made by the tenants, belonged to the landlord unless they had been
made with the landlord's permission and registered under the Landed
Property (Ireland) Improvement Act of 1860.[3] Many landlords, therefore, supplied building materials free to tenants who would do the
building themselves and would compensate them with a deduction
in their rent.[4] As a result, the landlord had no liability in cases where
dilapidated homes fell in on the tenants or where fire broke out.

Four of the five cases listed in the coroner's reports of tenants
being crushed by their homes falling in on top of them, involved elderly women, widows, well into their seventies, who were living alone.
Unable to perform the tasks necessary to maintain structural integrity of the home, these women appear to have relied upon the kindness of their neighbours to rebuild walls and repair roofs. In one case,
Biddy McGuiness of Skinnagin, an old woman living alone in a frail
old house, had just received help with well-needed repairs. Pat Meighan and Peter Connolly had begun work on the home and were in the
process of propping up the roof that appeared likely to fall in. Biddy
was in the house with them as they began measuring and preparing
for the job, when suddenly they heard a loud 'crack' and the roof began to fall in on top of them. Pat and Peter were lucky enough to narrowly escape before the rubble fell on their heads, but Biddy, being
old and infirm, was not so lucky. As soon as possible they dug her out
of the mass of rubble but she had been killed instantly. It was the
chimney brace that gave way and brought down the house.[5] Rachel
Tole was also unlucky. She was seventy-eight years old and living
alone in her home in Aghareagh and recovering from a fall which
had fractured her thigh near the hip joint. While working in the field
cutting corn, Thomas Dogherty was called to go and check on Rachel
as her roof had fallen in. When he dug her out from under the thatch
timber; her other thigh had been broken. Having been visited by Dr
Taylor who prescribed some medicine, as well as by members of her
family, she died early the next morning.[6]

One case published in the newspaper provided more detail of the
personal life and tragic death of Bridget Prunty of Ballybay:

Singular and Fatal Occurrence
On Monday last, an old woman named Bridget Prunty, who resided in what
was considered to be a rather substantial little cottage, in the townland of
Drumhamond, [Drumhaman] within two miles of Ballybay, came to her

death in the following singular manner – She had been at Ballintra chapel and after returning home desiring her nephew, who had lately returned from Scotland, and who was the only person dwelling with her, to go to a neighbour's house and hear the contents of a letter from America. She cautioned him against staying long as she was preparing dinner. He went as directed and had just sat down, when one of the inmates shouted, 'Lord! Biddy's house is down!' They all ran out and sure enough so it was – the roof and gable had fallen in burying the poor old creature beneath. Immediate efforts were made to rescue her, but when discovered, life was extinct. An inquest was held on Monday, before Hugh Swanzy, Esq., coroner of the district and a verdict in accordance with the above facts returned – Cor.[7]

Burned Alive: Deadly House Fires

An open flame from the hearth or a candle, although necessary for cooking, warmth or light, was dangerous given the often poorly-constructed stone and mud homes with thatched roofs that could easily ignite if a stray spark were to escape the embers. It is always a sad story, the loss of a home and its contents, but the loss of life which may be involved when a house surrenders to fire is tragic.

High Wind and Sparks Hit the Turf: Two Sisters Die in Bellanode
The Death of Margaret and Elizabeth Ann Martin, January 1869

On the evening of 2 January 1869, Henry Martin was making his way home from Monaghan town and stopped to buy some items from Mr Moorehead of Bellanode. He went home for a few hours and then decided to go back into the village to pick up his purchases. Before leaving, he put his two young daughters, Margaret and Elizabeth Ann, to bed. After the girls were safely tucked in, he secured the fire and then locked the door behind him until his return.

Edward McMahon was sitting at home that same evening when he saw smoke billowing from the home of Henry Martin. He hurried to two other neighbours for help and they all ran towards the burning house. Edward began shouting, 'Martin! Martin!' However, receiving no answer, he burst in the door. The whole back part of the roof was in flames and immediately after he entered, the front part of the roof began to burn as well. Realising the smoke, heat and flames were too great for just a few persons to put out, he hurried to the village for more help.

While in the village, Henry Martin was stopped and told that his home was on fire. He hurried home and on reaching the spot, he found the neighbours striving to get the fire under control. It was in vain as it had gained too great a hold and everything but the walls was consumed – including his two girls. Henry Martin's words to the coroner at his daughters' inquest describe what he found in the rubble:

> Nothing could be found of them, but charred portions of their bones, including a skull with some hair on it. I found it immediately under where they were sleeping. In the corner and very near the hearth, there had been a load of turf. The wind being very high that night, the draft under the door must have carried a spark from the fire to the turf and on no other principle can I account for the sad occurrence.

The verdict was death in consequence of their house accidentally taken fire in which the girls were burned to death. Margaret was seven years old and Elizabeth Ann was five years old.[8]

THE ELDERLY AT RISK
On the Farm and in the Home

Elderly persons living alone in the house were also at risk from being burned in the fire or drowned carrying water to and from the well. As they advanced in infirmity and age, many of the elderly liked to sleep by the fire and, as a result, were burned. For example, Mary Dawson of Drumcaw set up her bed in the house in the chimney corner, but the embers were too close to the bedding and she was burned severely down the right side of her body. She was seventy years of age.[9] Bridget McDonald of Garran was also burned sleeping too close to the fire. The feeble old woman died two hours later from the severity of the burns.[10]

Others were drowned as a result of not being able to perform daily chores and duties on the farm such as gathering water or even just walking along the land alone. Mary Keenan, a feeble old woman, went to the well to draw some water on Christmas Day 1857. Young Mary Caldwell found her; it appeared that the full can of water proved too weighty for her and drew her down into the well where she drowned.[11]

The heavy lifting and the unpredictable nature of the animals on the farm put the elderly at risk of fatal accidents. The age of the victims involved in farming accidents in the coroner's inquests was between sixty-five and eighty-six years old.

Falling off the Manure Heap: The Death of Robert Storey
Aghagaw, Tedavnet Parish, February 1867
Edward W. Storey was 'drawing home' turnips while Robert Storey

was reeling up the yard and working at the manure. When Edward went down the field for a load of turnips, he heard Robert ask for a shovel. By the time he returned, he saw Robert lying on his side in a gutter of water – dead. He immediately picked the old man up, cleaned him off and carried him into the house. The body was warm, but life had fled. Robert Storey was eighty-six years old and died as a result of accidentally falling off the manure heap.[12]

Crushed by the Manure: The Death of Thomas McArdle
Dunsinare, Monaghan Parish, April 1863
Bernard Trainor went out into the field to make conversation with Thomas McArdle, who was busy working at the side of his house. As the two men talked, Thomas was slowly digging up manure from the grip at the head of the field and throwing it up over his shoulder into a cart. After they had concluded their discussion, Bernard went off to tend to his own duties. Twenty minutes later, he heard a loud shout of distress and ran back towards Thomas. He found Thomas' wife, screaming and desperately trying to help her husband. Thomas was down in the grip and the end of the back-rail of his cart was pressing hard against his chest. The buck was close against his back and the entire weight of the heavy cart of manure was lying on him. Bernard realised immediately, as the cart had slid into the ditch, that 'twas utterly out of human aid to relieve him' as he was quite dead. It appeared that Thomas had tried to prevent it from falling. The verdict was death from injuries sustained accidentally caused from his cart, loaded with manure, sliding into the grip.[13]

Falling from the Haycock: The Death of Felix Began
Calliagh, Aghabog Parish, September 1860
James Carragher was working with Felix Began Sr cutting the hay. Carragher was gathering in the hay, Felix Jr was forking it to his father and Felix Sr was tramping.[14] When the haycock was nearly finished, the father called to his son and James to look around because he thought maybe the cock was sliding. Felix Jr moved his two children away and at the same moment it slid off and hit his father, a man of between sixty and seventy years of age, throwing him violently to the ground. He was lifted up, carried to his home and the doctor sent for. Dr Reid found Felix suffering from 'regular paralysis from the vertebrae of the neck downwards, in fact all extremities upper and lower'. Felix's neck had been broken and he died a week later. The verdict of the coroner's inquest was death from injuries accidentally sustain-

ed on 8 September by falling off a haycock that he had been engaging in building.[15]

Livestock, specifically cows, proved to be a danger to the elderly. Some were thrown down by cows as they did not appear to have the stamina to guide or direct them or the physical agility to remove themselves from their path. For example, while at the Ballybay fair, sixty-five-year-old James Duffy was thrown down by a young heifer. The hips of the cow slammed against him and as a result he broke his leg. He was taken to the Monaghan infirmary where a few days later he began raving from 'Erysipelas' and 'Mortification' and he died the same day.[16]

Thrown Down by the Cow: The Death of Shane (Shibby) McKenna
Kilnageer, Errigal Truagh Parish, July 1860
'The old woman's right eye is considerably blackened,' Dr Douglass told the coroner and his jury. 'On the right shinbone is a large ragged wound and I believe that the deceased's death arose from internal injuries caused by being thrown down and trampled on by a cow that was on the road at the time being baited by two dogs.'

The death of old 'Shibby' McKenna was an unfortunate accident. Ann Treanor was herding cattle on the evening in question near Shibby's house. While she was on the road, a jaunting car drove by with several acquaintances on it. Ann immediately recognised Mary Keenan and in play, threw a pebble at the car. Laughing, she continued walking down the road when she heard dogs barking and saw a cow running and excited. As she got closer she saw old Shibby lying on the road and bleeding from the mouth and nose. She screeched out, 'O God! O God! The cow has killed Shibby!' The old woman was then carried to her own house where she lingered until 10p.m. that night when she died. The verdict was death from injuries sustained by being thrown down and trampled by a cow – roused and excited by two dogs.[17]

OLD AND ALONE
Elderly Neglect and Abuses

The importance of strong family interpersonal relationships and adult children accepting responsibility for the care of their elderly and sick siblings, aunts, uncles, parents and grandparents was a matter of life and death for those too weak to take care of themselves. Without family members to care for them, some of the elderly either wandered around towns and villages, going from neighbour to neighbour, or relied on the kindness of strangers for food and shelter. The poorhouse was an option; however, it was a last resort – and a disgrace. The elderly didn't go to the poorhouse and come out again. Instead they went there to die.

The elderly were also at risk of violence, neglect and abuse particularly in situations when there was not a 'responsible' person available to care for them who would ensure their safety and well being; in short, truly *care* for them. In some instances, the feeble and weak were ignored and treated like a burden. It is clear that the negligence in many cases warranted legal action, however these persons had no recourse, no voice and lacked the support of the community when those closest to them were their abusers.

Great Destitution: Blind, Cold and Hungry
The Death of George Lee, Corravacan, Ematris Parish, February 1863

Ignorance and lack of nurturing appear to have contributed to the death of George Lee who spent the last days of his life blind, shivering on the damp dirt floor of his wretched cabin and lying on a bit of straw with very little covering for his bed. He was infrequently fed and the window in the house was left open. A cold wind blew through the house right where he lay. His friend, James Wells, had come into the house and found him gathered in a lump on the ground endeavouring to keep warm. His daughter, Elizabeth Donaghue, and granddaughter Mary Ann Duffy, were living with him as he was in their care. Poor conditions and their apparent treatment of him left much to be desired. As Wells stated, 'There was great destitution in the place.'

'I called in to see George and asked if he was better. He replied "not",' said Wells. 'He made no complaint to me of wanting food and I think he would had it been so. However, he was cold and the wind blowing on him, and he was lying in a most uncomfortable state.'

Mary Ann Duffy told the coroner at her grandfather's inquest that, on Monday morning, her mother left the house, leaving a stone of meal and some bread in the house. 'Of the meal, I made stirabout each day,' she said. 'On Friday, he took his breakfast but no dinner and died that night about 1 o'clock – I having sat up with him.'

Dr Moore had long known the deceased and was in the habit of visiting him as the dispensary doctor. Dr Moore said, 'Of late, George was subject to swelling in the limbs and joints from cold and want, being made exposed to the cold and the severity of the weather.' He continued, 'I most solemnly declare that I believe there was great and culpable neglect on the part of his daughter, Elizabeth Donaghoe.' The verdict arrived at was death on the morning of 7 February from insufficiency of food, exposure to the severity of the weather and much of culpable neglect on the part of his daughter, Elizabeth Donaghoe.[18]

There was no supporting documentation or evidence to suggest she was charged in connection with his death.

Left to the Elements: Thrown out before Death came to Visit
The Death of Rose Ginely, Kilnaclay, Drumsnat Parish, June 1871
Seventy-five-year-old Rose Ginely had been lodging with Rose Cassidy of Kilnaclay for several months. Cassidy, fearing the old woman would die soon of fever and wanting no responsibility for her care or burial, went to the Monaghan poorhouse to ask if she could have Rose removed before death came. An ass and cart were sent to the house to get the old woman, but Rose refused to go. Some neighbours (Catherine McMahon and Mary Sreenan) gathered while Rose argued in front of the house with the man sent from the poorhouse. Cassidy used this distraction as an opportunity to put all the old woman's clothing outside along with her. Rose requested that, instead of being taken to the poorhouse, she be taken to the house of her nephew, Michael Ginely, who lived a short distance off. The man refused and the cart was forced to leave without her. She now realised she had nowhere to go, no transport to safety and would not again gain entry into Cassidy's house. Rose remained outside all that night and the night after that. She was found dead the next morning on the roadside a little after 9a.m. The verdict at her inquest was death from natural causes.[19]

When Rose's body was found, it was discovered that the police had only just been informed of her condition and were planning to have her removed to safer lodgings that same morning. Additionally, although her friends would not take charge of her, the Revd John McKenna, PP at Drumsnat was encouraging them to do so. Mr Swan of Threemilehouse on hearing of this terrible occurrence, had Rose's body brought to his house and at considerable expense and inconvenience to himself, he had her waked and buried in a suitable manner.[20]

Religious Differences within the Family: The Death of Phillip Donaghy
Edenaferkin, Tullycorbet Parish, March 1857
On Monday, 23 March 1857, the coroner received a report that Phillip Donaghy of Edenaferkin had died under very suspicious circum-

stances on 15 March. He had been suddenly interred and neither a
doctor nor a priest had been called in to see him. W. C. Waddell
called in to some of the 'respectable' neighbours of the deceased and
learned that much ill-feeling and contention existed in his family.
Phillip's mother had died recently in the house of one of her daughters. That daughter had married a Protestant and conformed to his
religion. Some trifling property she had at the time of her death was
a subject of contention between the deceased Phillip Donaghy and
other members of the family. The consequences of the dispute resulted in warrants being issued by the Ballybay police against some of the
family.

Waddell also heard from W. Sam Brown of Edenaferkin that the
deceased man had worked in the mill of Mr Gordon Riddle in Edenaferkin. On Thursday he was in the mill as usual, but not being well,
Phillip was told 'he need not be there, as they wanted no idlers'. He
left and went home. He took to his bed and by Saturday he was in a
raving fever, receiving little if any care and neither a doctor nor priest
was sent for. Upon his death, Phillip was buried with the least possible
delay.

Although not stated in the inquiry, there is an implication that
Phillip was not living alone, but because of the heated dispute amongst
the family members, they simply let him die and buried him without
a proper wake and funeral. Though the conduct was extremely unfeeling and blameworthy, the coroner did not consider it would justify raising the body for the purpose of holding an inquest. The body
was not exhumed.[21]

The Reverend Mr Pounden's Charity: The Death of John Christy
Golanmurphy, Killeevan Parish, March 1870

John Christy was a very healthy man until his wife died and several
months later, on 21 December 1869, he suffered a stroke which left
him partially paralysed. Since his wife's death, he had lived alone but
had a man in his house sleeping with him – a man named Quinn.

On 2 February, John Keenan, a very close friend of John Christy,
heard the bailiff of the landlord tell Quinn that for the time past, his
landlord, the Revd Mr Pounden, would pay him for his past care of
Christy, but as of that day, the payment would cease.

Quinn exclaimed, 'My God! The man will be lost.'

The bailiff then again explained to Quinn that there would be no
more payments to him from Mr Pounden for the care of John Christy.

Quinn thought for a while and then said 'If you'll give me Christy's land (about one rood of a garden) then I'll take care of him as long as he lives.'

The bailiff would have none of it and told Quinn he would not get the land. Quinn said that he would now give up all care of the old man.

Five days later, Keenan called up to see John Christy. He entered the house and saw Christy lying on a wisp of straw that used to be his bed. The rest of the bed was burned and Christy appeared injured from the fire on the left side of his body. Keenan immediately asked the cause of the fire, and the old man told him 'his bed took fire and 'twas a great mercy he was not burned to a cinder'. Dr Reid called to see Christy a few days later. John Christy died on 15 March 1870 from paralysis but it was accelerated by the effects of a burn accidentally caused. He was sixty-years of age.[21]

BARE WOMBS AND JEALOUSY
Domestic Violence

Causes why girls become old maids
'Young girls may generally thank themselves and those who rear them if old maidens be their lot. Men will be found ready enough to marry if they find anything worth marrying; but the artificial useless daughters of a family, who neither know of, nor care for, the comfort of any but themselves, do not offer sufficiently attractive points to compensate for the loss of bachelor freedom and bachelor goodfellowship. Young ladies who deck their faces with the gayest smiles in society, very frequently hang up the fiddle at home and what is the consequence? Some deluded swain meets the fair one at a party; flowers deck her hair, smiles animate her face; she is the very personification of amiability; and he rejoices in the idea of having met with perfection and found a wife with whom he will be supremely happy, for man is but a selfish creature, and thinks first of his own happiness.'
– The Times, 12 June 1858

Domestic violence towards women in the nineteenth century was invisible. It was widely-known that some women were experiencing beatings, tortures and psychological abuse at the hands of their husbands, yet it went on without any community or governmental effort to prevent it, almost as if it were accepted as one of the probable pitfalls of marriage. Even Lady Wilde depicts such occurrences in one of her stories entitled 'The Fairy Child': 'an ancient woman living at Innis-Sark said that in her youth she knew a young woman who had been married for five years, but had no children. And her husband was a rough, rude fellow, and used to taunt her and beat her often because she was childless.'[23] There was no recourse in law for victims of domestic abuse except to file charges and be at the mercy of individual judges and juries. Very often, having pressed charges against their husbands, wives would ask the court for lenience or mercy, denying any real physical abuse, begging the court for their husbands' release or explaining away the incident. For many women, the risk of losing a husband's income was too great and, without that support, her family could be in great jeopardy should he be put in jail for any length of time.[24]

The Green-Eyed Monster
Eliza McElnea summoned her husband, William J. McElnea, for assaulting her on the 5th inst. Mr Reilly appeared for the defendant.

Mrs McElnea said that on the morning after she had sent the children to school, defendant called her 'out of her name' and accused her of improper conduct. He then caught her by the throat and thrust her back over a seat and threatened to break every bone in her body.

Defendant said she done some particular things which he did not like (laughter [in the courtroom]) – and he was just giving her a caution; but he did not strike her, or use any violence to her.

The Bench dismissed the case.

– *The Northern Standard*, 30 August 1873

The Green-Eyed Monster
A woman named Ellen Murphy, apparently about fifty years of age, and of by no means inviting appearance, made an application to their Worships to have a warrant issued against her husband, under the following circumstances: She stated that he had been absent from her for ten years, and now he had come back and ill used her, breaking several of her ribs, and locking her up in a room, and allowing no woman or girl to stop in the house with her. She stated that it was all jealousy (laughter [in the courtroom]). He had been 'mad jealous' of her for the last twelve years.

Their Worships directed her to take out a summons against him.

The Court then rose.

– *The Northern Standard*, 1 March 1873

A man's jealousy was a source of humour as well as humiliation in a court of law and a woman's behaviour, what she did to provoke him, was a standard question in such cases. From the reaction of the jury, the laughter directed at each woman's probable antagonism towards her husband depicts that their claims were not always taken seriously when they did try to confront their abusers. Other factors that were taken into consideration by the jury were comments on the physical appearance of the woman, such as in the case of Ellen Murphy ('and of by no means [having an] inviting appearance'). Her husband had not been living with her for ten years yet retained the right to enter her home, beat her, lock her up and prevent her from speaking to any of her friends.

Although verdicts were inconsistent, in some instances the justice system did sympathise with the abused women. It appears that when the evidence against the husband included not just the physical abuse, but intemperance, combined with a lack of income, juries were more sympathetic to wives and children. These men were viewed as dregs of humanity or rather 'dead beats' who should be reformed through the punishment of sobriety and hard work. From the many examples of cases in the nineteenth century and well into the twentieth century, the beatings a wife received would alone not have warranted guilty verdicts against many abusing husbands.

ABUSE AND MURDER
The Homicide of Wives

Clones Petty Sessions
Wife Beating
Ann Boylan charged her husband John Boylan with assaulting her on the 28th of August. The defendant did not appear.

The complainant said she had lived upwards of forty years with the defendant, but some time ago she was obliged to leave him owing to his intemperable habits. On the 28th ult., he met her, and without any provocation struck her several times on the head and shoulders with a stick.

Mr Wall – I think the defendant was in jail before?

Complainant – Yes, but it was only for drunkenness. He often struck me before, but I never prosecuted him. He does nothing to support me, and he will not even allow me to support myself. I am willing to support him by my industry if he would only allow me.

Mr Wall – Did you give any provocation or bad language?

Complainant – No more than I could help – (laughter [in the courtroom]).

Constable McDonald said the defendant was a confirmed drunkard.

The defendant was ordered to be imprisoned six months and kept to hard labour.

– *The Northern Standard*, 10 September 1875

There were several cases in the newspaper reporting incidents of the homicide of wives at the hands of their husbands (e.g. 1868: John Crow charged with the murder of his wife, Mary) but unfortunately, many conclusions of criminal trials can't to be located. The documentation is incomplete for many of these murders and therefore no background information of the husband's trial is available. In criminal reference files (National Archives, Dublin), these murderers might be referred to only by name but no further evidence can be found. If they were convicted, their name might appear in one of several prison registers; if acquitted, there is barely a trace of their whereabouts.

In the coroner's casebook there are two inquests suggesting the deceased, a wife, was a victim at the hands of her abusive husband. These cases have disappointing conclusions as well. In one instance, the coroner admits he would not be able to provide enough evidence to pursue a conviction. In the other case, he does charge the husband yet there is no trace of his trial by jury in a magistrate's court in any source that can be traced. One can only suppose that the charges were dropped.

Co. Monaghan was not unlike the rest of the country in regard to domestic abuse. This was a society hesitant to acknowledge charges brought against men abusing their wives when they were alive and lax in pursuing a conviction against the murderer upon the woman's death. Additionally, even through people could read almost daily reports of harrowing incidents of the abuse of women, there was virtually no outcry against wife-beating and domestic violence in Ireland.[25] Although the Ulster suffrage movements became organised in the 1870s, counties Cavan and Monaghan remained largely untouched by the campaigns for women's enfranchisement well into the twentieth century.[26] Domestic violence simply was not acknowledged.

The Cruel Treatment of Jane Gordan
Dundrannan, Ematris Parish, January 1867
Fifty-four-year-old Jane Gordan died on 24 December 1866. Her husband, William, registered her as dead on 9 January 1867 and the cause of death was valvular disease of the heart, six weeks certified. However, the coroner began to investigate the circumstances of her death and recorded the following note in his casebook:

> From the 12th to 19th January 1867 several persons spoke to me on the subject of death of Mrs Jane Gordan, wife to William Gordan of Dundrannan, parish of Ematris, stating that her death was the result of violence sustained at the hands of her husband. Having made all possible inquiry on the subject, I find I could not have sworn depositions such as would justify me in having the body of the deceased exhumed or would lead to incriminating of the husband, but fear the reports made to me were not altogether without grounds for belief in harsh if not cruel treatment.

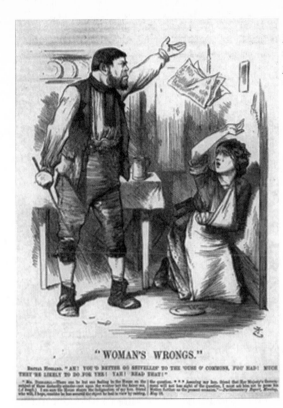

*Domestic violence
is brought to the
public's attention.
(Punch, May 1874)*

There were no criminal records or index references to this crime in any court or criminal documents, no mention in the newspaper. William Gordan was never charged.

*Tortured and Beaten to Death by her Husband
The Murder of Mary Magee
Derryvolan, Co. Fermanagh, Clones Parish, September 1866*

> Ellen Mullen deposed that on night of last New Year's day, January 1, 1866, 'I heard Mary (deceased) shouting "Murder" and at the time no person but her husband was in the house with her.'
> – Testimony relating to the beating to death of Mary Magee

Thirty-four-year-old Mary Magee had only been married for about two years when John Madden of Hilton Park took her death-bed deposition of the events leading to her death:

Mary Magee of Derryvolan said on her death-bed that in or about the month last, the defendant, my husband, having returned from Monaghan after selling pigs, knocked me down, kicked and abused me in a most cruel manner ... Sometime after, he again knocked me down, kicked and abused me in a most inhuman manner ... Shortly after, in or about the same month, I was out in a field at Derryvolan helping my husband to carry manure and he then and there knocked me down and gave me several kicks in the ribs, side and back in the most brutal manner from the effects of all which several beatings I am now dangerously ill and do not expect to recover.'

On a former occasion, some time since I told Dr Knight who was attending me that my husband had not beaten me because he was standing beside my bed and I feared his ill usage.[27]

Mary Magee died on 10 September 1866. The verdict of her death was injuries caused and inflicted by her husband, Charles Magee. The details of the events in her unhappy life and the vicious abuse by her husband were told to the coroner's jury by her sisters, neighbours, local police, doctors and friends. Their individual accounts provided vivid details of her inhumane treatment at the hands of her husband, and the gruesome injuries that resulted.

Ann McCabe, Mary's sister, deposed that before May 1866 she had heard that Mary was ill and she went to see her. Ann told the jury, 'Mary showed me her side and her belly where there were marks of severe injuries. About four or five weeks after, she went to the Monaghan infirmary. Her husband had forced her to work out in the fields, creeling ashes and at spade work; but she, already in a state of weakness, became worse and worse, and had to go to the Monaghan infirmary,' she said. 'She was there for seven weeks and where I went to see her five times. While there, she told me that her injuries were caused by her husband – one time after selling butter in Monaghan and another time when they were creeling ashes.'

Catherine Quigley provided a background to the history of abuse of her sister Mary. In April 1866, Mary told Catherine that Charles had beaten her twice. 'I asked to see where she was hurt,' said Catherine, 'and she showed me her side and her belly, where there were marks of violence, as well as a cut on her navel.' He had beaten her with his fist and kicked her. She was immediately taken to the Monaghan infirmary, where she lay for seven weeks in consequence of these beatings.

Catherine continued, 'After her return from the Monaghan infirmary, she was still very weak but her husband left her – going to England to the harvest. She was unable to move about or do anything for herself and her husband left no money, no food in the house save stone meal, tea, sugar and flour – about enough for two days use. Charles instructed her that before she died, not to use any of the sheets for a shroud as he had left word with Mr Whitside of Roosky to give what calico would be required.

'When I saw the state she was in, I stayed for several days with her. As there was no suitable nourishment in the house, I provided the food for her myself. My sister, Ann, and I took turns taking care of Mary,' she said. When the sisters realised Mary wasn't getting any better, they had her removed on 12 July to the Clones workhouse to receive proper medical attention. She added, 'Mary blamed her severe illness to the beatings she received from her husband. The last time I saw her, she said she had not many days to live and she laid her death on her husband.'

Constable Michael Clark of Newtownbutler had been called to visit the Magee home on 9 July 1866 by Catherine Quigley and Ann McCabe. The two women asked Clark to come in order for Mary to report the crimes that had been perpetrated against her. He said, 'When I arrived, Mary was on a bed of straw with clothes on it. She was assisted to sit up to show me her emaciated state. Her arms and legs were mere skin and bone. She said she was daily getting worse,' he said. 'I asked her what the cause was, and she replied from abuse by her husband.'

Clark continued relaying the facts told to him by Mary Magee. 'One time on return from Monaghan market for advising him against getting drunk, he caught her by the hair of the head, pulled her to the ground out of the chair she was sitting in (high upon the cart or carriage) and then kicked her. On turning on her belly, he kicked her on the back and side from which for some time she was unable to rise; but when she did rise, he caught her by the head striking it severely against the wall.

'The second beating was for having made a shift out of a bed sheet. On her husband counting and missing the sheet, she said it had been washed and while drying at the fire was accidentally burned. For this he took her down to the room and there, while lying on the floor, beat and kicked her severely,' he said.

Clark continued, 'The next time was while they were creeling out ashes. The loads being too much for her to carry, in consequence of her previous injuries, her husband beat her, knocking her down and kicking her on the back and sides.'

Charles' conduct on several occasions was harsh, cruel and unfeeling. She was deterred from giving earlier information from dread of her husband killing her. She did not tell the truth to Dr Knight as to the cause of her illness because her husband had been present (in the past) and she feared worse treatment. Mary told Clark that her husband did not support her, but that her sisters provided help. Clark was so affected by the physical state of Mary Magee and her testimony, that he immediately reported the case to his superiors and Thomas D. Maxwell, sub-inspector of the police at Lisneskea, went to visit the Magee house on 11 July.

Maxwell met Mary's sisters who led him into the bedroom where Mary was lying. On asking her as to her illness, she said she was suffering from the effects of bad treatment from her husband who on three separate occasions kicked and beat her severely on the back and ribs. One of her sisters pulled down the bedclothes, exposing her arms and legs – they were emaciated to skin and bone. Mary told that her husband had left for England, leaving her no provisions. Maxwell told her to go into the union poorhouse where she would be properly taken care of and attended.

Mary was received into the Clones poorhouse. George Little, Master of the Clones poorhouse, told the jury that Mary was received into the house on 12 July 1866 in a very weak and emaciated state. When he asked her the cause, Mary said, ''Twas the ill usage by my husband.' She was at once placed into the sick ward where she was seen regularly by Dr Henry until the day of her death on 8 September 1866.

Dr Henry explained Mary's physical state upon the day of her admission. 'She was weak and emaciated and suffering from an abscess in the parietal area of the abdomen which was discharging at the umbelica [sic] (navel). She stated that it had burst when in the infirmary. Having been sometime in the house, another abscess formed on the right hinch (hip). After it was opened, she sunk rapidly. I never had hopes of her recovery after her admittance. Both abscesses continued to discharge until her death.' He also performed the post-mortem examination.

'I found strong adhesions in the lower part of the bowels. The result of previous inflammation and which might be the result of previous severe injuries,' he said. 'The deceased told me that her husband had beaten her severely and kicked her. She had not told the truth to Dr Knight as her husband was present and she feared to tell the truth lest he would ill use her still more.' Dr Henry considered that the abscesses were the cause of her death.

Dr Knight had taken care of Mary in May. 'Feverish and complaining of a tumour over her abdomen,' he stated. 'I asked her the cause which she said was from carrying manure – the husband at the time was in the house. I saw her twice and recommended her to go to Monaghan infirmary. I saw her after leaving the infirmary. She was very low and weak. She then told me abuse from her husband was the cause of her illness and that her previous statement was from fear of his further ill treatment.' The verdict of her death was injuries caused and inflicted by her husband, Charles Magee. Her death was recorded at the Registrar's Office by the coroner. The cause of death was 'malicious injuries; 4 months certified.'[28]

Upon the conclusion of the inquest, Charles Magee was arrested and held for trial at the next Monaghan assizes.[29] The sad and deadly story of Mary Magee was run in *The Northern Standard*, Saturday, 15 September 1866. It recaptured the details of the inquest in Clones; however, no follow-up as to an indictment or trial was ever published. There was no documented cry for justice from the community. Life went on as if she had never existed.

Possible explanations for Charles' behaviour can be offered. Marriage in the post-famine years of the nineteenth century was a union between two persons both bringing a financial package to the 'deal'. The husband was to provide a home and land. The wife brought a dowry and the natural ability to provide heirs for her husband. As many women were getting married later in life, there were more cases of infertility. Many men, in particular those with a propensity for violence, became angered by their wives' inability to give birth. The couple had been married for eighteen months when the abuse first started and it became increasingly more violent. This may have been a result of his frustration at their inability to produce an heir. It is worth mentioning that some of her injuries occurred in her abdomen, suggesting that it had been kicked repeatedly.

Additionally, Charles Magee was a migratory worker – one of a group who were the most documented women-beaters as recorded from that time.[30] This was a chronic dilemma in England and Scotland, and although reported in Ireland, little prevention was taken. Many reasons have been offered for this problem. The Irish migratory worker was treated poorly when working the farms and fields in England and Scotland. They were displaced and many had 'identity' problems upon returning, finding it difficult to conform back to life in Ireland.[31]

'Domestic violence is always different from other violence, however, there's always a fine line between men taking out their anger and frustration on their wives and a blatant disregard for human life,' says forensic psychologist, Cristy Ettenson, who, in an interview with the author, offered a more challenging analysis of Charles Magee's behaviour: 'The murder of Mary Magee is indeed disturbing. Nothing here indicates to me that this is a man who is just stressed and taking his anger out on his wife. This is a man who has no remorse. He abuses Mary, tortures her and lets her die. He was likely upset because she was infertile and because he would never have an heir to his farm, but this man would be capable of far worse crimes. In contemporary terms, a profile of Charles Magee is that of a psychopathic personality.'

It may never be understood why Charles Magee tortured and beat his wife, but it is important now to acknowledge the treatment that she endured, as it is a mirror image of a society becoming increasingly violent and uneasy. Mary Magee is just one representative of a larger body of women beaten, abused and killed by their husbands within the home.

NEEDING EYES IN THE BACK OF YOUR HEAD
Minding the Children

It was in the home and the nearby fields that children were involved in fatal domestic accidents, usually occurring while a child was on its own, not being monitored by the principal caretakers: the mothers, fathers, grandparents, aunts, uncles and guardians. These persons, in their desire to tend to the children and simultaneously carry on with their work, could not always protect them from danger. Almost all the child fatalities occurred when an adult was not watching the child for a period of anywhere from a few moments to twenty minutes. One extreme example is provided in which a lad of seven told his aunt he would go to his grandmother's house. The aunt, satisfied that he was safe, left two days later for Scotland. She did not discover his disappearance and death until two weeks later upon her return.[32]

Men did not usually mind children, feed them or change their nappies – that was women's work. However, to prevent the suggestion that Monaghan men of the nineteenth century were not good caretakers of their families, it must be understood that this was a society in which work was divided into 'women's' work and 'men's' work. Just as women may have been excluded from what were perceived as 'manly' tasks, so also were men 'prohibited' by society's collective attitude and convention from 'women's' work.[33] A man would never participate in work that was the duty of women as it would be considered degrading. If he did perform such duties as, for example, handling eggs, milking the cow and in some cases, feeding his children, he would thereby become a 'woman', who was considered his inferior at the time. In Ulster, a man who did a woman's work was called 'an oul' jinny', which amounts to being called a woman – a derogatory slagging.[34] However, there were men mentioned in the inquests that 'kept an eye on the children' while working on other tasks. Sadly, similar to their female counterparts, these men sometimes lost track of their children – and the results were fatal.

As children grew, they too would become responsible for the care of even younger siblings. The inquests provide insights into the jobs and responsibilities of the young children involved in these tragedies. Children as young as five and six years of age were in charge of taking care of younger children or siblings, including infants. Some were responsible for kitchen duties that involved tasks such as working in and around the fire.

Another aspect of the life of children younger than five was that they were often left alone, although only for a short amount of time; by today's standards this would be considered much too long, if at all acceptable in the first place. In one such case, while the father, Pat Barkey, went to work in the fields of their farm at Carnbane and the mother walked to the market in Monaghan, the care of the children was the responsibility of six-year-old Susan Barkey. Pat went into the house to check on the children and each time found them all secured and the infants in their cradles. After the last time he went to check on them and then returned to his work, within ten or fifteen minutes his little boy came to him saying, 'Sister's clothes are burning'. He was so terrified that he could barely speak the word 'Run!' to one of the shoemaker's apprentices and they all began running towards the house. The apprentice reached and entered the house first, and according to Pat Barkey, 'On his entering [the house] a shout from him roused me to exertion. When I entered the home I found my six-year-old daughter lying on the floor and her clothes burned off her.' Soon after, several of his neighbours were with him but, despite all they could do for the 'little sufferer', she lingered but three hours before she died.[35]

Younger children under the age of three or four were always close to their mother as she performed her duties in and around the home, especially infants. Most homes consisted of three rooms: a bedroom, a room for the livestock and a living room/kitchen where the hearth fire was located. All activities of the house usually occurred in the

'kitchen' where the mother was busy with her chores as well as keeping a mindful eye on her children. The old saying, 'A woman's work
is never done' is an accurate description of the responsibilities of our
female Monaghan ancestors. Within the home, as described in the
inquests, these women were responsible for, at the very least, nurturing, feeding and clothing the children, doing laundry, pulling water
from the well or nearby lake or stream, making soap, candles and
butter and milking and feeding the animals; outside of the house she
would be responsible for herding the animals, clamping and drawing
the turf, working in the garden 'weeding', cultivating the crops, gathering herbs for remedies, or taking eggs and butter to market. After
breakfast, the man would leave to do his work in the field and about
the farm, while the woman was remained in the home to tend to her
duties and the children. It was in the home, while she performed her
duties and her back was turned, that the disastrous accidents occurred.

HOME IS WHERE THE HEARTH IS

The hearth was the location in the home that was used for cooking,
heat and in many cases acted as a primary source of light. Infants
were usually fed and then left in the cradle by the hearth fire, as most
of the activities of the mother took place here. In many inquests,
evidence was given that infants were burned as a result of an accident in front of or near the hearth fire. Traces of a belief in the power
of fire can be seen in the superstitious dread many people had of
allowing the fire to die out. It has been said that there are houses in
Ulster where the fire has not been out over many years. In some mys-
tical fashion, the life of the fire is believed to be bound up with the
life of the family. The same idea is responsible for the belief that it is
wrong to allow a fire to burn low when there is illness in the house.[36]

There are several instances in which cradles, being left too near
the fire, capsized, spilling out the infant child right into the flames
and hot embers.

A Different Kind of Crib Death
The Death of Patrick Smith, Caddagh, Tullycorbet Parish, December 1859
Thomas Smith told the coroner the tragic story of what had befallen
him and his wife just six days before Christmas. His wife was engaged
in nursing the infant and attending to the rest of the family when
one of the cows got loose and came to the house door. Fearing the

heifer might go where the rest of the cattle were, the wife got up and went to secure the animal. Upon returning, she entered the door of the house and saw that by some terrible accident the cradle had over-turned and the child had fallen into the fire. As quick as possible, she caught it up and saw that his face had been severely burned. Every-thing that Thomas and his wife could do was done, but the injuries were so terrible that the child died just a few hours later.[37]

The Hand that Rocks the Cradle
The Death of Mary Ann and Francis Kerr,
Milltown, Ematris Parish, January 1865
John Creighton was working in the corn kiln in Milltown when a person called at the door and told him that the children in the little house above were burned. He ran immediately to the house and could see smoke billowing out from inside. With great difficulty, he got into the house but because of the intense hot and dense smoke, he could manage only to grab the shape of the young child, who was lying near the door in the cradle. When he made it out of the house, he looked down and saw the burned and black body move a little and then no more. The infant was Mary Ann Kerr. Her head and the upper part of her face were completely charred and the bones at the back part of her skull were exposed. Her tiny body was crushed, the back and abdomen severely burned. From the extent and severity of the in-juries, death was presumed to be instantaneous.

After the fire was put out, her slightly older brother, little Francis Kerr, was found in the rubble. His lower body and the back part of the body were quite hard, stiff and severely burned. The tip of his tongue was black and his burned lips protruded. The extent and severity of his burns were believed to have caused instant death.

How the fire originated was never determined. However, the lit-tle boy left in charge of the two still-younger children said that when he was rocking the cradle, it over-turned into the fire. The verdicts were death on 17 January 1865 from being accidentally burned to death.[38]

Often children were left playing on the floor in the kitchen and crept too near to the fire on the hearth. The following is an example of the many inquests in which a child left unattended for just a mo-ment died:

10.829, McCabe, Mary Ann
16 October 1866
In the townland of Corrinshigo in the parish of Currin an inquest was held on view of the body of Mary Ann McCabe 11 October 1866. Mary Mc-

Cabe, mother of deceased, deposed that '[Mary Ann] was about 2½ years of age and on the morning of 16 October last, I went to a neighbour for a can of milk leaving deceased in the house. With so little of fire on the hearth, I had no fear of danger. I was about 20 minutes absent and when returning observing a great smoke, I hurried as fast as I could. On reaching my house, I saw my child's clothes all in flames. I quickly extinguished the fire and then used such remedies as I could till better arrived from Dr Taylor of Drum (I had sent for him by messenger). But all was of no avail as she died within 1½ hour.' Dr Taylor deposed to being 'called on to prescribe for Mary Ann McCabe on which I did. I saw her next day but she was then dead.' The verdict of death was severe burns caused by her clothes accidentally catching fire.

Children, Changelings and Sympathetic Magic

There are several possibilities as to why these infants and children in their cradles were at risk of burning in the fire and superstitions are at the root cause of some of these cases. There was a belief that when a sleeping infant was laid in the cradle by the hearth, the fire should never be allowed to die out, in order to keep the fairies from taking the child.[39] Tongs (used to place the turf in the fire) were placed across the infant's cradle so that the fairies could not touch the child.[40] If the fairies did 'take' the child, the child would become a *changeling* – an imitation child, sickly, or chronically crying, a fairy child that replaced their own. One legend from Co. Monaghan says: 'There was a woman one time who went out one day and forgot to put the tongs across the cradle. When she came back in, her child was gone. There was a little deformed fairy child lying in the cradle in its place. It yelled and cried day and night and the mother did not know what to do about her child.'[41] The cures for dealing with changelings included children being placed on a hot griddle, branded with the sign of the cross, left out on a shovel on the manure-heap all night,[42] set on top of a fire,[43] or the changeling being taken to a nearby fairy fort to exchange it for the real child, hitting the real child with a 'wand' and bringing it home.[44] These remedies were believed to replace the changeling and bring back the healthy child.

14.978
Cox, Jane
28 September 1870
An inquest was held on view of the body of Jane Cox on 28 September 1870 in the townland of Bagher in the parish of Ematris. Martha Anderson, grandmother of deceased, deposed Jane was in care of her at the time of her death. 'On the evening of the 24th, the deceased was put into her cradle by me. When asleep, I left her to take turf out to the hill for drying flax. I was

absent about four minutes but on my return I found her sitting close to the
fire crying. Her feet were a little burned, having somehow got out of the
cradle during my absence. All the care we could was taken of her, but she
died on 27th. She had been poorly for some time past, 'twas 19 months old.'
The verdict was death from burns accidentally sustained; taken in consideration with her previous delicate state of health.

As gruesome and unfortunate as was the burning of Jane Cox's feet,
it is possible that these were not accidental burns, but the result of
such a 'cure' for a changeling. Angela Bourke, author of *The Burning
of Bridget Cleary*, has written the account of the true story of a Tip-
perary woman killed by fire in 1895 at the hands of her husband and
family. They believed that she had been turned into a 'sick fairy' or
'changeling' and performed several ritualistic measures, including burning, to cure her. Bourke states that, 'Changelings' behaviour is often
intolerable as they take the form of sickly babies who never stop crying, or adults who take to their beds, refuse to speak when spoken to,
or otherwise conduct themselves in anti-social ways. A last resort is
to threaten a changeling with fire. This is said to banish it for good,
and so force the return of the abducted human. Legend after legend
recounts how what has seemed to be a baby in a cradle smartly takes
to its heels and leaves the house when some adult, usually a visitor,
builds up the fire and announces that the baby is to be placed on
top.'[45]

In most burning inquests, the witnesses provide vivid descriptions of the burns and provide a good amount of detail. In the case of
Jane Cox, her grandmother simply states, 'her feet were a little burned' yet this was a leading cause of death. Is it possible the child was
held over the fire by the grandmother in an attempt to cure it from
its 'previous delicate state of health'? The grandmother also says the
child was 'poorly for some time past' yet no doctor was called for and
the child lingered with the burns for three days. It is possible that this
was such a case of trying to rid the house of the changeling and bring
back the healthy infant Jane Cox.

The overwhelming message of the fairy-legends is that the unexpected may be guarded against by careful observance of society's
rules. These stories are important components of child-rearing practice, establishing the boundaries of normal, acceptable behaviour, and
spelling out the way in which an individual who breaches them may
forfeit his or her position.[46]

CRIMES AGAINST CHILDREN
Child Abuse

Cases of child abuse as with domestic violence against wives were seen as a daily, petty occurrence and most incidents of children being abused were dismissed and ignored. It was only when children turned up dead that authorities acted and an inquest and investigation were carried out. Offenders were usually not prosecuted owing to a lack of confidence in the evidence. Physicians drew different conclusions as to the nature of the physical evidence and, without witnesses, most cases were impossible to prove. Juries and judges were reluctant to convict men accused of beating and murdering a child in their own home as it occurred in the private domain. Even when children were living in a public facility, abuse and neglect were difficult to investigate. For example, in 1855, two inquests were held on the bodies of two pauper children living at the Clones workhouse who appeared to have died from starvation and neglect. The evidence was contradictory. On the one hand, Dr Moore stated that although the children presented a very emaciated appearance, he would not take it upon himself to say what contributed to their death. Dr Hoskins however, testified that the children died from insufficient and improper food.[47] As one might suspect, justice for murdered children was rare.

Ultimately, children living in a non-traditional family were most at risk of abuse. Children sharing a home with a stepparent or caretaker might be perceived as a threat to the inheritance. The 'rightful heirs' of the new couple's natural children or other close relations might see themselves as having a right to the farm and therefore become threatened by the stepchild, the misfit. Another group at risk were orphans. Children living at the workhouse were sometimes matched with a family and offered an opportunity for work on their farm or in their home. Before the turn of the century, there was very little follow-up by the board of guardians of the workhouse, to check in on the welfare of these children. Very young children were hired out to employers that often treated them badly – like slaves – subjecting them to poor living conditions, lack of proper diet and beatings when work was not accomplished to their liking. These children were seen as vulnerable, weak links in society and, as they were likely illegitimate, they were viewed as a scourge. Ultimately children without families, either lacking one parent (usually the father) or orphans from the workhouse, had no legal recourse and no one to protect them from the pressures of exploitation through excessive labour, neglect or abuse.

Did the Stepfather Kill Him?
The Death of Hugh Croarken, Shanroe, Clones Parish, October 1857
Having asked around the community and spoken to neighbours and relatives, the coroner had heard enough about the suspicious circumstances involving the death of eight-year-old Hugh Croarken to order his body to be exhumed from the grave. The evidence gathered implicated the boy's stepfather, John McGuiness, as having beaten and killed the boy. The exhumation took place at the Roslea chapel graveyard and the body was taken to Dr Knight's for autopsy.

The coroner's inquest began on 9 October 1857. The first witness called was Rose Croarken, the boy's grandmother. The boy lived with her from time to time and the last time she'd seen him – about a month prior to his death – he was in his usual good health. On the night the boy was due to return to her, John McGuiness, the boy's stepfather and his servant girl, Kitty McKeary, called to her door and asked her to hurry to their home. Her grandson was throwing off blood and was very ill.

She told the jury, 'I hurried up to the McGuiness' when near the house I heard the deceased's mother call to her husband, "John, come up fast for Hugh is dead!" On entering the house, I went to the bedside and saw the child lying there dead.'

Rose continued, 'The boy was buried the following Saturday, 19 September 1857 and on the following Tuesday, when in conversation with McGuiness' servant girl, she told me that a few days previous when the cows were being milked, the boy had put his finger in the milk and then to his mouth. This act so provoked McGuiness that he ran violently at him and gave him a kick with such force as to knock him over against the dung heap. She told me that he was not able to stir till they thought fit to carry him into the house.'

Rose was then asked several questions by the coroner. An issue was raised that the grandmother might be lying and had offered Kitty McKeary a bribe to relay the detail of the boy's abuse at the trial. To this she said, 'I never promised the girl a bribe to encourage her to tell anything respecting the treatment of the boy.' She added, 'I never knew the boy to be under medical treatment.'

The next witness called was Kitty McKeary. She stated that she was the servant of John McGuiness. On the night of the boy's death, she was sent by her master to his grandmother to retrieve her. She added that this was not the first time the boy had been sick. 'The boy had been ill with a pain about his heart for three weeks prior to his death,' she told the jury.

Again, Kitty's story varied greatly from that of the grandmother in regard to the boy being abused by McGuiness and shed light on the matter of a bribe being offered to her. 'I never saw McGuiness kick the boy, though I'd been with him for several harvests. Also, Rose Croarken did offer me a kerchief and money if I would swear that McGuiness gave him a kick, knocking him into the dung heap. I refused, saying I would not damn my soul to gratify her. The old woman applied to me on the same subject over again but I had nothing to tell.'

Kitty concluded by revealing that she herself had been ill with the mumps for a month and her mistress had been at the dispensary respecting the boy, Hugh.

Hugh's aunt, Sally Croarken was the next to give evidence: 'I heard that the child had been sick prior to his death. Shortly after which, John McGuiness called on me and told me "little Hugh is dead". I accompanied him home and assisted in washing him and when doing so, observed a slight swelling on his private parts. They did not present a black appearance and the grandmother, although present, passed no remark,' Sally stated.

She did admit that she had reported to the grandmother that McGuiness was abusing the child. Sally had asked Rose, 'Why do you not go up to see your grandchildren for they are getting bad treatment from McGuiness?' However, she stated that it was a long time since she had made that comment.

Dr Alexander Knight performed the post-mortem examination. He told the jury that he had carefully examined the body and could detect no marks of external injury. Dr Knight could form no other opinion but that the boy's death arose from natural causes.

The verdict handed down by the jury was 'death from natural causes and not from any injuries inflicted by his stepfather, John McGuiness, who in this case has been most unjustly charged.[48]

It appears that the grandmother gave false evidence as to the boy's abuse. However, it is difficult to come to a definitive conclusion as to the boy's fate. Was this boy murdered? No information was provided to determine if the boy had indeed been seen by a physician, the dispensary doctor, and was suffering from an illness. What illness was he suffering from? The grandmother, clearly protective of her grandson, appears to have been willing to do anything to prove the stepfather a murderer. It was the elderly woman's son who was Hugh's natural father and after his death, the daughter-in-law had remarried. Was Sally Croarken desperate to portray John McGuiness as an abuser or was she bitter about this second father taking over where her son left off? One valuable piece of information is that the body was exhumed. Given these facts, would W. C. Waddell, with years of experience as the coroner, dig up the body of an eight-year-old boy if he did not feel that there was evidence and a basis for a possible conviction? Child murder, just as with infanticide, was difficult to prove and therefore many cases were just ignored or dropped for lack of evidence.

The Practice of 'Renting' Children

Orphans living at the workhouse with no family, financial support or future opportunities were sometimes given the chance to live and work in the nearby neighbourhood and countryside. They were an enormous expense to the taxpayer and very often such children were put into domestic service as soon as they were considered old enough to perform such duties. With the approval of the board of guardians of the workhouse, farmers and other employers might offer food, shelter and a small wage to orphaned pauper children to satisfy their need for inexpensive labour. These schemes did afford the child the chance to live outside the workhouse as well as to learn different trades that might provide an income for them at some point in the future. However, this economical solution for labour did come at a high price. Although the children hired out of the workhouse were supposed to be provided the opportunity for work, food and shelter, these require-ments were not always met.

One prominent case occurring several years after the last inquest of W. C. Waddell, illustrates how children were subjected to abuses at the hands of their 'surrogate' families. Eleven-year-old Anne Daley was beaten and killed by her employers. Before her death, she gave the authorities a deposition, describing the abuse she received at the hands of Patrick and Anne McCabe; yet more evidence was needed to get a conviction. The issue in question was whether or not the beatings she suffered, directly accelerated her death or if she was already of a weak constitution and that she might have died from her pre-existing condition. As with all domestic abuse, judges and juries were quick to disbelieve the victim, usually requiring more direct or 'sufficient' evidence to convict a killer.

Measles or Murder? The Death of Anne Daley
Clonacullion, Aughnamullen Parish, March 1884

Eleven-year-old Anne Daley, an orphaned pauper girl was hired by Patrick McCabe and his wife, Anne, to work about their home and farm. The couple made the arrangement through the Cootehill work-house, with the approval of William Gardiner, master of the workhouse and the board of guardians. The McCabes assured them that the girl would be given work, proper food and shelter and would be well looked after. Within six months of commencing her employment with the McCabes, Anne Daley was dead.

The little girl began working for the McCabes on 24 August 1883. Her duties were to clean the home, mind an infant and another young child, as well as working on the farm. By December, the authorities knew there was a problem. McCabe had visited the home of John Primrose, a guardian of the Cootehill Union, to complain of the unwillingness of the little girl to work and that she was untrustworthy. He threatened to send her away but Primrose warned him not to, as if anything happened to her, that he (McCabe) would be responsible. A week later, McCabe dropped her back to the workhouse and left.

On the day Anne Daley arrived back to the workhouse, Dr Henry Moorehead examined her. She had been his patient while an inmate of the house and he always considered her to be a girl in good health. Upon seeing Anne this time, he immediately had her sent to the infirmary where he could more closely examine her. He found the young girl covered in bruises. There were cuts on different parts of her body. Her feet were swollen. She was in a filthy condition and her general appearance was that of a child that was neglected. He also noticed that Anne had two patches on her head where the hair appeared to have been pulled out by the roots. There was an abscess on her left knee. She was also greatly emaciated, looking as if she had not been fed in a long time, and very feverish.

The police were informed of the girl's state of health after only four months of employment with the McCabes. Mr Brabazon, JP, for Co. Monaghan went to Anne Daley's bedside, and took a statement from her. As she lay in her bed, the girl spoke of how Patrick McCabe had beaten her with a leather belt on the legs and arms, kicked her and pulled her by the hair some days before she re-entered the workhouse. A few days later, Mr Brabazon returned and got more information from her. This time she explained how Anne McCabe had pulled her hair and on the same day slapped her on the cheek. The woman then caught her by the wrist with a pair of tongs used for the fire, burning her hand. All the wounds and bruises to the girl's body corresponded with the testimony given.[49]

Anne Daley died on 1 March 1884. Patrick and Anne McCabe were indicted for feloniously killing and slaying the girl. The charge was manslaughter.

The first trial was held in July of 1884. Many witnesses were called to testify. Witnesses for the defence explained that they had never seen the girl abused in any way by the prisoners. One man called was Thomas Monaghan, father of Anne McCabe. His explanation for some of Anne Daley's bruises was that the McCabes kept a goat 'which was very cross'. He told of how he saw Anne Daley and the goat fighting one day and he had to separate them. In an attempt to be humorous he quipped, 'I did not see the goat burn the little girl's wrist, pull her hair out or beating her with a strap.'

After all the evidence was heard, the jury was instructed to return a verdict. Before they were to deliberate, the judge stated that 'whatever aspect the case assumed, that [he hoped] it would induce the authorities who had the regulation of the children of the workhouse who were sent out at tender years to service, to have some supervision over them and that some person would go and see how these poor, helpless little outcasts were treated by their employers.' The jury returned a verdict of not guilty for prisoner Anne McCabe. There was a disagreement in relation to Patrick McCabe and another trial date was set for December 1884.

In the second trial, Patrick McCabe stood alone charged with the manslaughter of Anne Daley. Much of the same information in the first trial was provided, but the focus appeared to be on the physical state and medical history of Anne Daley prior to her employment with the McCabes. The prosecution contended that Anne Daley died from consumption as a result of the ill-treatment she received at the hands of McCabe. The defence claimed that Anne Daley died as a result of long-standing illnesses and that many of the marks on her body could be explained as a result of those conditions.

Dr Moorehead was questioned. He was again asked about Anne Daley's physical state when she returned to the workhouse. Again he explained the cuts, burns and bruises covering her tiny body. She was also suffering from consumption.

'I found on making a post-mortem examination a tubercular deposit in the lungs and generally in the system, and the opinion I gave at the inquest was that the disease from which the girl died might have been caused by, or aggravated by, bad treatment. She died in March 1884,' Dr Moorehead said.

When cross-examining for the defence, Mr Smith asked if Anne Daley had been examined in the past for tubercular disease, prior to entering work with the McCabes. Dr Moorehead said, 'No. I did not, but if she had been suffering from it I would have taken note of it.'

He did offer that Anne Daley was in the infirmary in 1879 from October to December and that in 1882 she was in the infirmary again for measles.

He concluded by telling the judge, 'I formed the opinion with reference to her condition when she was brought back from the prisoner's house that the bruises were nearly all inflicted at the same time.'

The most controversial witness of the trial was Dr John Crystle, who assisted Dr Moorehead in making the post-mortem examination. He corroborated with Dr Moorehead about Anne Daley dying from phthisis or consumption. However, when Mr Smith for the defence asked Dr Crystle if the girl might be emaciated even if given good food, Dr Crystle replied, 'I think the emaciation that I saw might have existed even if the girl had been receiving good food. A scrofulous constitution when measles had occurred would have a tendency to produce lightness of the head, however it would not explain the bruises which I saw.'

The judge then asked one question of Dr Crystle, 'Would ill treatment and bad food bring on tubercular disease?'

Dr Crystle answered, 'In many persons it would and more rapidly in the case of a person who was delicate.'

Mr Smith now called Head-Constable Hall of Cootehill. Constable Hall told the court he had arrested the prisoner on a charge of seriously assaulting Anne Daley. When he cautioned him Patrick McCabe stated that he'd never laid a hand on the girl and that she fell several times in the lane as she had 'lightness' in the head.

Michael Dempsey was then called to testify. He stated that he saw the girl at the house of Patrick McCabe before she was taken to the workhouse. Anne Daley had told him that she suffered from lightness in the head. 'She was sitting at the fire in McCabe's house with a shawl on her head,' said Dempsey. 'I did not see any "patches" on her head where the hair had been pulled off.'

The prosecution then asked, 'How did she come to tell you she had a lightness in her head?'

'I overheard her telling it to Mrs McCabe,' Dempsey said.

The judge then asked, 'What brought you to the prisoner's house that day when you saw the girl?'

'I was there to thresh corn for Mr McCabe.'

'Did he say anything to you?'

Dempsey replied, 'He said he was going to bring the girl to the workhouse and that, perhaps, he would not go on with the threshing and he would go into the house to see if the threshing was to go on.'

The judge then asked, 'Did you not then know that if he went to the workhouse it was to take the girl there?'

'No.'

'What did you do then?'

'I went into the house.'

'And you saw the girl there?'

'I did.'

'And did you speak to her?'

'No.'

Surprised, the judge then asked, 'Did anyone speak to her?'

'No,' said Dempsey.

'And none of the three spoke to the girl? The only one who spoke was the poor girl herself?'

Demspey replied, 'Yes.'

Anne Daley was in a very bad state, weak and tired with a shawl wrapped around her. The three adults, Patrick and Anne McCabe and Michael Dempsey stood discussing her while she sat there disregarded and their primary concern was that the corn threshing might not be taking place that day on account of her. Patrick McCabe was angry that he might have to take the girl back to the workhouse.

Thomas Monaghan was called to testify about a conversation he'd had with Anne Daley. He claimed that Anne Daley told him that Patrick and Anne McCabe (his daughter) were good to her and that she would not like to go back to the workhouse. At this time, Monaghan observed that her feet and legs were swollen. He could tell as she did not own a pair of shoes and was in her bare feet. Monaghan also saw that there were a few bare patches on her head but that Anne had told him her hair had fallen out. He advised her to go back to the workhouse for the winter.

He was also asked about the character of Patrick McCabe. In reply to this he told the court, 'Mrs McCabe is my daughter and Patrick McCabe is my son-in-law. I always regarded McCabe as a man that was not wise (laughter in the courtroom). I thought him to be a simple, quiet and easy-going man.'

'Would it be evidence of his simplicity if he pulled that hair out of the poor child's head?' asked the prosecution.

'I never saw him do anything to her,' Monaghan responded.

'Did you think it a kind thing for Mr McCabe to beat that little child with a strap on the head?'

'I never saw her being beaten by him.'

Dr Boyd continued his questioning. 'I am not asking you what you saw. Do you think it a sign of his quietness to beat a little girl such as you saw on the feet?'

'I would not, but I did not see her being beaten by him.'

'No, he nursed her all the time,' quipped Dr Boyd and the court-room erupted into laughter.

By the end of the trial, it was clear that Patrick McCabe had not called a doctor or in any way attempted to accommodate the needs of Anne Daley, if her condition was pre-existing. The fact that even friends and relatives made note of her ill-health only strengthened the foundation of the case against Patrick McCabe. If they had not beaten the girl, why then did they not get a sick young girl, entrusted to their care, medical attention?

The jury returned a verdict of guilty. The judge made a lengthy statement addressing the prisoner, Patrick McCabe.

'Patrick McCabe, you have been convicted on the clearest pos-sible evidence in this, what appears to me at least a very atrocious crime. This poor, friendless child was taken by you out of the work-house in order that it might perform such services as were suited to her age in your house. The Guardians thought they might safely en-trust her to your charge and she left the workhouse apparently a very healthy child. Four months and one fortnight she was under your roof, and at the end of that period she is brought back by you and left in the porter's lodge at the workhouse – an awful spectacle from the ill-treatment she had received; broken down and emaciated, all the health of youth gone, black and bruised from head to foot as the doc-tor describes, filthy and in a wretched state, left there and notwith-standing the great care bestowed on her in the workhouse infirmary, she never recovered from the condition which she was then in,' stated Justice Barry.[50]

He continued, 'You are answerable before God and you are ans-werable to the law of this country for the death of this child and no other person in these counties shall, taking example, with impunity, follow such crimes or inflict similar treatment on any poor creature that gets under their charge. They must know that if they are in their service they are not their slaves and you must be kept in penal ser-vitude for a period of five years for this abominable crime.'

Patrick McCabe was convicted on 11 December 1884. Prisoner A929 arrived at Mountjoy Prison on 27 December 1884 where he remained for four years. While serving his sentence he was in trouble on several occasions for not picking his proper quantity of oakum and was eventually given two days solitary confinement in the pun-

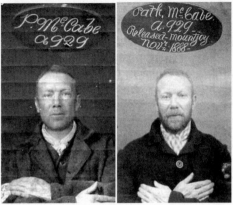

Convicted murderer Patrick McCabe. He was described as having sandy blond hair, grey eyes, fair eyebrows, a small nose and mouth, a fresh complexion and oval-shaped face. He was of medium build (or make) and 5 ft 4 in in height. After four years of imprisonment, he was released on 19 November 1888. He returned to Rockcorry, Co. Monaghan. [Patrick McCabe, GPB, PEN 1884/929, National Archives, Dublin]

ishment cell on only bread and water. He was also charged with being 'noisy' in his cell and had many altercations with other prisoners such as wrangling and fighting with them. His medical record from prison states that he was 'febrile' and treated with 'turpentine formentations'. On 19 November 1888, Patrick McCabe was released from prison on licence and returned to Rockcorry, Co. Monaghan.[51] According to research of the Outrage reports, Patrick McCabe received the longest sentence for killing a child servant during the post-famine years.[52]

COOKING FOOD AND DOING LAUNDRY
Watch Out for Boiling Water

Water was brought into the house to be boiled for many different chores and activities such as cleaning the laundry – an arduous task. In addition to several trips to the well (children were usually sent to fetch the water), the water had to be boiled first to steep the clothes. Then another pot of water was boiled to wash the clothes in, and finally, the last pot of water was needed to put the clothes into a boil (to rinse them).[53] Every drop of water carried into the house for washing, cooking, churning and doing dishes, had to be boiled. Several deaths resulted from open pots of boiled water or food being accessible to young curious children.

Curiosity Killed the Baby: The Death of William Gibson
Cornasoo, Kilmore Parish, March 1862
Anne Gibson was in the house with her one-year-old boy, William.

While in the midst of stirring about the house, he pulled a bowl of boiling water down on himself. She immediately attended to him but he was not progressing favourably. Anne went to the dispensary at Slieveroe to see Dr Reid and received some salve for the child. Unfortunately, when she went back home and applied it, she could see it was doing little good. She went back the following week, but as she told the coroner, 'Dr Reid being intoxicated could not attend to the deceased, but said he would visit. He never did.' Young William died a week later on 11 March 1862.[54]

Blow on your Tea – First: The Death of Robert David Phillips
Carrigans, Donagh Parish, January 1862
Margaret Phillips was making breakfast for her husband, a gardener to Mr Murphy of Truagh Lodge. She had just wet the tea in the teapot from the boiling kettle and was turning around to put back the remainder of the tea, when her young child, Robert, got hold of the teapot and took a slug or draft from the spout of the teapot. He immediately gave a loud scream. She caught him up and gave him some milk, hoping it would cool his throat. She took him on her knee and put him to sleep, but upon waking he began to vomit and continued to do so for some time after. She sent to Dr Douglass of Glaslough for some medicine and direction, which she received, but the child died the next day. The verdict was death on the morning of 26 January 1862 from internal injuries sustained the morning of 25 January 1862 from having hastily and incautiously swallowed a mouthful of scalding hot tea.[55] Robert was two years old.

Cattle Food Can Kill You: The Death of Mary Finley
Drumbin, Tedavnet Parish, January 1873
Mary Finley was a baby girl, sixteen months of age. On a Saturday afternoon in January, her mother, Ellen, was busy in the house preparing a pot full of boiling hot food for the cattle. The infant sat at the table next to her mother. The mischievous baby attempted to climb up on the table and when doing so, she slipped down and landed feet first into the scalding-hot pot of food. As quickly as possible Ellen lifted her out and did everything in her power to heal her wounds from the blistering, but the child died two days later. The verdict was death from falling into a pot of boiling food prepared for feeding cattle – falling accidentally.[56]

Cooking for the children was the duty of the mother or the 'babysitter', who was most often a young child in charge of even younger children. Whether it was stirabout, potatoes or cabbage, the meals were cooked in a pot over an open fire – a dangerous endeavour for anyone, but especially a small child. Even with parents present or even two babysitters, accidents were likely to happen when a child went too near to the fire. For example, a young daughter of Margaret Corly was left in the home to be taken care of by two older children while Margaret went to mass. After she had left the house, her young daughter went to stir the breakfast over the fire when her clothes caught the flames. She died as a result of the burns a few days later.[57]

One babysitter, seven-year-old Sarah Reilly, was in charge of several children when her mother, Catherine, left the house to go to Newbliss on business. Later that day, neighbour Ellen Clarken received a visit from little Mary Jane Reilly, one of Sarah's younger sisters, who asked her to come over and help. While she was linking the pot on the fire, Sarah's clothes had caught fire. Ellen rushed over to find the children all unattended and their big sister, Sarah, lying on the bed without any clothes on. They had all been burned off her. Ellen immediately ran into Drum and got a bottle of castor oil, and smeared it all over her body. After six hours of severe suffering, Sarah Reilly died.[58]

While Putting on the Cabbage: The Death of Mary Jane Willis
Aghadrumkeen, Ematris Parish, February 1865

Young Mary Jane Willis was left in charge of several younger children on a Sunday evening, 22 January 1865. Some time later, neighbour John Glen saw the young girl running towards his door with her clothes all in flames. As quickly as possible he extinguished the fire and he and his wife, Cecelia, began removing her burning clothes. She was charred on the arms, face, breast and belly; some of the burns were severe. They put her to bed and sent for the doctor. Dr Moore attended to her, prescribing some necessary washes, salves and wadding. The next morning, the Revd William Cooke was called to see her. As there was no older person present, it was she who told the story of what had occurred. While she was alone in the house with the little children, she was engaged in putting cabbage in a pot on a large fire when her dress was caught up in the flames. Although all Dr Moore's directions were followed, it was in vain. She lingered and died ten days after the accident on 2 February 1865.[59]

WATERY GRAVES
Children Drowning

Water or any fluid that was in any way deep enough for a child to fall into and be submerged was a serious hazard in the home. In fact, death by drowning was the third leading cause of child fatalities as recorded in the coroner's casebook (infanticide was first [64]; burning was second [52]).[60] There was a total of 43 children killed having been submerged in bog holes, lakes, streams, wells and other pools of 'liquid'. The following are just two examples of death by drowning in the home under unusual circumstances.

Submerged in the Pot of Milk: The Death of Susan Donaghy
Corduff, Aghabog Parish, September 1859
On 8 September 1859, Phillip and Mary Donaghy enjoyed breakfast together along with their young daughter, Susan. Phillip left the house to go to work on the farm and Mary was left to attend to her chores in the house with Susan at her side. Having looked after the house matters, she began to feed the calves. Realising that she had milk for some of them, which was held in a large pot, she went to look for a vessel to fill with milk for the others. She was out of the house about ten to fifteen minutes, and upon returning, she found little Susan with her head downwards in the pot of milk. Mary quickly snatched her out of the pot and used every means in her power to restore animation to her lifeless body but without avail as life was gone. She called Phillip into the house, and he found his daughter, dripping with milk in the arms of her mother – dead.[61]

Drowning in the Potato Puddle: The Death of Hugh Calaghan
Creeve, Monaghan Parish, May 1873
Catherine Calaghan was running about her home, busy with her affairs, with her fine stirring, eighteen-month-old boy, Hugh, following her much of the day. After a while, having missed him from her side, she went outside to look for him. She could not find the child, began to tire and decided to head back to the house. The sad conclusion unravelled as Catherine told the coroner of her son's fate: 'When almost at my very door, in a small puddle of a hole made for washing potatoes, I found my dear lying dead. Quickly I caught him up and carried him into the house but life was gone.' The verdict was death from accidentally falling into a small pool of water and when found, life was extinct.[62]

Small children needed to be supervised while parents, as well as grand-parents worked in the fields simultaneously. This was a challenge for everyone with small children without the help of a servant or arrang-ed caretaker. For this reason, some women when working in the fields alongside the men would put their infant child into a horse's collar and leave it in the field.[63] In some cases, the women built fires to keep the child warm while waiting for the work to be done. Some mothers nursing infants even had their children brought down to them to feed while they were working in the bog.[64] The children were taken away and the mother continued to work. Most of the children who drown-ed, did so while the parent or caretaker endeavoured to work in the fields. On these occasions, the children usually wandered off for a short amount of time, until it was discovered that they were missing.

In the Fields of Leitrim: The Death of Margaret Kelly
Leitrim, Tyholland Parish, November 1856
John McGee was in the field digging potatoes alongside Pat Kelly, while Pat's mother herded the cattle just a short distance off. Little five-year-old Margaret, Pat's little sister, was in the field as well and her mother had just made a small fire for her to keep warm until she was done with the cattle. A few moments later, the two men heard a loud scream, and turning saw young Margaret running towards them across the field, screaming with her clothes on fire – a human torch. The men began running towards her across the field and caught her. Pat frantically extinguished the flames. At this point, Pat's father appeared and carried his daughter back to their home. Her clothes were black and charred. Her body was burned all over, especially her belly, chest, arms and face. The men were distraught and went into Middleton for Dr Watters but, not finding him, went to Dr Loughran. Having heard a description of Margaret's injuries, Dr Loughran told them there was no use in his going out to the house as the child would not recover. He sent some oil to anoint the child and it was applied upon their return, but she died later on that evening.[65]

A Grandfather's Heartbreak: The Death of Ellen Brides
Knocks West, Currin Parish, May 1860
Thomas Brides was the grandfather of Ellen, a fine two-year-old child. He had been engaged in scouring a ditch and she was beside him, being very fond of him. She brought a tiny shovel with her and a neigh-bour boy wanted as a joke to take it from her. To avoid him she ran off. She then returned with her shovel and told her grandfather she

would 'help him'. He smiled and allowed her to pretend to help. After a little while, she left his side and when he hadn't seen her a little bit longer, he went to a neighbour's house to search for her. Not finding her there, he started to become nervous and proceeded to his own house, hoping that she would be there. On his way home, he was passing near the well and looking towards it, 'saw [his] little darling floating on the surface, but her wee head down.' Quickly as possible he caught her up out of the water but alas and alas, life was gone.[66]

While Stacking the Turf: The Death of Thomas McCaffrey
Lurgachamlough, Aghnamullen Parish, June 1864

Pat Fitzpatrick and Mick McCudden were making turf while two-year-old Thomas McCaffrey ran around along the bog bank with his mother nearby. His mother needed to go back to her house and asked the two men to keep an eye on the boy. As they continued working, they lost sight of the little boy and forgot about him. When his mother returned asking where her son was, a search began, and a short distance away Mick came upon the boy who had fallen into a bog hole. His tiny body was floating on top of the water.[67]

Two Young Brothers Drown in a Well
The Deaths of Richard Alexander Martin and Thomas Samuel Martin
Correvan, Aghabog Parish, August 1863

Jane McMahon told the coroner and his jury the following sad story: 'On 31 July 1863, my master and mistress, Mr and Mrs Martin, went to Cootehill leaving the place and two children in charge of myself and Margaret McCloy. Margaret was the children's nurse. About 2 o'clock, I saw wee Richard and his younger brother, Thomas, among the beans in the garden. About a quarter of an hour later, I called to Margaret who was in the barn, and asked had she seen the children. She immediately called for them and was answered. They were calling from the field with the calves. Another fifteen minutes later I again went to see about them, but did not find them and when returning to the house I met Mr Richard Martin, the master's brother. I asked him to see had they gone over to Mr James Martin, which they often did. He suddenly exclaimed, 'It's in the well they are!' There is a large, open, unfenced well within a few perches of the hall door to which he ran to at once. Just a minute later I heard a shout and I ran forward to see the two children lifted out of the well by the labouring men now gathered around. They were dead. The two lifeless bodies of the two young brothers were carried up to the house and everything done to restore life into them. Dr Taylor of Drum was sent for but it was all in vain. They had drowned. Richard was three years old and Thomas was two years of age.'[68]

Children were responsible for retrieving water from the well, taking care of ducks, herding the cows as well as tending to milking and cleaning the 'outhouses' or barns. These were the mothers' duties, however, when a child became old enough to work the farm, he or she was required to make his or her own contribution to the family holding. The following inquests detail how death came as children attempted to perform their chores.

On Gathering Water, Two Young Children Drown

Young William Maguire was sent by his mother to the well for water. When he delayed longer than he should, his mother went to see about him. Seeing the can standing full of water, she took it up and brought it to the house. Some time after, realising he had still not returned home, his father, Pat, went looking for him, accompanied by several neighbours. They could not find the boy and began searching bog holes with a long shovel. Sadly, they at last succeeded in finding William. His small body was raised from the bottom of one of the bog holes and he was dead. The search had gone on for about an hour and the result was finding only his tiny corpse.[69]

In another similar story, eleven-year-old Mary Hughes had been sent by her grandmother to fetch a can of water. Since she was out longer than usual, her sister, Ellen, went searching for her. On reaching the spot, she saw her sister lying on the surface of the water. Bernard Casey heard Ellen shrieking that Mary was in the water and he began running down to find her. He pulled the body out of the water but when she was taken out, 'life was clean gone'.[70]

Bringing in the Ducks: The Death of Patrick McGinn
Drumacreeve, Ematris Parish, June 1860

On the evening of 17 June 1860, Mary McGinn was on her way to the bog to bring the ducks home when she saw her younger brother, Pat, coming towards the house carrying a creel of grass. He immediately offered to go and help his big sister. The two children walked together on the land and reached the bog. There had been some flooding, but they knew well the passes amongst the bog holes which were scattered underneath the water like a hidden maze. They carefully and successfully drove the ducks out off the water.

Now that the ducks were back on shore, it was more difficult to remember the path back to the shore. As they reached the banks of the bog, Pat slipped and fell into a deep bog hole and sank immediately. He began screaming and crying, 'Oh Mary! Oh Mary!'

Mary told the coroner, 'I immediately shouted out to my Dada who was very convenient and he ran quickly over. Dada began to search for him and I kept calling till scared neighbours came and joined to look for him. After an hour, the body was found and got out of the water.'

Richard Harper was one of those neighbours. 'I was sitting in my house when I heard Mary shouting and at once hurried to the place. Learning the cause, I got a drag and commenced to search for the body. The first hole I searched, I caught hold of the boy and raised him and got him out, but life was quite extinct.' The verdict was death from having accidentally fallen into a bog hole and thereby drowned.[71]

STRANGER THAN FICTION

There were other strange accidents which occurred while children were performing their chores:

Suffocating in the Dung: The Death of Owen Slevin
Coolcorragh, Kilmore Parish, October 1875
On a quiet Monday morning, a lad of twelve years of age, Owen Slevin, met his death under peculiar circumstances. Although Owen's father was a man named Slevin, who resided in Drummuck, the boy resided with his grandfather, Owen McEntee of Coolcorragh. On the day in question, Owen went to the cow house to put out the cattle.[72] He was alone and shortly afterwards was found quite dead, lying on his face in the gripe (soft dung) behind one of the cows. It is supposed that the animal kicked him and knocked him insensible; he was smothered as he lay. Every effort was made by his sister, Bridget, and the grandfather to restore animation but to no avail. The coroner held an inquiry and Dr Reid testified that the deceased came to his death accidentally – by suffocation in cowdung.[73]

Running an Errand for Da: The Death of Mary Cushlan
Urbalkirk, Monaghan Parish, May 1856
One can only imagine the anguish and guilt of the father of Mary Cushlan who requested his daughter run an errand for him – that of gathering some hot embers and coals from the fire to light the pipes

of the men in the field. Frank McMahon and Mary's father were in the field ploughing with their horses. While yoking,[74] Cushlan sent Mary home for some hot coals for lighting their pipes. Young Mary ran to the house to gather the load of coals for her Da and McMahon, and, while on her way back with the bucket at her side, her clothes caught on fire. They heard the screaming, then saw her in the distance. Mary's clothes were in flames as she ran towards them for help. They rushed to the child, extinguished the burning clothes and carried her home. She was attended by Dr Temple for over two weeks, but she died from her injuries on 8 May 1856.[75]

Hanging in the Byre: The Death of James McKelvey
Anaclar, Clones Parish, March 1863

James McKelvey had just started working as a servant for Mr and Mrs Moore of Anaclar. He was of good temper and attended to his duties. The Moores were quite satisfied with his performance. After dinner one evening, James left to clean out the byre. Jane Callaghan was working in the house and, needing James' help, went to fetch him. When she reached the byre, the door was open and, in the upper part of the pathway, she saw him in a hunkered position. The shovel he had been using was under his arm and there was a rope hanging above him. She began screaming and drew the attention of another servant, Joseph Cordon. They stood staring at the boy suspended from a rope kept in the cow house – his head in a noose. The rope had been used to tie a kicking cow when it was being milked and it appeared that, quite accidentally, it must have got tied around him. As a result of the rope slipping, he was hanged. An inquest was held to determine if possibly the boy tried to commit suicide, but based upon the testimony of all that knew him, he was quite content and happy in his new position. Also, the rope kept in the byre was kept on a pin about six feet from the ground, while the noose of it was about three feet from the ground. The verdict was death from accidental strangulation.[76] James was 14 years old.

Natural Disasters or Acts of God? Killed by 'Electric Fluid'

On occasion, people were struck down by 'electric fluid' or lightning. A single bolt of lightning may carry over 100 million volts of direct current and reach 50,000°F. The main bolt causes massive tissue damage, burning and charring, sometimes causing a limb to swell, burn and split open. William Guy, in his book, *The Principles of Forensic Medicine*, in 1868, stated, 'as a general rule, it may be stated that the electric fluid prefers and seeks out good conductors; and as the human body is a very good conductor, it is as likely to be struck as any object similarly situated, unless perhaps, that object be of metal ... the clothes may be torn and burnt; the shoes struck from the feet; metallic bodies fused and forcibly carried to a distance ... bodies are often black, bruised and torn at the spot where the electric fluid has entered.'[77]

On 30 May 1859, a thunderstorm raged over Co. Monaghan. In the townland of Golanduff in the parish of Killeevan, John Moorehead was sleeping in bed with his wife when, about midnight, they were startled awake by the glass of their bedroom window shattering and a vivid flash of lightning entering the room. As the thunder died away, John called to his young nephew, Charles, a lad of fourteen years of age, whose bed was at the foot of his own. Receiving no answer, he called more loudly. He scrambled to get a lamp to check on the boy and, in the dim light of the room, he found Charles dead where he lay. The hair on the left side of his head was black and burned, his thighs were blackened and blood was trickling out from his ears. A terrier dog, the boy's pet that slept under the bed, was also killed by the same flash. There is little doubt of the acrid smell of burning flesh stinging the air throughout the house. The coroner determined that the death came by 'electric fluid'.[78]

That same night in the village of Milltown in the parish of Monaghan, the lightning touched down on yet another home. In the early hours of the morning, James Carson and his wife were awake and getting ready for beginning the day and going to work. Suddenly James was struck violently 'as if a by a cannon ball' and knocked down. On recovering, he found his wife Jane lying beside him insensible. He carried her out into the open air where she revived. It is likely that James and Jane were struck by stray currents and not the main bolt of lightning. Both would have suffered from sore muscles and slight burns where the current exited. For every person killed by lightning, there are at least three who are struck by currents that are not lethal.

Feeling anxious about the rest of the family, James went to check on his married son, William, and his wife, Jane, who slept in the loft above. He began shouting their names and heard no reply, no stirring. As he climbed the ladder to the loft, James noticed the electric matter appeared to have entered at the top of the gable. A line of entry descended into the wall for about six feet when part of it broke through into the room. It continued farther down the wall and close to where the couple were sleeping. He surmised it must have touched the floor continuing through the house where he had seen it burn a bonnet hanging on a peg in the room downstairs whereupon his wife was struck.

Upon reaching the top of the loft and entering the room he saw that the young couple were lying in their bed and quite dead. William and Jane's faces were black and their hair burned, but their infant child of five weeks was still lying in its mother's arms – unharmed and untouched.[79]

Later that year, the electric fluid struck again in the meadows of Henry Armstrong of Clones. John Kalaghan and John Dodson were in good health, clearing and cutting the brush. About 5p.m., Kalaghan noticed John Dodson suddenly fall forward over his scythe. He paused for a moment, shocked and then ran forward to help him. He called for help and Henry Armstrong came to raise up the injured man. Dodson had been struck by lightning. A black streak covered his body from head to foot – incurred when the lightning, appearing to come from nowhere, struck as he raised the scythe. They did everything in their power to restore animation to his body; a mustard poultice was immediately applied over the body by Dr O'Reilly but to no avail. The verdict of the inquest was death from the effects of electricity.[80]

The Lone Thorn Bush: The Death of John McCarn (Medecurne)
Corclare, Errigal Truagh Parish, July 1867
A young boy of thirteen years, John McCarn, was working as a servant to Andrew Murray, luring cattle through the fields in Corclare. A neighbour, Charles McArdle, was watching the young lad from a distant field as he tended to the cattle. Young John was standing underneath a thorn bush when suddenly a great clap of thunder was heard overhead. McArdle saw the boy lying in the bush and ran to his side. He found him lying dead on the grass but his body was still warm. Dr Douglas examined the deceased and saw no marks on his person except a small scratch such as from a thorn mark on his face. It was determined that death was caused by lightning.[81]

The veneration accorded to whitethorn bushes – fairy thorns – certainly outlived the nineteenth century and is by no means forgotten. The power of the lone thorn still rivals that of the priest in the mind of some people.[82] There are a number of stories of taboos and superstitions associated with the fairies and lone bushes. Bad tidings would come to those who interfered with a fairy fort or lone bush as the following stories illustrate only too clearly:

If anyone touched a lone bush they went mental afterwards. You daren't touch it. Something always happened to them. There was only a thorn out that way on the lone bush, you'd never see side thorns and the old people told me that people would lose their limbs after interfering with them.[83]

LET THERE BE LIGHT ... BUT NOT FIRE
Candles and Lamps

Before the days of widespread electricity, introduced to Ireland by the Shannon Scheme in 1926, the hearth fire, candles and lamps were the only sources of lighting in the homes around the country. Candles were made using several different methods, one was using rushes called 'rush-lights.'

> Candles were made from rushes. They put fat on a grisset beside the fire and when it melted they got rushes and took the covering of them [they covered them with fat]. Then they dropped them in the gravy and hung them up to dry. They put them in stands for the purpose and they burned for a while.[84]

'Stands' were circular rings or holders, such as the holders seen on Christmas trees of long ago with the candles burning in them. The following inquest of John McMahon provides an example of how these primitive sources of light were a fire hazard.

Three Children go to Sleep: Only Two Wake Up
The Death of John McMahon, Newbliss, Killeevan Parish, October 1864
Bernard McMahon had tucked his three young children into the bed they shared, lit the candle in the socket above the bed and left the house for a walk. About fifteen minutes later, he heard a shout from his house. He ran forward and found the bed in the house on fire and the three children screaming inside it. He caught two of them up in his arms and rushed from the house. A neighbour grabbed the other child. One of the children Berny picked up in his arms was his infant son, John, who was about twelve months old. The baby was suffering from severe burns on the arms, belly, head and breast and Dr Andrew Robinson was sent for. He arrived and stayed with the child till its death the next morning. At his child's inquest, the only way Berny could account for the fire was that the candle was placed in the socket, and, as the stand was open at the bottom, the candle must have dropped through to the bed after it burned down, setting it and the children on fire.[85]

Paraffin Lamps
Burning the Midnight Oil and the Children
Paraffin lamps were oil lamps; a reservoir of oil was contained in the base of the lamp, while a cotton or flax-woven wick was lit and covered with a glass cylinder. In two cases, paraffin lamps were blamed for igniting a couple of children and inflicting burns which caused their death.

In November 1866, John Hearst was thrashing vats in his barn with his son James, a young two-year-old child, at his side. The boy wandered away from his father and went into the house. Within five minutes John heard a horrible scream. He ran straight into the house and found his young son with his clothes in flames. He put out the fire, tried the usual remedies but, not trusting them, sent for Dr Coulter of Scotstown. Dr Coulter did all he could for the boy, but little James died the next evening from his injuries. John believed the accident occurred from the boy's clothes accidentally catching fire after he'd spilled a lamp on himself with paraffin oil in it.[86]

Several years later, in the town of Clones, a similar accident occurred.

Martha Kane lived with Mary Ann McGorman and her young child, Agnes. On the night of 27 February 1875, Martha heard the child cry in the room above her. She ran upstairs and found the child standing in the middle of the room with her clothes all ablaze. She immediately wrapped her clothes around young Agnes to extinguish the flames, then went for the child's mother.[87] Mary Ann was at the pump waiting for water when Martha arrived and told her that her Agnes' clothes had caught fire and that she was nearly burned to death. Mary ran home, caught the child in her arms and ran with her to Dr Henry's.

Dr Henry heard violent screaming on the street and went to the door to open it. Before he reached the door, Mary Ann rushed through with the child in her arms saying that she had been burned. He advised her to take the child back home immediately. Mary Ann was frantic and with some difficulty, he got her to return home. Agnes' side, chest and under her arm were burned; however, her face was so severely burned that he determined there was no possibility of recovery. He went the next morning to see the child, but she had died. The poor child had lived another nine excruciating hours before her pain ended.

The unfortunate occurrence had happened while little Agnes was playing with a cord that accidentally caught the burning paraffin lamp suspended against the wall. The cord by chance pulled the lamp down and the oil spilled all over her, then ignited.[88]

CHAPTER FIVE

DEATH BY MISADVENTURE
TRUE TALES OF BAD LUCK AND STRANGE AND UNUSUAL DEATH

ad•ven•ture: (n). 1 a: an undertaking usually involving danger and unknown risks b: the encountering of risks <the spirit of adventure>. (v). 1.
to expose to danger or loss: venture; 2. to venture upon: try; 3. to proceed
despite risk; 4. to take the risk. mis•ad•ven•ture: (n), Middle English
mesaventure, from Old French, from mesavenir to chance badly, from
mesmis + avenir to chance, happen, from Latin advenire.[1]

Lurking, waiting in the shadows as children played in the grass or
foolishly threw stones at one another, while men chatted by the fire
with shotguns resting at their side, and even as drunken fools stum-
bled home along the roads of the county, death was there – ready to
snatch them from this earth.

CHILDREN TAKING CHANCES
Children At Play

Don't Play with Matches – or You'll Get Burned
The Death of John Morris, Clones, Clones Parish, July 1870
Mary Ann Morris woke up on the morning of 21 July 1870 and check-
ed in on her three-year-old son, John. He was lying there asleep, safe
and sound and so she went about her usual chores. About an hour later,
she was startled by the wails and screeches of her boy coming from
his bed. She rushed into his room and found him in flames, flailing
his burning arms and legs. Having extinguished the blaze, she immediately sent for Dr Gillespie to attend to the small child who was covered with extensive burns all over his body. No remedy could be applied to save the child and he died at 7p.m. that evening. Mary told
the coroner, 'I can only account [for the burns] for as he had a box of
matches he was playing with.' The verdict was death from accidental
burning – aged three.[2]

Impalement of an Unusual Kind
The Death of Thomas Corbitt, Corrinshigo, Currin Parish, May 1856
On 8 May 1856, Catherine Corbitt sent her daughter, Jane, to call the family in to dinner. Her son, Thomas, came running through the field and took his usual shortcut leading through the garden. As he came up to the gate he had jumped many times before, he leapt, but in mid-air he was surprised by a broken stick that had nestled in the 'hurdle'. The pointed edge caught him by the trousers and he was instantly impaled. The family, hearing his screams and cries came rushing to his aid. They carried him into the house, put him to bed and waited for Dr Taylor to arrive. Dr Taylor found Thomas in great pain and suffering from a wound in the side of his anus. The stick had entered there, penetrating the rectum, lacerating the intestines and entering the bladder causing retention of urine and violent inflammation. A laceration of the rectum, intestines and bladder, such as the wounds sustained by the boy, may have caused sepsis, peritonitis or other types of infection and was likely to have been extremely painful. Thomas lasted for two days, but he died on 7 May 1856 from his injuries.[3]

Keeping Warm in the Field: The Death of Two Young Girls
Catherine Thompson and Mary Ann McKenna
Young Mary Steen was playing with several children in a field near her home. They were amusing themselves as children do, when they decided to build a little fire at the back of a ditch. The fire was started and all the young ones sat around it in a circle. Mary took a seat in front of the fire and another little girl, Catherine Thompson, took a seat on the side of the fire above the ditch. As the fire was being kindled, Mary looked just in time to see Catherine's clothes go up in flames and within seconds she was ablaze. Mary tried to grab Catherine to put the fire out, but Catherine was uncontrollable. In her terror and panic, she would not wait and started running home yelling, 'Mammy! Mammy!' She had a distance of sixteen perches to travel before she reached the house.[4]

By the time Catherine reached home, her clothes had been almost completely consumed. Jane Berny was sitting in the Thompson's home when Catherine arrived. 'Her clothes were burned off her and her whole person from her thighs up to her eyes was burned black,' said Jane. Everything was done by the family and the neighbours to comfort the child, but she died at daybreak the next morning.[5]

In a similar case, one Saturday afternoon young Mary Ann McKenna was playing outside her grandmother's house with a group of children. They were amusing themselves in an outhouse by making a fire with some loose straw, when suddenly the fire caught Mary Ann's clothes, setting them on fire. Jane Campbell, a friend of the family, heard the girl's screams and cries, ran out, and caught her up in her arms and carried her out of the flames. The child was given to her father who took her home. Unfortunately nothing could be done. The young girl lingered until the morning when she died. The verdict was death from injuries caused by her clothes having accidentally caught fire.[6]

'Hound and Hare': The Death of James McConnell
Drumsheeney, Drumsnat Parish, October 1860

Peter Murphy was sitting in his neighbour's house on a Sunday evening when word came in that nine-year-old James McConnell was missing and his family was searching for him. Peter and the others decided to go out and participate in the search for the child. After fifteen minutes, the boy's body was found in a deep bog hole and life was extinct. It appeared that young James and the other children were playing 'Hound and Hare'. Hound and Hare was a game played by boys. One boy is selected as the 'hare' and gets a headstart of a couple of fields. The others follow and try to catch him. They run after him until he is caught and then 'kill' him by giving him three blows on the head.[7] James, as the hare, went off to hide among the clamps of turf and, descending from a higher to a lower band, missed his foot and fell into a bog hole. When the evening became dusk, the other children were still looking for him and realised he was missing. They had turned home without him and raised the alarm, leading to the search and the discovery of his body.[8]

'Duck!'
The Death of George O'Reilly, Clones, Clones Parish, July 1875

George O'Reilly's granny sat and watched while he and some other boys were playing the game 'duck' – another game played by children, requiring the throwing of stones. George had thrown his stone at one boy and then he bent his knees to duck. It was James Carr's turn next. As James threw his stone, George was in the act of rising to his feet from his stooping posture. The stone struck the boy on the head. It was a deep wound and George began bleeding severely. His granny took him home immediately.

Dr Gillespie was called and told that his nephew had been hurt. When he reached the house, he found the boy unconscious with a severe contusion on his head. His pulse was intermittent and his breathing laboured. On closer examination, he found a soft swelling on George's head that appeared to be a 'concussion on the brain'. It was this swelling that caused his death. The verdict was 'death from injuries accidentally sustained whilst engaged in play and no blame attaches to the boy who threw the stone causing the injuries'.[9]

Stoned to Death: The Accidental Death of James Smollen
May 1868, Monaghan Town[10]

> A famous pastime of the giants of Irish legends was hurling boulders at each other, and that this was a projection of a prevailing custom is suggested by the persistent habit of stone throwing, whether as a game among country school children or with more serious purpose in the streets of Belfast and other towns.[11]

> The Irish are quicker and more expert than any other people in flinging, when everything else fails, stones as missiles, and such stones do great damage to the enemy in an engagement.
>
>   – Giraldus Cambrensis, 1185AD

James Hamill was walking down the jail hill in the town of Monaghan on a Sunday afternoon in the spring of May 1868. He had attended mass in the morning and was now looking for his friends, as was the usual routine. Hamill met a few friends who included Stephen Smith, James McKernan, Patrick Hoey, Bernard Manlin and several others. After they had gathered, a younger boy, James Smollen, approached them to play as well.

While they were just beginning their game, Hamill noticed Smollen running away quickly. He didn't know what to make of it except to think that possibly he had just done something that would warrant some type of retaliation. He then saw Stephen Smith begin throwing stones. Although the stones were hurled into the air backhanded, they were moving swiftly. The first hit a tree but the second hit Smollen in the face. There was no blood drawn on Smollen's cheek, but the young boy started crying. Smollen accompanied the group further down the road and then sat down on the grass with them. Smith told Smollen he was sorry for the incident and to take his advice and play with his equals'. As Smith and Smollen talked, it appeared that the situation was resolved and James Hamill left the group for home.

Later in the afternoon, about 4p.m., Bernard Smollen was in bed when he heard his son James arrive home. He was woken by the sobbing and moaning of his son. He asked the boy what had happened and heard the story of the stone thrown by Stephen Smith. James complained of pain in his head and of being very sick. When he began to throw up and said he was going to die, his father went at once for Dr Temple and Dr Rush. Fourteen-year-old James Smollen died that same evening between five and six o'clock.

At the inquest, Dr Temple said that he had performed a post-mortem examination and found that externally there was no wound. However, upon removing the skull and opening the head, he found a fracture of the skull over the left ear, about an inch in length, and observed a clotting of blood. It was this clot of three ounces of blood that put pressure on the brain and caused his death. The verdict of the jury was that death came from a blow of a stone accidentally inflicted by Stephen Smith.

The Northern Standard carried this story a few days later on 9 May 1868 in a news article entitled 'Melancholy Accident'. Along with the details of the incident, it offered an additional comment: 'It is worth observing that the young people of Monaghan are too fond of throwing stones: and if we consider how light a blow is sufficient to take away human life, it really becomes a duty incumbent on parents to punish severely this dangerous amusement on the part of their children, and on the Police to look more closely after it.'[12]

Boating at Annaghmakerig
The Deaths of James Sheridan and Francis McDermott
Doohat, Aghabog Parish, August 1866
David Daly was walking one quiet evening at Annaghmakerig Lake when he encountered young James Sheridan, who said he was going for a pair of oars to take a boat out on the lake. Daly looked down and saw Francis McDermott sitting in the vessel waiting for his friend. The boys were preparing to go out on the water and so Daly continued on his way.

Thomas Armstrong was the next to see the boys out on the lake. He saw the two of them amusing themselves with the boat at the side of the lake, where there was a shallow strand. They were pushing the boat forward towards the shore. Breaking off some branches from a plant in the water, the two friends played with the sticks, hitting each other and dipping them in the water while sitting in the boat. How-ever, when trying to move closer to shore by plunging the branches in the water, they instead pushed it out further into the lake. The boys began to panic and became alarmed. Armstrong heard one of the boys say, 'O boat, will you not go back to the land?' and immediately the two figures jumped into the water. He heard the splash and saw the water rippled where they had jumped in. Immediately, he ran home to tell what he had seen. A search was commenced but within three or four hours, their corpses were recovered and life was long gone.[13]

Swinging in the Barn: The Death of John Caulfield
Killynenagh, Currin Parish, March 1866
On a quiet March evening, Mary Ann Caulfield was playing in the barn on a swing with her sisters and brother, all ranging in age from four to ten years. Her big brother, John, said he must go and meet mamma coming home. On this, all dispersed, one to look about the calver, another to warm herself.

The children's mother, Mary, came home from Cootehill and was looking for her eldest son, John. One of the girls told her he was in the barn and she walked in to speak with him. On entering the barn she was shocked to see him hanging by the neck and dead. While John was getting out of the swing, part of the rope broke and another smaller piece that was loose got entangled about his neck. As there was no one present to render help, he was strangled. The verdict was death from being accidentally strangulated while amusing himself on the swing. John was ten years old.[14]

Fighting in the Schoolyard: The Death of William Nichol
Mullaglasson, Clones Parish, April 1870
William Nichol woke up in the morning complaining to his mother of pains in his back and belly. He ate breakfast, but could not keep the food down and soon vomited. Later that evening after dinner, he again threw up his food. He told his mother and father, Sophia and Hugh, that he had been fighting at school a few days earlier with another pupil. When he was on the ground, a lad named Brian Dogherty kicked him in the stomach. Since that time, he had the pains and could not keep food in his stomach without vomiting. His mother immediately took a look at his body and found his stomach was black where he'd been kicked.

William died the next day. When the coroner's inquest commenced, the boys involved were questioned. John Sloan told the jury that William was out during play hour on 1 April and when running about, tried to kick another schoolboy named McQuade. William's foot got caught in McQuade's clothing and he fell. He did not state that he saw anyone kick him. Thomas Graham, the National School teacher, stated that William never made any complaint of being sick or having taken place in any altercation.

The verdict was death by 'natural causes'. William was eight years of age.[15]

Don't Get Stuck in the Sandpit: The Death of Edward McCaffrey
Monaghan, Monaghan Parish, February 1858
Peter Carroll was working for the Revd Mr Blackly near a sandpit when he heard the crying of a young boy. Young James McCaffrey stood sobbing and asked if Peter had seen little Neddy, his brother, because the sandbank had fallen in. At once, accompanied by another man, Peter started off to find the boy. They began digging carefully through the fallen debris and soon uncovered the boy's head. They dragged the body from the sand and removed him to the nearby house of James Adams. Dr Henry of Clones who was visiting Mr Blackly immediately attended to the boy and used every means possible to restore animation, but it was all in vain. Little Neddy was dead.

The authorities inquired as to why the two young boys were at the sandpit. Edward McCaffrey, the boys' father, was engaged in plastering his house and requiring some sand, so sent his son, James, to get him a little. He cautioned him to remove the sand from the top of the bank lest it should fall on him. After a short time, he'd heard the alarm that the bank had fallen and ran off to it fearing that somehow his son might be in trouble. He was present when the body of his child was dug up and found dead. The young James McCaffrey, crying over the loss of his little brother, said that the little boy had followed him to the sandpit and 'when the bank fell, he was partly covered by it, and Ned had disappeared'. The verdict was death from a bank of gravel falling on and killing the deceased, on Saturday 6 February 1858 whilst playing near it.[16]

BULLETS AND BUCKSHOT
Accidental Gun-Shootings

Accidental gun-shootings were likely when a loaded gun was kept about a house in a 'safe place', but happened most often when the person holding it was not focusing his attention on the direction of the barrel. Nineteenth-century single-action revolvers, rifles and blunderbusses were easily discharged. In fact, they were likely to go off just from being dropped. For these reasons, there are several accidental gun-shooting deaths recorded in the coroner's casebook.

When a gun is discharged, there is an instant explosion of gunpowder and flame and a hot cloud of gas shoots from the barrel. When the gun is in close proximity to the victim, the flame might set the victim's clothes on fire. At very close range, if the gun is actually touching the skin, the gases can actually rip the skin apart, bursting it open. If the bullet or shot did not instantly kill its victim, they might run the risk of another complication – *tetanus* or *lockjaw* from the bacteria entering the wound that had penetrated the skin was much-feared. This dreaded disease was accompanied by violent spasms and the rigidity of certain muscles, especially in the face, and was usually fatal.

Widowmakers: Mishandling Guns
The Death of Foster Dunwoody, Tully, Monaghan Parish, January 1868
William Carroll, Esq., County Surveyor of Co. Monaghan, accompanied by Mr Foster Dunwoody, Deputy-Surveyor for the Barony of Monaghan, were out on 10 January 1858 for a day of snipe shooting. They had been shooting for some time along the Castleblayney road and decided to drive to Mr William Crawford's house with the intention of shooting over the bogs in the neighbourhood.

The two men got out of their car and were greeted by Joseph Crawford, Mr Crawford's son. Carroll removed his cape and gave some parcels to the boy for his father. The gun Carroll had been using was rolled up in a cover in the well of the car and a dog whip was placed over the pillars to prevent any accident. As he began to unravel the cloth around the gun, it suddenly went off. To everyone's shock and horror, the discharge shattered the lower portion of Foster Dunwoody's left hand. In the midst of the confusion, the horse had been startled and began to run away. Foster stepped forward as if to stop him, while at the same time exclaiming, 'Oh!' as if he had just realised that he'd been hit by the spray of the gun. Immediately, Carroll caught Foster in his arms exclaiming, 'Oh my! Oh my!' The wounded man was then quickly brought into the house.

Carroll, shocked and dismayed, wrapped his friend's hand as quickly as possible and set off for Dr Irwin's house so that he could dress the wound. Foster being a healthy, strong young man was not too concerned. Just to be safe, Dr Irwin and Surgeon Rush attended him daily. The wound was not considered to be dangerous and appeared to be healing quite well.[17]

The bad news came a week later. On Friday, 17 January 1868, Foster appeared to have tetanus or lockjaw. Dr Young was called in but the fatal disease had got a death-hold on the young man. He died two days later and was buried in the Presbyterian graveyard in Monaghan. Foster Dunwoody was cut off in the prime of life at thirty-five years of age leaving a pregnant wife and a small child to mourn him.[18]

Calling for Da: The Death of Jane Parks
Ardgonnell, Tynan Parish, Co. Armagh, April 1872
Thomas Parks was working out in the fields at a rig of beans with his thirteen-year-old daughter, Jane. He told Jane she might as well go inside the house until he set the beans again. Obeying her father, she left to go into house. Several moments later, he heard a gunshot. Instantly, Thomas could hear his daughter screaming, 'Da! Da! Da! I'm shot!' He raced as fast as possible towards the house and coming directly at him was Jane, screaming his name with her clothes on fire. Her mother, Mary, who had been at the well gathering water, grabbed Jane before her father could get to her and put the fire out. The back part of her dress was smoking. The two distraught parents then carried her into the house to have a better look at her wounds and find out exactly what had just happened.[19]

As Jane was put into her bed, her mother and father saw the gun lying on the floor. The gun had been lying in Jane's way. She had taken it by the muzzle and it accidentally went off. Thomas and Mary immediately started on their way to the county infirmary where Jane could be seen by Surgeon Young.

Dr Young saw Jane that same night. She was suffering from a gunshot wound in the left armpit. The ball had passed out through the shoulder blade shattering the bone. There was not much he could do for her. The shock and irruptive fever caused by the wound accelerated her death. The unfortunate young girl died on the morning of 14 April 1872 just one week after the accident.

At her inquest, Constable McDermott read a statement made by the deceased to him which was read as follows: 'I was standing at the fire at 4p.m. on 5 April. The gun was standing against a bag in the corner. I touched her and she went off. There was no person in the kitchen at the time.'[20] There was no suspicion in the case.

Shooting Birds and Each Other
The Death of Merideth Scalon, August 1862 and
Elinor Dinny, November 1857
On 26 July 1862, two young lads about fifteen years of age, Master McKinstry, grandson of Mr Johnston, and his cousin, Merideth Scalon, nephew of Henry G. Johnston, Esq., asked the elder man if they

might go out into the garden to shoot birds. Fearing that an accident might happen, Mr Johnston gave them a small gun, rather than a pistol, to amuse themselves. Unfortunately, while they were passing through a hedge, the gun went off – most likely as a twig caught the trigger – and the contents passed through young Merideth's arm. As quickly as possible, Dr Douglass of Glaslough and Dr Young of Monaghan were called. Merideth appeared to progress very satisfactorily until in late August. Tetanus or lockjaw had set in and he died on 26 August. He was buried in Glaslough Churchyard on 26 August 1862.[21]

In a similar case, James Dinny of Aughnacloy was in the garden shooting birds early one morning in November 1857. He entered the house putting the gun in its usual place. Shortly after, James heard the gun go off. On looking around he saw the gun had fallen down and his mother standing near it exclaiming, 'I'm done!' He ran out of the house for two neighbours, Mrs Taylor and Mrs Hewitt, and then sent a messenger into Smithborough for Dr Moorehead who came immediately. The doctor found her stretched on the kitchen floor just where the accident had occurred and helped put her into bed. On probing the wound, he found it was a gunshot to the left side of the spine. She complained of great weakness and loss of power in her limbs. She died later that evening at 7.30p.m. The verdict was death from injuries caused by the accidental discharge of a gun in her kitchen. She was said to be 'a smart woman of about 55 years of age.'[22]

Chatting the Face off Him: The Death of William Doran
Cornawall, Ematris Parish, May 1862
Moses Little received a visit from William Doran who wanted to chat and ask Moses for a favour. They agreed to work together the following day to harrow some flax. They continued their conversation with William standing on top of a ditch chatting to Moses who worked below. William had a loaded gun in his hand. As William talked away, Moses noticed that he often shifted the gun up and down in his hands and it appeared to be slipping. After several minutes of adjusting the gun and while talking away, it went off, without any apparent cause. It appeared that the trigger may have caught on the twigs of the cropped hedge which were at his feet causing the discharge.

William fell directly off the ditch into the arms of Moses. To Moses' horror, the man's face was shadowed, black and bloody. The muscle was blown off the skull and hung a little below his face. The gunshot had also carried away a portion of the upper lip, passing up the right side of the nose and through the orb and entering the brain.

The ball passed out through the top of the head, shattering the brain, muscles and bones and carried a considerable portion of the brains out through the orifice. This was the wound that proved to be the cause of death. William survived for two hours after the accident.[23]

DEATH AND DRINK
Misadventure after the Pub

Death from Drunkeness
On Tuesday evening the body of a man named Keenan, a blacksmith, was found in the townland of Killydonnelly. It appeared on investigation that Keenan had been one of a runaway party* and that while engaged on that expedition had drunk an overdose of whiskey, from the effects of which he died.
– *The Northern Standard*, February 1858

A runaway party was where a man and woman ran off to get married together – or eloped. In some cases, many persons participated in the party.

Freedom in Drinking
We wish some one town would try the experiment of abolishing the sale of liquor to be drunk on the premises altogether except at hotels and allowing any shopkeeper to sell it, provided it was taken home. The lower classes would then be placed by law exactly in the position in which the well-to-do place themselves voluntarily. There would be genuine freedom, yet all enticements to drink would cease.
– *Spectator*, 9 February 1867

Seventy-one of the deaths and murders in the coroner's casebook for Co. Monaghan were recorded as being influenced by or directly resulting from alcohol consumption. If alcohol had been mentioned as a contributing factor to death in the inquests, this figure would be higher. Although such terms as hearty or merry helped indicate the intake of alcohol of the victim, other circumstances, for example, if they died in or near a public house, would have helped identify just how prevalent alcohol was in many unfortunate fatalities. Alcohol-related deaths reflect verdicts such as death by accidents, death by misadventure, alcohol poisoning, suicide, domestic violence or different forms of *recreational violence* – when drunk men began fighting, the violence escalated, tempers flared and restraint was absent.[24] Concern for drunkards existed in terms of moral reform as was carried out with vast temperance movements, institutionalisation and preaching God and teetotalism, yet the attitudes towards the drunken dead, or the inebriated murderer or victim, are revealed in the verdicts of death.

Those who died as a result of involvement with alcohol brought about contempt and shame. For example, in November of 1872, Bernard Reilly had been drinking for forty-eight hours in mourning and celebration at a wake held in Clones town. While singing songs the second night, he drank several pints of whiskey. After his last whiskey at 6a.m., he passed out on the floor in the house of John Eager. After he had been lying on the damp floor for six hours, his wife put him in the back of a cart and brought him home. By the time Dr Henry was called, Reilly was described as 'pulseless'. Dr Henry prescribed treatments for the dying man such as putting heat around him, warm bricks, a boiler, etc., to keep him as warm as possible. Reilly did make a short recovery, asking for a glass of water, but, by the next morning, he was dead. Dr Henry stated, 'I consider his death arose from lying on a cold floor for about seven hours *while stupidly drunk*'.[25]

Examples of doctors being called on to attend to drunken patients in the early hours of the morning were common and it appears some doctors held contempt for those whom they needed to call on for such reasons. In another case involving Dr Richard Henry, George Welsh had been in a drunken altercation at Phillip McCabe's pub in Clones where he was either pushed or fell down the stairs. When Dr Henry was called, the constable retrieving him told him that Welsh was in no danger. The doctor told the coroner's jury that he'd planned to see Welsh in the morning as he was retiring to rest 'as a result of being repeatedly called out late at night to see drunken people'.[26]

During the post-famine years, temperance movements swept across the country. They created animosity between Protestants and the Catholic church, who would not embrace the movement for fear that it might appear too close to the values of Protestantism. Waddell made an inquiry into the death of Joseph McMahon in 1859 which may reflect contempt for those who chose to imbibe, when well known in the religious community. Only a few notes were taken, but the coroner made a record that Captain McKelvey of the Monaghan police told him Mr Edmondson, the organist of Monaghan Church, and three others had spent a night in William Cunningham's public house in Monaghan town, drinking and playing cards. Edmondson and McMahon got into a drunken brawl which poured out into the streets of the town. McMahon later died, but the coroner determined it was his chronic inebriate habits rather than this one particular incident that caused his death. The body, which had already been buried at a Roman Catholic graveyard in Warrenpoint was not exhumed and no inquest was held.[27] Is it possible that the notation of Edmondson's occupation reflected Waddell's view of temperance in relation to the politics of the time? Other mere inquiries rarely, if ever, provided so much detail about the parties involved, especially their occupation. It appears that Waddell may have been allowing us a window into his personal political views in regard to alcohol via his commentary and note-taking in his casebook.

Alcohol-related deaths occurred very often after a night at the pub. Those imbibing in spirits and chat with friends attempted to make their way home alone, staggering along the roadside. Whether it was the fresh air combined with too much alcohol, fatigue, dizziness, alcohol poisoning, dangers of the deep grips along the roadside, horses and carts moving quickly through darkness or simply, the risks taken from being intoxicated, many braving the crooked journey home never made it to the comfort of their beds. The inquests that follow are only a sample of inquests where drink was the major contributing factor of death.

Greeting the Mailcoach at Midnight
The Death of John Byers, Carrigans, Donagh Parish, December 1857
Edward McEnally was the night driver of the mail coach that regularly made its way through the darkness between Monaghan and Omagh. One very black December night, Edward was passing through the town of Emyvale when he met a section of road shaded with trees. He was travelling at his usual speed, but the road had become much darker and impossible to see up ahead. Suddenly the horses began violently swaying and plunged to one side of the road, dragging the wheels after them. Edward pulled as hard as he could at the reins. With his eyes wide open in an attempt to see what lay ahead, he spotted a man lying on his back on the roadside. The coach wheels and horses were about to make contact and before he could pull them up or steer away, the lead horse dragged the coach over the body. Three or four perches past where the man lay, the driver was able to stop the horses, get down, and run back towards the body. Assisted by his guard on the mail coach and a gentleman passenger, he was able to carry the wounded man into a nearby house. They left the man in the charge of the owner and rode off to Emyvale to give word of the circumstances to the police.

The man injured was John Byers. Earlier that night, Byers and several other men were in and out of different pubs throughout the town. After a night of drinking, he and a few friends finished a bottle of whiskey while standing outside on a bridge near their homes. John was well known and it was common knowledge that he was not a man of temperate habits. He was walking home, heavily intoxicated, fell down on the side of the road and did not get up.

Dr McKinstry examined the body of Byers.[28] On opening the body, he found the sternum crushed and the second rib on the left side, broken and driven into the lung. There was also a quantity of dark blood surrounding and pressing upon the heart. This was quite sufficient evidence to cause the deceased's immediate death. The verdict was death from being accidentally run over by the night mail coach from Monaghan to Omagh, the night being very dark and the deceased lying drunk on the road the night of 9 or morning of 10 December.[29]

Tipping over in Mr Brian's Millrace: The Death of Thomas Salmon
Monaghan, Monaghan Parish, October 1861
Allen Mitchell was on his way to work at Mr Brian's mill, Faulkland, when he looked down into the millrace (the channel of water which feeds the mill's water-wheel) and saw a cart had overturned. Lying next to cart was a dead horse and the body of a man. The deceased was lying partly on the horse's neck with his limbs submerged in water that was about ten or twelve inches deep.

Constable Trimble was informed of the discovery of a man lying dead and quickly arrived on the scene. He found the body of Thomas Salmon in the race. The man was lying on his back, his hand on his breast. There were no marks of violence on his body and £4.5.0 of change in his pocket. The bank from which the cart fell was about seven feet above the water. It was difficult to say what brought the man to the spot where he lay as it was entirely out of the way. One could only assume that as the cart had passed along the bank of the millrace, and at a narrow part of the road, one of the wheels passed over the edge of the embankment throwing horse and driver deep into the ravine.[30]

Thomas Salmon was very well known as a civil car driver in Monaghan town and for many years he belonged to Mr Campbell's posting establishment. Mr Joe Campbell was questioned in the investigation. He explained that Thomas was one of the car drivers that left his yard for Aughnacloy at 6p.m. the previous evening with a gentleman passenger. He should have returned sometime between 11p.m. and 11.30p.m. Joe had sat up most of the night waiting for his return, yet he never arrived.

Dr Young examined the body and, finding no marks of violence, concluded that death resulted from exposure. The verdict was death from the accidental overturning of the cart that the deceased had been driving into a millrace and exposure therein on the night of 17 October 1861. There was one additional comment – he was most probably drunk.[31] Although he was known as a sober man, he was believed to have been drinking at the time of the accident.

The Sound of Spirits in the Air – Glaslough Street, Monagahan
The Burning Death of Mary Kelly, Monaghan Town, August 1869
One dark night in Monaghan town Richard Tweedy, the town watchman, was working his post on Glaslough Street when at about one o'clock in the morning he heard an eerie sound that stopped him in his tracks. It was a heavy moaning. Tweedy and the second watchman, Mick McCormick, walked down the street listening to the strange hum hidden amongst the crowded houses. They strained to hear over the sound of their own footsteps and the thumping of breath and heart and allowed it to pull them forward. Soon they reached a house where the sound was the loudest and began pounding with their fists on the front door. Receiving no reply, Tweedy went to the police barracks to report the circumstances. He returned bringing the help of a few policemen and all resumed knocking on the front as well as the side door. At last, the man of the house, Mr Kelly, leaned out of the upper window and asked why the crowd had gathered. They yelled up to him to hurry downstairs and open the shop door as someone was downstairs, either ill or injured. The crowd outside watched as the door was flung open, a voice called out 'Fire!' and the alarm was sounded.

Great black smoke came billowing out of the shop door, curling up into the night air. Constable John Keeran was one of the men who raced inside the warm glow to find the moaning woman in the midst of the fire. It was Mary Kelly lying on the floor of the shop with her clothes on fire. Another woman, Catherine McDonald, ran forward and splashed some water on Mary's smouldering clothes. After the flames were doused, the burned woman did not move nor speak. Mary Kelly was already dead. She was immediately removed to the parlour where witnesses could see that her right hand, arm and breast were all badly burned. The right side of her body and across her chest to the left breast was scorched. It appeared that the boards of the floor beneath her body had been burned and the conclusion was drawn that her clothes had accidentally taken fire. She had thrown herself down on the ground in an attempt to smother the blaze.

The cause of the fire was not determined but Catherine McDonald explained the events of earlier that evening. Catherine was sleep-

ing in the upstairs quarters of the Kelly's residence with Mr and Mrs
Kelly's daughter. The two girls were lying in bed when one of the other
children began to cry. Mrs Kelly had come up to investigate and check
on the children at which time Catherine smelled spirits on her. She
concluded by stating that recently, Mrs Kelly had fallen into intem-
perate habits. Mary Kelly, wife and mother, was thirty-seven years of
age.[32]

Neither Sober nor Dead Drunk
The Death of Thomas Murphy, Clones, Clones Parish, March 1871
A body was found floating in a pond near the Clones Railway Station. It was a man about forty years in age and it appeared that the
corpse had been in the water for some time. When the body was
being raised from the water, two coils of telegraph wire were entangled around it and it was assumed that it was the coils that kept the
body submerged. This is why it had not floated to the surface for
several days.

Earlier in the week, the Murphy family had been searching for
Thomas who was last seen on 23 February 1871, a fair-day in Clones.
Fair-days were days of work, trade and especially drinking. Two weeks
passed as the family made inquiries all over town. On 6 March, George
Murphy received information that a body was found floating in a pond
and hurried to the site. Sadly, he immediately identified the dead man
as his brother. Dr William O'Reilly examined the body and found no
marks of injury, except an old wound at the back of the left thigh,
another at the back of the head and a blue mark on his shin bone.
None of the marks was considered to have contributed to the death.

At the inquest, several friends serving as witnesses explained
that they saw Thomas in town on the night after the fair. The best
clue as to his whereabouts came from information given by John Ferguson. He had indeed been drinking.

Ferguson said, 'It [the body] was on the plot of ground between
the paling and pool of water. When the farmyard gate is open, there
is nothing to prevent a person falling into the pool of water and they
are generally open of a fair-day. He was neither sober nor dead drunk.'

The jury was unanimously of the opinion that it was the duty of
the owners of the pond to surround it with a fence sufficient to ensure public safety. The verdict was the deceased came to his death by
drowning.[33]

Hallow's Eve: The Riderless Carriage Returns from Caledon
The Death of Francis Halfpenny
Gibraltar, Tyholland Parish, November 1859

Francis Halfpenny was sitting atop his cart filled with a heavy load of wheat while his horse pulled him towards the road to Caledon. His sister, Ann, watched from the doorway until her brother and his cart disappeared from sight. It was early in the morning on 31 October and although she wasn't aware of it at the time, it was the last time Ann would see her brother alive. At 7p.m. that evening, Ann was shocked to see Francis' horse and cart at the front door of the house – but no sign of Francis.

The alarm was raised, the neighbours were informed and a search continued through the night. It was a particularly cold, dark, and stormy night and the search parties turned up with no clues as to the location of the missing man. It was ten days later when the body of Francis Halfpenny was discovered in a hole in Garran bog about two perches from the public road. His pockets contained £6 in cash, a little bottle of spirits and some tea and sugar.

Only two people believed they saw Francis the evening of his disappearance. Francis McDonald believed he saw a horse and cart like that of Francis Halfpenny's on the road that night, but he could not identify him because it was a very dark and wet night. The last man to see Francis alive was Pat Finegan. Francis arrived at Finegan's Forge that evening about 6p.m. to light his pipe. He chatted for a while, got into his cart and left. Pat claimed that Francis was 'in liquor but not incapable of taking care of himself'.

Whether it was the spirits of Hallowe'en or those sipped from the bottle, Francis Halfpenny came about his death having fallen into a bog hole on his way home from Caledon. It was Hallowe'en night 1859, the night having been dark, wet, cold and very windy.[34]

Outrageous from Drink: Falling out the Bedroom Window
The Death of Henry Smith, Monaghan Town, October 1867

Henry Smith had been drinking at John Irwin's public house when John Rusk found him. Rusk, a long time friend of Smith, persuaded him to go home to the house of his master, Mr Ben Skelton. With some difficulty he finally got Smith home and into bed and remained with his drunken friend until he thought he was asleep. Just after Rusk left the room and quietly crept down the stairs, he heard a crash of glass. He went running back up the stairs and threw open the bedroom door. There lay an empty bed. The window of the room was broken and the curtains blowing in the wind. He raced to the window and on looking down, saw his friend on the ground, lying partly under a cart. Rusk assumed that Smith must have fallen or jumped out of the window. Owen McCleary who was on the ground standing nearby had been startled as the body of Smith suddenly plummeted from the sky. The men immediately took Smith to the infirmary.

Dr Young, the surgeon of the Monaghan infirmary would not accept Henry Smith as a patient. He found him to be outrageously drunk, angry, unpredictable and a possible danger to the other patients. In fact, there was one man in the ward whose life was in great jeopardy and any disturbance might be fatal. Dr Young felt that it was unfortunate that Henry Smith needed the medical attention of a private institution and that the injuries to his head were of a serious nature; however, he did not have a spare bed and he did not want to risk injury to other patients for one drunken man.

Henry Smith was taken back to the home of Ben Skelton who was shocked to learn of the events occurring in his absence. Smith was a militia man who was to receive his pay and Skelton had gone to Bessmount to pick up his money for him. Dr Temple was called to attend to him. He began coming round the house every day to tend to Smith, but his health continued to decline. The sharp blow to the head was considered to have caused brain damage. He had gone deaf in his left ear and was declining daily. Henry Smith died on 22 October 1867. His death was a result of injuries to his brain caused by falling out of the window of his bedroom.[35]

Walking Home from the Pub can be Dangerous
The Death of Phillip McCague, Milltown, Monaghan Parish, April 1863
On 7 April 1863, Phillip McCague went to the Monaghan fair. He saw his brother-in-law, Pat Corgan, chatted for about two hours and then went to see some friends off by train about 4p.m. The two men met up again at 6p.m. and walked to Milltown to have some drinks at Francis McCleary's public house. Phillip left at 7p.m.

The next morning, a man named James Quigly was out looking for fowl and when walking towards a quarry, saw the legs of a man sticking out of a nearby well. He ran immediately to the man and pulled him out, but he was dead. He had £2.5.0 in his pocket and it was determined that his death had not happened by violence, as he had not been robbed. The verdict was death by accidental suffocation. The pub owner stated that Phillip McCague had only 2oz of whiskey.[36] Was alcohol a contributing factor in his death?

What Lies Beneath the Grip?
The Death of James Andrews, Clones, Clones Parish, March 1860
Richard Andrews was scared and worried when he arrived at the police station to report his brother, James, missing. Richard found James' cart and horse on the side of the road, but no sign of James. John O'Hare, constable of police, accompanied Richard to the site where the cart and horse were found and began searching further down the side of the road. They had not gone far when they found the body. It was lying in a deep drain at the roadside, facing up, staring at them from underneath the water. They got him out quickly, but life had been gone for some time. Beyond some slight bruises about his face, there was nothing to indicate a struggle or violence. However, the coroner investigated the case.

James Johnston told the coroner's jury that he'd seen his cousin, James, the night before in the Oats Market in Clones. He'd been there until 11p.m. and when James left, he was very tipsy. Johnston wished his cousin to stay with him for the night, but he'd refused. Instead he helped him to his own house, but James wished him to go no further.

Dr Henry performed the post-mortem examination and concluded that the body presented all appearances of one who died from drowning. There were some slight scratches on his face such as would arise from falling on the gravelled road.

The verdict was death from having fallen into a pool of water on the roadside on the night of 30 March and the morning of 31, being thereby drowned.[37]

Wandering too Close to the Canal
The Death of Francis Cumiskey, Point, Kilmore Parish, April 1858
Anyone walking along the Ulster canal was taking a risk. There were many sections and patches along the sides of the water where there was no fence to protect them from falling in. Even the most diligent and cautious might find themselves in the water. Such was the case of Francis Cumiskey. On 20 April 1858, Francis and Richard Hanna ran into each other in Monaghan town. They spoke briefly and parted ways. Richard found Francis to be quite sober and just going about his business. Later that same evening, Francis had not returned home. Hanna and several others became concerned and decided to begin a search for their friend.

Francis went missing for a week. His body surfaced in the water on the Monaghan side of the Brandrum bridge. It appeared to have been in the water for several days and Richard Hanna was one of many who witnessed its retrieval from the water. The coroner's report was the only document providing an explanation. 'The day after the deceased was in town, his stuff was got on the canal bank. Beside it were marks of where a person had fallen, all which was considered to apply to deceased.'[38] The newspaper suggested that where Francis fell into the water there was 'no fence between the bank and the footpath' thereby creating a dangerous situation.[39]

Briars and Thorns: The Death of James Graham
Smithborough, Clones Parish, February 1869
Joseph White, Station Master at Smithborough, watched as James Graham got off the number five train coming from Monaghan at 8p.m. He was in good health and appeared to be perfectly competent to take care of himself under any circumstances. White also watched him delay in the village for about twenty minutes before heading for home.

A short time later, Henry Williamson, the constable of police, received the grim information that a man was lying in the grip alongside of the road. Upon arriving at the spot in the townland of Templetate, he saw the body floating in the water. The road and fields had been under water after several days of continual rain. It appeared that he had gone off the road into the grip and was unable to free himself in consequence of briars and thorns growing there. Williamson said, 'With difficulty, I got the body out of the water. When I searched the pockets, I found £9.17.6 of money and a silver watch, which had stopped at 9.50p.m.' The verdict was death from accidental drowning when on the way home. James Graham was 54 years old.[40]

THE LAST NIGHT OF CHARITY
Dying from Exposure

Beggars, travellers, gypsies or tramps were treated well in Co. Monaghan in the nineteenth century. These were persons depending upon the charity of the people of the countryside for food and temporary shelter. These travellers were quite welcome as they were a source of news from near and far. Below are two such persons who spent their last days and found their final resting place in Co. Monaghan.

The Unknown Stranger: The Death of an Unknown Man,
Cortober, Ematris Parish, June 1865
A traveller had arrived at the house of Mary McGeough one summer

afternoon and, thinking he appeared hungry, she offered him some food. He sat, ate and went away shortly after. About two hours later, being down on the road, a little girl called Mary's attention to a man lying in the grips on the roadside. It was the traveller; he was dead. The neighbours helped retrieve the body from the ditch. Dr Moore examined the body and determined – as there were no marks of injury – that he accidentally fell into the roadside filled with mud and water, and drowned.

At the coroner's inquest, the jury earnestly desired to call the attention of the country survey to the very dangerous state of the public road leading through the townlands of Cortober and Cookill East and also as they are convenient to the railway, Coolkill viaduct and bridge.[41]

Wild Arabs of Society: The Death of Patrick Smith
Corraghy, Clones Parish, August 1875
Patrick Smith knocked on Mary Cunningham's door on an August evening in 1875 asking her if he might sleep in their shed for the night, as he had no place to put his head. Mary told him he could not since that was where the ass lay each night. Nothing further was said.

The next morning, a neighbour of Mary Cunningham, James McCaffrey, awoke to prepare for the day and made his way to his lime-kiln for work. Upon arriving, he found Patrick Smith lying dead inside the kiln – his head on the rim of it and the rest of his body on the stones. James knew that Patrick was a wanderer and said of his character, 'He was one of those "wild Arabs of society" who settle no where and sleep anywhere. He would not stop with his own father or family.'[42]

Dr Alexander Knight examined the body of the deceased and concluded that he had no doubt that death came from inhaling the gas given out from the burning lime.[43]

BAD LUCK
Unusual and Unfortunate Accidental Deaths

Picking Plums can be Fatal: The Death of John Holdsworth
Carrickmore, Clones Parish, September 1870
Mary Ann Holdsworth and her sister were riding with their father, John, in a cart on their way to Clones town one September morning. John was seventy-nine years of age, a stout and generally healthy man. As the horse pulled the cart along one of the laneways, they came

upon a plum tree. While in the act of passing it, he stood up and reached to pick some plums from the trees that shadowed and lined the
lane. It is likely this was an activity of habit that John had done for
many years and now, well into old age, he was still limber enough to
reach for the fruit. Unfortunately, this would be the old man's last
pick from the trees. While he was standing retrieving the plums, the
horse turned suddenly into a gap in one of the fields. The wheel came
in contact with a stump, raising the cart so suddenly and so high that
it threw John to the ground. The old man fell directly on his head.

Quickly his two daughters raised him up into a sitting position
and began speaking to him, but their father could only move his lips.
No sound came from him. Help soon arrived. He was carried to a
neighbour's house and a messenger was dispatched for Dr Knight. Dr
Knight was not at home and in turn Dr O'Reilly was sent for. Time
was running out. By the time Dr O'Reilly arrived, John had drawn
his last breath.

Dr O'Reilly told the coroner's jury that having examined the
body of John Holdsworth, he found a concussion of the brain and
spinal marrow. The verdict was death on 22 September caused by the
turning over of his cart and he landing on his head.[44]

Bathing in the Canal: The Drowning Death of John Stalker
Tully, Monaghan Parish, July 1872
John Stalker woke up on a warm July morning and decided to take a
quick bath in the canal before breakfast. He had planned to go on a
fishing excursion for the day with some friends and, as he was not in
the habit of bathing, John would have his first bath of the season.
Although his sagacious pet Newfoundland was always at his side, this
morning he ventured off on his own down to the water. Leaving Tully
House – where he rented a room with Mrs Campbell – he reached the
canal bank, removed his clothes and plunged into the water. The spot
he chose was under the bridge where the water was seven feet deep
and extremely cold.

Another renter at Tully House, Mr Philip O'Carroll, postman and
student of Trinity College, saw John walk down to the canal for his
bath. After breakfast was eaten and finished, Phillip was surprised that
his friend had not returned. He went to investigate and saw the dis-
carded clothes at the side of the bank. On looking down into the
water, he was shocked to see John's body at the bottom. It was face
down underneath the water. Terrified, Philip began running towards
the house screaming for help. Joseph Mayne, another inhabitant of

the house and a close friend of John, came running down to see what
had happened. Philip went immediately to the lock-house to find a
drag and the two men removed their friend's body from the bottom
of the canal.

Surgeon Rush deposed that he was taking a walk when he heard
of the accident and went to the scene at once. The only thing extraordinary he observed at the time was that there were some worms
from the bottom of the canal in John Stalker's eyes. It appeared from
the curling of his toes and feet that he had got a cramp and accidentally drowned. He was not believed to have been a powerful swimmer.

Stalker, O'Carroll and Mayne had been lodging together at Tully
House and his friends were devastated by John's death. Everyone in
the neighbourhood was said to be saddened. At the inquest, Joseph
Mayne was described as deeply affected. He told the jury the events
of the day and also that John Stalker was a twenty-seven-year-old native of Scotland working in Monaghan as an excise officer. Joseph
and John had been good friends for the past two years since John
moved to Monaghan.[45]

The newspaper carried some of the details from the inquest and
noted that there was deep regret expressed by the town as well as the
jury. Two very sad circumstances were also added. There was a schoolteacher who usually passed in the morning beneath the bridge at the
precise time the accident would have occurred, but unfortunately went
in another direction that morning. The other was the mention of John
Stalker's dog – that he invariably accompanied him everywhere and
it was believed that if the animal had been with him during the accident, the alarm would have been raised in time to save him. Death
came with the sudden and silent certainty of fate, and the community deplored the loss of a generous and amiable young gentleman.[46]

The Skeleton in Clonkeelan Bog
An Unknown Man found June 1869, Clonkeelan, Drummully Parish
John McKiernan was the first to find the body as he was cutting turf
in the bog. When he had dug down about three feet deep, to his surprise he came upon the skull of a human being. Shocked and bewil-
dered as to how the skeleton would have come to this fate, he immediately contacted the police in Clones. Dr Henry examined the
remains concluding they were those of a male person of middle age.
The bones were perfect and entire. He could not form any opinion
as to what would have been the cause of death. Considering the nature of the bog (it could preserve anything entrapped in it for hun-

dreds of years) he could not determine how long the body had been there.[47] The newspaper carried the story stating, 'The whole thing is strange and we have no recollection of any sudden disappearance or foul play having taken place, and this locality is quiet and peace-able.'[48] Who was this man?

DANCING BY THE FIRE
The Tragedy of Oscar Wilde's Two Half-Sisters, Mary and Emily Wilde, November 1871

Sir William Wilde, father of famous author and playwright, Oscar Wilde, was also the father of two illegitimate children, Eliza and Mary Wilde. The girls were raised by William's eldest brother, the Revd Ralph Wilde.

On 31 October 1871, the girls attended a Hallowe'en ball at the home of Mr Reid at Drummaconor House, a large manor house loca-ted off the Clones-Monaghan road. The two girls had stayed behind after the party with their host, Mr Reid. The gentleman took Emily for a last dance around the floor. As they glided past the open hearth, the girl's crinoline dress swept by the embers and instantly caught fire. As she began to scream, her sister Mary came to her assistance. As both girls swatted and fought to put out the flames, Mary's dress caught fire as well. Mr Reid wrapped his coat around one of the girls and carried her outside to roll her in the snow in an attempt to ex-tinguish the flames. The other sister, panic-stricken and on fire, rush-ed around in screaming terror until she collapsed, exhausted.[49]

Both girls lay at Drummaconor House and were attended to by Mr Reid. Mary Wilde lingered more than a week and, after nine days of suffering, she died from the results of the burns. An inquest was scheduled to be held in Carrickmacross on 10 November 1871, but William Charles Waddell received a letter from Sir William Wilde of Dublin. In it, Sir William requested that the coroner hold only an *inquiry* into the death, as a full inquest might be of fatal consequence to Emily Wilde, who was now dangerously ill. One can presume Emily was not told of Mary's death and that Sir William was trying to pre-vent her inevitable demise. However, there was another ulterior mo-tive. His daughters were illegitimate, hidden from public view and kept as a secret from the children in his 'legitimate' family. Any pub-lication or exposure of their situation would draw attention to the prominent Wilde family and enhance the scandal.[50]

The scandal was discussed in high society. John Butler Yeats wrote a letter to his son, W. B. Yeats, relating a story told to him by a local woman, Mrs Hine, who had left the dance before the crinolines caught fire. There are several gaps and errors in his facts, such as that the Revd Mr Wilde's name was Ralph, and that he was a brother, not the father, of Sir William. However, it does shed light on the story of the girls. His letter appears as follows:

May 30, 1921
317 W. 29. S.

My dear Willie,
Here is a story about Sir Wm. Wilde, that I got from old Mrs Hime, mother of Maurice Hime, headmaster of Foyle College. When she and her son lived in Monaghan, they had a neighbour the Rev. –Wilde, D.D. father of Sir William and with him, lived two pretty girls, his nieces, and daughters (illegitimate) of Sir. Wm. There was a dance one evening at the house, to which the Himes went. After Mr Hime left, one of these girls in her muslin dress and crinoline went too close to the fire and the dress was instantly in flames – after some cries of agony, they died. While they were dying, their mother, who had a small black-oak shop in Dublin, came down [went to Co. Monaghan] and stayed with them. After all was over, even to the funeral, Sir Wm. came down and old Mrs Hime told me that his groans could be heard by people outside his house. There is a tragedy, all the more intense, because it had to be buried in silence. It is not allowed to give sorrow words. Sir Wm. Wilde's vivacity and stream of talk had its source in this kind of [word indecipherable] – perhaps like the bubbles that appear on the surface when the water begins to boil. Had Oscar known of them, he would not have been so scornful of his poor father – successful, parsimonious, and bedevilled, yet Oscar benefited by his parsimony. I wonder what Lady Wilde thought of her husband ...
... Tolstoi was perhaps a weak husband, and then again so unlike many of us who if we have not genius, have virtue and dignity and can maintain our dignity as husbands and men.

Yours Affectionately,
J. B. Yeats.[51]

The coroner complied with Wilde's request and held only a brief inquiry. When Emily Wilde died on Wednesday, 21 November 1871, her inquiry was handled in the same manner and again, no official inquest was held. The girl had lain as an invalid at the residence of Mr Reid for three weeks after the accident.[52]

The Northern Standard only published a short mention of their deaths stating that Mary died on 8 November and 'Emma' [Emily] died on 21 November.[53]

The two girls were buried at St Molua's graveyard in the parish
of Drumsnat. Their headstone reads:

> In memory of two loving and beloved sisters, Emily Wilde aged 24 and
> Mary Wilde aged 22, who lost their lives by accident in this parish in Novr.
> 1871. 'They were lovely and pleasant in their lives and in death they were
> not divided.'

CHAPTER SIX

DEATH IN THE WORKPLACE
RISKING LIVES FOR EMPLOYMENT

One poor little girl persevered in attending the Sunday school, and had no sooner sat on the bench than she was fast asleep. The teacher chided her and she replied, 'Please Sir, I can't help it for I am so tired. I works from daylight to dark all the week, you see, but I'll just stand up and try to keep awake.' Often the children are so weary at the end of the day that they are unable to drag themselves home, and have to be carried by the men.
            – Report of the Children's Employment Commission
                by Mr H. W. Lord, *Belfast Newsletter*, 10 September 1866

Industry and development presented various employment opportunities for men, women and even children, yet those engaged in such work often put their lives at risk when executing the duties and tasks necessary to perform the job. The work-related deaths recorded in the coroner's casebook illustrate the very dangerous nature of trades and manufacturing industries in nineteenth-century Ireland. They demonstrate the unique challenges and hidden dangers for the physically and legally unprotected worker engaged in constructing buildings, roads and railways as well as the manufacturing of textiles. Often the very nature of the work combined with the poor conditions, lack of safety-procedures and dangerous machinery, proved fatal.

Factories and mills were often dimly lit and the heavy and fast-moving machinery caused some to lose arms, legs and lives when flesh intertwined with metal. Dust in the air during the process of making linen or cleaning and sifting corn and flour caused respiratory problems that were a contributing factor in the deaths of many. The absence of safety-procedures to protect the integrity of the railway work-sites put members of the railroad workforce at risk while they administered explosives to blast through earth and rock in the construction of tunnels and rails. Another ever present danger was the chance of collisions, as a multitude of wagons and cars carried men and materials to and from the construction site. Accidents were frequent. Builders erecting churches and other buildings often risked falling from great heights. Even farmers bringing their goods and cattle into town for fair-days risked injury and death when animals could not be controlled in such a tightly-packed area filled with noise and confusion. Regardless of the employment or trade, workers needed to be alert and at all times aware of the dangers they faced.

Although legislation attempted to keep up with the growing need for the protection of workers, enforcement proved difficult until the latter part of the century. Those workplace fatalities listed in the coroner's casebook in Co. Monaghan represent deaths occurring at a time when the justice system lacked due diligence to hold the employers and companies legally responsible for these fatalities. There are several examples of inquest verdicts making clear that the jury's opinion is that the worker was at fault for his own demise, not the employer or the poor conditions under which they were engaged. Such was stated in the inquest of Mary Benner, a mill-worker who became entangled in the cogwheels while looking for flax. The verdict of the coroner's jury was death from injuries accidentally inflicted in Mr McGlone's mill in consequence of deceased having gone into a part of the mill *where she had no business*.[1] Although committees reviewing conditions within factories and mills recommended the enactment of safety provisions designed to prevent accidents (putting fences around dangerous areas within the mill) and to provide some degree of compensation in the event of injury or death, the bills or Factory Acts throughout the century contained few safety or compensation provisions.[2] When an inquest verdict in Waddell's casebook was returned stating that the employer was at fault for the conditions that contributed to the worker's death, it was impossible to find a source containing one single instance where charges were pressed further and brought against them in a court of law. Other family members were likely employed by the mill and could easily be discharged should there be any trouble. In most cases, workers were unaware of their rights and nothing was done except mourning and burying their dead.

Widows and families of those men contracted to work at the time of the construction of the Great Northern Railway received no compensation if a fatality befell their loved ones. These were simply contractors, not permanent employees of the railway. Some never returned from work, crushed by the carts or earth in the removal of the land or struck down by the engine travelling along the 'Permanent Way'. One might imagine that, as many of the men building the railways in Ireland and England were often hired by local contractors along the

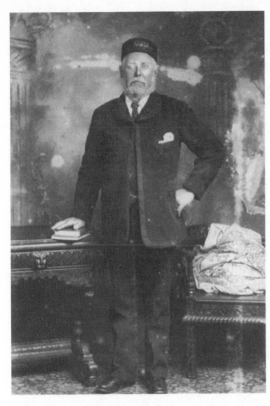

Mr William Taggert,
Station Master
at Essexford,
Co. Monaghan

miles of track, their names were likely to be unrecorded and they were paid their wages upon completion of a week's work. Compensation for their deaths eluded their families and they received only what money was in the men's pockets or owed to them at the time of their death.

In contrast, permanent railway workers employed by the Great Northern Railway appear to have been in a different situation. If injured while at their work, they were offered either a 'job for life' or lump-sum compensation. One example of this is the station master at Essexford, Killanny Parish, Co. Monaghan, Mr William Taggert. His toes were cut off when a cart on the rails passed over them. His wife went to the headquarters in Dublin to ask them for the 'job for life' which was granted. Taggert, born in 1841 was employed with the railway from an early age and worked his way up to station master until he died in 1922 at the age of 81 years.[3]

Railway employees appear to have been acknowledged with an inquest in the event of death and juries did, in some cases, find fault with the railway company when conditions contributed to the death of the deceased. When Michael Crolly was killed in a blast at a construction site, the jury at the inquest pointed out that there had been great neglect in not having a man specifically appointed to act as a lookout man during such explosions. In contrast, at the inquest of Edward Molloy, a man whose legs were severed by a train, the jury made mention that Mr Mitchell of the Irish North-Western Railway Company was 'only fulfilling his duty (directing Molloy towards the train) and completely exonerate him from any blame.'[4] Although negligence existed in both cases, the verdicts were unpredictable as to whether the jury would view the railway and its employees as in any way responsible for the fatal accidents which occurred there.

The mere existence of industrial and construction sites created a hazard not just for employees, but for the general populace as well. Millraces and canals that cut through the countryside and towns presented danger for any small child, elderly person or inebriated individual who lost their footing and fell into the fast-moving water. Construction sites not properly secured proved fatal to pedestrians unaware of the hazards beneath their feet or above their heads. Another man-made danger was the use of the railroad tracks as a shortcut along the line by neighbours travelling to nearby towns and villages. This new clear pathway was sometimes the fastest way to a destination, but many started and finished their journey walking the tracks. Some were caught as the train passed over their bodies leaving them to be found by the railway workers the next day, or by the engine drivers who leapt from their posts in the hopes that their fears of a horrible fatality were not realised.

The persons listed as being killed while at work or as a result of the industrialisation of the countryside are often unremembered for their efforts. As time progressed, these fatalities carved the path for greater legislation and the accepted need for employers to take responsibility for the dangers in the workplace. Some of those people recorded by the coroner, who died on the job, are remembered here.

MILL ACCIDENTS

Mutilations and fatalities occurred frequently in and around the mills of Co. Monaghan. The lack of safety features on mechanised mill equipment and the absence of secured fences or barriers restricting public access to the areas around the mills resulted in many accidental deaths. Additionally, long hours and the wages system were contributory factors in many of these accidents. The wages system in mills and factories meant that workers would get paid according to their output rather than the work completed within the course of their workday. The average mill-worker began the day at 5a.m. and ended work between 7 and 8p.m. Not until 1874 was an act passed laying down a maximum workday of ten hours, Monday to Friday, with no more than six hours on Sunday, and the average work week limited to fifty-six hours.[5] Wages of linen industry workers consistently fell below the cost of maintaining a minimum standard of comfort. In the 1850s, the most industrious and active spinners could not earn more than twopence per day. The price of weaving was also proportionately reduced. For example, Mr Davidson of Laragh Mill employed weavers who could, on average, weave a piece 52 yards in length in 15 days for which they received six shillings and board and lodgings during that time.[6]

Poor conditions, bad lighting, loud and deafening machinery, equipment hazardous by design, and long hours contributed to the following deaths. The deaths listed in Waddell's casebook probably represent only a fraction of the accidents and tragedies that occurred.

DEATHS IN THE LINEN INDUSTRY

Linen manufacture in the nineteenth century was a complicated process involving several different stages of production. Flax was first grown and harvested by hand with scythes from the fields [a method also known as pulling] and then stacked. One case records the death of Owen McKenna at this early stage of production when he fell from the top of a flax heap while stacking it in the barn, breaking his spine, thus depriving him of the use of his legs and the ability to pass urine. One can only imagine his suffering five days after the accident as urine had to be drawn from him by Dr Scott.[7] Another man was crushed by his own horse and cart while transporting flax from one location to another. The verdict of death was that the flax-laden cart, which he was in charge of, accidentally inflicted injuries that caused his death.[8]

The flax was next soaked in water so that its bark would rot away from the plant fibres and could be more easily removed. Deep holes were dug in the land around the mill and filled with water to soak the flax for approximately ten to fourteen days. These open, water-filled craters were not fenced in or sectioned off to prevent public access. Some unfortunates met their fate by drowning in these pits filled with rotting plants, unable to pull themselves out of the tangle of bark, mud and stagnant water. There are five such flax-hole drownings recorded by the coroner.

Mrs Molly Skeath, daughter of Charles McCluskey, former owner of Crumlin Mills, explains the features of flax-holes. She describes walking the road boarded on either side by flax-holes on her way home to the mill in the parish of Tyholland. 'The smell of the rotting plant was so bad that we used to have to put a handkerchief to cover our nose and mouth until we passed the spot.' She also explained that the flax-holes were '... not very deep, possibly about three or four feet. However, if one accidentally fell in, it would be difficult if not impossible to get out.' The sides of the 'pits' were high, muddy ridges making it even more difficult for someone to escape. Such was described in the inquest of Thomas Hughes of Sillis. Witness Henry Bradley explained that when 'kneeling down on the bank, I stretched into the hole. I caught the body of deceased by the hair of the head ...' He was unable to lift the man from the hole until help arrived.[9] The fact that he describes himself as stretching *into* the hole shows the incline that presented a problem for the drowning victims and their potential rescuers. Such a person entangled in the rotting plants would find it difficult, if not impossible, to manoeuvre out of such a fate.

After the flax was soaked, it was dried either by laying it out in a field, leaving it open to the natural element, or by fire-drying – a process frowned upon in Scotland and England as it dried up the natural sap of the fibre on which the strength, softness, elasticity and even durability of the flax depended.[10] When flax was being fire-dried, it was taken to a kiln and set over a fire where the flax was dried quickly and then removed to be bundled. Kilns were dangerous places where the utmost care was to be taken in keeping the fire at the right temperature and also to ensure that the flax did not stay on the heat too long and catch fire. Patrick Larkin, a servant of Mick Smith's at Faltagh in the parish of Aghabog, was assisting in drying and rolling flax when the kiln collapsed. A woman named Rose Smith and her two children barely escaped; however, Larkin was buried beneath the rubble for forty-five minutes and was dead when found.[11] The heat produced from such continuous fire easily wore down an already impoverished structure. It contributed to other health problems as well. Alexander Wallace of Hillhall died suddenly in the flax kiln as he was stoking the fire with some coals. He was found with his face blackened, trembling violently and died moments later.[12] It is likely that the heat, combined with the smoke, brought about damage to his heart and lungs, thereby accelerating death.

Scutching Procedures
Breaking Flax and Body Parts
After flax was dried, the process of breaking or *scutching* began – a complicated process of separating the fibre from the unwanted part of the plant to prepare it for spinning.[13] The early machines used for scutching were crude and depended largely on human muscle for the desired effect. The flax was laid across a notched, upright board, fixed a few inches from moving blades and fast-moving wooden rollers to be thrust through by the workers. The rollers (sometimes known as the scutchers or bruising machines) were machines used to continue the breaking process by moving the flax through three fluted rollers to break the woody part of the flax plant. It was this close association between worker and machine which was the major cause of accidents.[14]

There may have been several scutching machines at a particular mill, but probably only one rolling machine with one operator. The operators of rolling machines were in danger each moment that they performed their duties. Besides the difficult working conditions – the mill was unheated (fire was a constant danger) and badly lit and working was often in excess of ten hours a day for about one shilling per day – one simple error could cost them a finger, an arm or even their life. William Greig, who prepared the *General Report on the Gosford Estates in Co. Armagh* in 1821, claimed that 'the scutcher (machines) in Irish mills are merely vertical arms fixed at right angles to the axletree; in applying the flax to these the workman has not sufficient command over it and [it] is so dangerous that it requires great care to prevent serious accidents.'[15] The workers at the rollers were required to introduce the stick of flax to the machine and also, as they saw fit, to shift it to ensure that the bark would be removed from the plant and not damage the fibres. Working at the rollers was a laborious, tedious job that required the worker to perform a detailed rhythm of movement – or dance – that did not allow for a single lapse in concentration as it could lead to horrific results.

Crushed Between the Rollers: The Death of Bridget McEnally
Seaveagh, Tyholland Parish, December 1858
Thomas Little had just begun his work as a scutcher early in the morning on the first day of December 1858 in Thomas McGlone's flax mill

at Seaveagh when he heard shouting coming from the rolling-house. Thomas was aware of the possible hazards and dangers of the machinery in that part of the mill and that Bridget McEnally, the feeder of the rollers, had just started her day. He heard horrible sounds of agony and began running in her direction. As he approached, he saw Bridget with her arms drawn into the cylinders – one of them up to the shoulder and the other near to the elbow. There was a great deal of blood on her face and the side of her head. He immediately reversed the rollers, got her torn and bloody limbs removed, to the horror of all those who watched, and laid her down on a bench. She never spoke a word and died a half-hour later.

Ellen Daily, who assisted in washing the body of the unfortunate woman, observed that the left arm was quite shattered and drawn from its socket. It was held to the body merely by its skin. The right hand was injured and the left side of the head was bruised with a great cut on it. It is likely that Bridget McEnally, just starting her workday, was still waking up and one small misjudgment or slip of concentration led to her death.[16]

Mutilation in the Cogwheels: The Death of Mary Benner
Seaveagh, Tyholland Parish, January 1864

Mary McKenna was engaged in her work along with Mary Benner at Mr McGlone's mill making streeks, long stretches of fibre later to be used for spinning, when they were in need of more flax. Benner left McKenna to walk to the rolling-house to retrieve the flax to continue the work. When Benner didn't return after a short time, McKenna was not immediately concerned as she was in the habit of taking a short break when retrieving more flax from the rolling-house. As more time passed, McKenna became curious and went looking for her co-worker. While walking around the mill and passing through the rolling-house, she saw Benner lying down and screaming that her clothes had been caught by one of the small cogwheels. With such loud machinery surrounding the suffering woman, other workers had not heard her cries for help. McKenna now began shouting and getting the attention of all that the mill needed to be stopped. The mill was promptly stopped to extricate Benner from the cogwheels.

Arthur McGlone, the owner, became aware that the mill had stopped and ran forward to learn the cause. He found Mary Benner caught by one of the wheels of the mill. He disengaged her body from the wheel, but by this time she was already dead. Her clothes had been partly torn from her body, and her arms and breast tightly crushed within the wheel. Under deposition to the coroner's jury he explained that where her body was retrieved, neither Benner nor any other employee had any business being there, except himself.

Margaret Boyland washed the body of Mary Benner. She found that the left-side shoulder and breast were 'much torn', particularly a large piece of her body beneath the left breast. The verdict of the coroner's jury was death from injuries accidentally inflicted in Mr McGlone's mill in consequence of deceased having gone into a part of the mill where she had no business.[17] This verdict reached by the jury clearly represented the attitude towards workers and employer's liability. Regardless that safety features were not in place, the employer was not considered to be responsible for barricading or using preventative measures for the dangers existing in his mill.

Owner of Ballynacanty Mill Killed by his own Machine
The Death of Thomas Macklin, Carnbane, Drumsnat Parish, January 1860
Thomas Macklin, the owner of Ballynacanty Mill at Carnbane, left his house for the mill on 19 January 1860. He returned home a half-hour later with his left hand holding his right arm and exclaiming, 'Oh Heavenly Father! I'm destroyed!' He took off his sleeved waistcoat and tore open the arm of his shirt, showing his servant, Margaret Smith, where his arm was torn, mangled and shattered from his wrist to near his shoulder. He frantically explained that the accident occurred when he attempted to adjust a strap or band without stopping the mill. His hand was caught and his arm dragged in between two cogwheels. Dr Moorehead attended him immediately and then took the patient to the infirmary to see Dr Young. The injuries to his arm resulted in a great loss of blood and he died three days later.[18]

Another danger in the process of scutching was the dust that came from the breaking of the flax fibres. It is possible that at least one of the deaths recorded was as a result of inhaling too much of the *pouce*, or dust, while working as a scutcher. Twenty-two-year-old Ellen Bready from the neighbourhood of Roslea was hired to scutch in the townland of Listellan with her friend, Ellen McKeon. For a few days she complained of not feeling well, that she had 'a great pain in her head'. She died suddenly on the morning of 4 December 1875. The verdict of death was apoplexy.[19] It is possible that, having been a scutcher for many years, the dust inhaled over time may have played a larger part in her death than described at her inquest. Many mill-workers suffered and ultimately met their fate as a result of lung-related diseases caused by the *pouce* that filled the scutch rooms at the mill.

Children in the Mill

Prior to 1875, children of any age were allowed to work in the mills around the country. The Factory Act of 1874 was the first to determine that the minimum age for child-employees was nine, and that children between the ages of nine and eighteen were allowed to work in the mills, but for *only* ten hours per day.[20] Very often, these children working near dangerous machinery were at risk of losing fingers, arms, legs and even their lives. One young boy named Patrick Mc-Geough received severe injuries to his right arm when it came in contact with a hackle (metal combs used to soften the flax fibres) at the mill at Emyvale. In the same mill, two of the middle fingers of Mary Anne McKenna, aged thirteen, had been torn off by machinery. Luckily for these two children, Mr Young at the county infirmary was able to treat them and save their lives.[21] Not all children were so fortunate.

Arm Ripped from a Seven-Year-Old Boy
The Death of William Bailie, Dunraymond, Kilmore Parish, June 1870
In the following inquest, it is unclear whether seven-year-old William Bailie was working in some capacity at the mill or if he was just on the premises visiting with his father. If he was working, it would have been illegal and, for this reason, it is likely that his purpose for being present is not mentioned in the following inquest explaining the circumstances of his death.

James Bell stood with the rest of the scutchers at the front of the mill at Dunraymond, when William Bailie, an active stirring lad of seven years, went into the scutch mill. Shortly after, a great scream was heard from the little boy upon which all the hands rushed back into the mill to find the cause, the boy's father, John Bailie, among them. As they got to the rear of the machine, James found the boy's tiny arm dragged in between two of the rollers. The boy screamed and shrieked as the rollers were reversed to free him and, when it was done, they could see that the arm had been drawn from the socket and blood was flowing freely. James had the boy in his arms trying to keep his arm near the socket as it was being held to his body by only a small piece of skin.

Dr Reid was called immediately to attend to the boy and John, his father, who in his frenzy to pry his son from the machine, had his own arm drawn in and had broken it a little below the shoulder. Both father and son were taken to the Monaghan infirmary. Little William Bailie lingered from the effects of the accident for three more days until the morning of Wednesday 29 June when he died. The verdict was death on 29 June from the effect of injuries sustained in Dunraymond Scutch Mill on 25 June 1870.[22]

Finishing the Process
When the scutching process was completed, the linen fibres were subjected to increasingly finer combing to clean and sort them by quality, and then to straighten the fibres. The first stages were called roughing; the later stages were called hackling and involved combing the fibres until they were fine enough to be spun. These fibres were then spun into linen. Having been spun and woven, the linen was then bleached at the bleaching mill. There were several bleaching mills in Co. Monaghan, although there are no coroner's reports which mention deaths at these locations. The dried material was then spun into yarn, and the threads woven together to make linen. The linen could then be bleached at a bleaching green or dyed. No deaths were recorded by the coroner during these last phases of the linen-making process.

DANGERS OF CLEANING THE CORN
Dust in the Air Kills

An old agricultural tool called a *riddle* can best be described as a large sieve, with mesh netting over it and a large ring to hold it down. It was used to clean corn and sift flours. One rare inquest records the dangers in the profession of 'riddling'.

Riddling is no Joke: The Death of Peter McKenna
Aghagaw, Tedavnet Parish, March 1860
Mary McKenna told the coroner what had happened in the few days leading to her father's demise. Peter McKenna was a man of about sixty-five years of age and generally very healthy. One Wednesday in March, he had performed the task of cleaning the corn. Later that night, he complained of a pain in his throat which he attributed to the dust from this riddling. The pain continued from day to day and increased in his chest and he believed that his heart was seriously affected. On Friday night at 11p.m. he retired to bed, where he slept with his brother, John. Not much sleeping took place. Peter tossed and turned and was restless throughout the night.

Towards the morning, his daughter, Mary, was alarmed by the strange sound of his strained breathing and arose to light a candle.

She walked towards his bedside and in the candlelight saw her father trying to speak to her, but he was unable to make a sound. Within fifteen minutes, he was dead. The verdict of the inquest was death from internal pain of some days standing, with death coming very suddenly in the end.[23]

DEATH BY DESIGN
Dangerous Structures in Industry

Most textile mills relied on water power for mechanisation. For example, a typical Irish scutch mill was built next to a stream that powered a water wheel, which turned a horizontal shaft with blades attached to it. The stream was diverted by a dam, through an artificial channel called a mill lead or millrace. It was then either sent to a mill pond to fill up before pouring on to the water wheel, or was sent to the wheel directly.[24] There were several deaths recorded by the coroner as 'death by drowning in the millrace'. They were not necessarily a danger to workers during a typical workday, but were a hazard to the public as they were not fenced or marked properly.

Drowning on Main Street in Emyvale: The Death of Thomas McRoberts, Emyvale, Donagh Parish, November 1864
In Emyvale, a millrace running under the bridge and through the centre of town proved fatal for several people in the community. The case of Thomas McRoberts raised issues for the community as others, previously unrecorded, had died as a result of its 'dangerously unprotected state': Edward Connoly (date of death unknown) was found 'lifeless between the mill-wheel and the wall [of the dam]' and John McAllen in 1855 narrowly escaped with his life as the police rescued him before drowning.

James McGurk observed a young boy of two years of age, Thomas McRoberts, while the child was playing in the main street in Emyvale. He kept an eye on the boy as two horses approached, to ensure that no accident occured. The child carefully avoided the animals, yet later word swept through the town that the boy was missing and a search began.

McGurk suddenly recalled that where the millrace passed under the street was a very dangerous place He had heard of several persons falling in; in fact, the last person who did so was carried under the wheel and torn to pieces. With this in mind, he at once feared that the child had fallen in and began searching for him where the millrace falls into the lake. This was the spot where the tiny body of Thomas McRoberts was found.

Several others gave sworn depositions at the coroner's inquest about the dangers posed to the public by the millrace. There were many who had been drowned and others nearly killed because of the hazard. The jury made a note that 'the millrace next to the public street should be made known to the proper authority ... that necessary steps should be taken to guard against future accidents as they consider the deceased's death resulted from said unprotected state of the race.'[25]

Slipping in the Millrace while Delivering a Message
The Death of Mary Tierney, Bellanode, Tedavnet Parish, December 1866
Mrs Sarah Wright sat in her home at Bellanode in the evening on the first day of December 1866 when a servant, Mary Tierney, came with a message for Mr Wright from her master. Mary's sister worked for the Wright family and the two sisters chatted for a bit; after which her sister went to walk her down the road but Mary insisted she would walk back to her own master's home without difficulty.

About two hours after the sisters had parted, Sarah Wright had retired to her bedroom when there was a knock at her bedroom door. As she walked to open the door, she could hear her servant girl in the hallway saying to another person, 'Oh she would go nowhere else'. Alarmed by what she was hearing, Sarah opened the door and discovered that the girl's sister had never made it home that evening. Sarah began to get dressed to go and look for her sister.

A search party was organised to look around the premises and the route between the Wright's home in Bellanode and the house of Mary's master. After a few minutes of searching, they first discovered her shawl and then her body in the millrace which flowed close by the gable of the dwelling-house. When recovered, she was dead.[26]

The Collapse of the Oats Store in Clones
The Deaths of Patrick and Alice Goodwin, Clones Parish, January 1862
Each season, farmers had to take their oat crop to the weighing house (or storehouse) to weigh the oats. This seasonal event was regulated by the landlord and fair prices were not always given. In many instances, there were disagreements between the tenants and the store owner as to a fair price and weighing procedures. In the following inquest, it was stated that such a dispute had broken out when the building itself gave way. Some persons were injured, while Patrick and Alice Goodwin, a mother and son, were killed.[27]

Thomas Brown was the manager of the oats store in Clones where he purchased oats from local farmers and stored them at the house before they were shipped. The building was rented from Dr O'Reilly, a local physician. Thomas Brown explained to the coroner's jury upon their investigation into the deaths that when the accident occurred on 11 January 1862, there were approximately 334 bails in the house, including the 180 he was purchasing from Patrick and Alice Goodwin. He was unconcerned with the amount of weight for the storage house floor since on 11 October 1861, there had been 345 bails in the same store.

Patrick McCabe was in Mr Brown's oat store at the time of the collapse of the building. He was assisting Patrick Goodwin in emptying his oats when some difference arose between Patrick and Mr Brown as to the quality of the oats. This caused a slight delay and, while the two men argued, the loft suddenly gave way and all fell to the floor beneath, about 15 or 16 feet. 'There were five or six people on the loft at the time of the collapse. There was a greater depth of oats where the floor sunk, than at either end of the loft. I consider that the cause of the loft falling,' he stated.

Dr O'Reilly saw a rush of persons into his yard and ran out to see the cause. He saw that the floor of Mr Brown's store had fallen down and a large quantity of oats had fallen to the ground floor beneath; and beneath that, several persons. He saw Pat Goodwin as he was taken out from beneath a quantity of the oats and at that time, to all appearances – dead. His mother, Alice Goodwin, was still alive and Dr O'Reilly attended to her for the next seven days as she had a lacerated wound on one of her thighs from falling off the loft. Her death occurred on 18 January from lockjaw arising from the accident.

At the coroner's inquest held on Patrick and Alice Goodwin, one man, John Irwin, testified that Mr Brown was correct in thinking there was no perceivable danger in the store and that he 'never doubted the strength of the loft'. However, others gave testimony that Mr Brown's oats store was dangerous. George Fitzgerald said he never desired to go into the store heavily loaded as he felt the loft would not bear it. Even the testimony of the owner of the building, Dr O'Reilly, was damning. Although he claimed that he considered the building quite suitable and safe to be used for that purpose, he would not say how much it would be able to carry, nor that he ever considered if Mr Brown was putting too much on it.

The verdict was that the deceased parties came to their deaths on 10 January 1862 from the accidental falling of the store floor on which Patrick Goodwin was emptying his oats. The jury stated that they greatly regretted that Mr Brown, the occupier of the store, had not seen to the greater security of the store before putting so great a quantity of oats in it. And the jury regretted that Mr Brown, or some competent person on his behalf, had not made a proper inspection of the store.

Falling into the Boilers: Accident at the Monaghan Poorhouse
The Death of Ann McDonald, Kilnacloy, Monaghan Parish, June 1872
Inmate Ann McDonald awoke on the morning of 17 May 1872 to perform her duties of washing the clothes of the inmates of the Monaghan poorhouse. She knew exactly what to do as she had been living at the poorhouse since September 1865. Suddenly a violent scream was heard by others who came rushing in to see the cause. Ann had fallen into one of the three boilers, giant vats of boiling water up to her waist, scalding her legs.

Ann Burns, an inmate of the house for eighteen years, heard the wild screams of Ann McDonald and hurried to the boilers. She found Ann standing on the lid of one of the three boilers; having just crawled out of one of them, screaming that she was scalded. The master of the house, Thomas S. Martin, came running in, picked up Ann in his arms and placed her on the table. He ran back into the surgery, took a web of lint and a bottle of limewater and oil and went back to Ann, saturating the lint with the oil, then rolling it over the wounded areas. Mr Martin then had her removed to the infirmary and placed in a bed. He immediately wrote a note to Dr Daniel McClure Ross explaining what had occurred and that his attendance was promptly needed.

When Dr Ross arrived, he found Ann McDonald in excruciating pain with severe scalding on her legs up to her thighs. He asked her how she got into the boiler, but she was so confused and appeared to be in so much pain, she could not tell. A brush was found where the accident occurred and it was now believed she was sweeping the top of the boiler.[28] Over the next few days, he visited with her four or five times a day. About three days after the accident, she developed an inflammation of the lungs from which she recovered; but then an inflammation of the bowels set in, from which she eventually died. Ann McDonald was 38 years old.[29]

THE PERMANENT WAY
The Workers of the Great Northern Railway

Most railway fatalities occurred during the construction of the railroad. Of the twenty-seven inquests reporting railway deaths, fifteen involved employees of the Great Northern Railway.

The employees who worked along 'The Permanent Way' (the railway track and the strip of land it sits on) ranged from general labourers to skilled engineers and each position involved varying degrees of skill and risk. Each jobsite was a flurry of activity: a mixture of men with varying responsibilities most often removing earth, excavating the path for the railway, building bridges and tunnels and laying down new lines of railway. Although *navvies* (workers who travelled far and wide to work the railways) were an available labour source, general labourers were also recruited locally along the lines being built in a particular neighbourhood. Wives and mothers of the employees visited regularly, bringing their husbands and sons their afternoon meals. As described in one inquest, Ann Mooney of Glaslough regularly walked the line to bring her husband and son their meals where they were working.[30]

The fatalities recorded in the coroner's casebook occurred during the construction of the Armagh to Monaghan, Dundalk to Enniskillen and Clones to Cavan lines. The highest number of deaths reported took place during the building of the Armagh to Monaghan line resulting in much criticism from the local paper and the coroners' juries, who were responsible for reporting and evaluating the incompetence of those in charge, although rarely were names of responsible parties provided. Even more rarely was anyone prosecuted.

Other 'employees' of the railway were doctors. There appears to have been such a frequent occurrence of injury and death that Dr William Henry of Clones was sub-contracted by the railway to attend to such cases. In one particular case, when Dr Henry was unavailable, Dr William H. Gillespie of Clones was called upon to attend to a man whose legs had been cut off in a railway accident. He refused to come to the man's aid, declaring that he was tired and that the Ulster Railway refused to pay his bill the last time he attended a wounded man. He was resolved never again to attend a case for them. Edward Molloy died a few hours later.[31]

There were few safety procedures, if any, at the jobsite and, as a result, many men were crushed between or under the wagons and many killed during the blasts of explosives used to carve out the drumlins of the countryside to make way for the tracks. The procedure of using explosives to cut through the landscape dictated a look-out man to be assigned daily. This man assigned to the duty of look-out would yell to alert all the workers before an explosion or accidental fall took place. Very often, unsuspecting workers were buried in the rubble or crushed amid the rush of earth and heavy stone.

Crushed by the Wall of Clay
The Death of Bernard Clarken, Mullaloughan, Donagh Parish, July 1856
Joseph McGuire had just finished his dinner and was back at work on the Armagh to Monaghan railway. He was engaged in filling a cart with large stones when he heard a shout, looked up and saw a man sliding down the face of a cutting where he'd been working. A wall of clay began falling after the man and part of it had struck him on the way down. He could only watch as, while the man was in the act of raising himself up, another lump of clay struck him. All men at hand began running to the aid of the injured. By the time McGuire reached the fallen man, he was already dead. The verdict was death from injuries accidentally sustained when a wall of clay fell on him whilst engaged in working on the Armagh to Monaghan railway.[32]

No Look-Out Man for the Blast
The Death of Michael Crolly, Clones, May 1857
Thomas Hamill worked side by side with Michael Crolly, a stout, healthy young man, as the two helped excavate a site of earth while working on the Dundalk and Enniskillen railway. Thomas left to go to the 'tip head' and, when he returned, saw Michael being carried away to his lodgings in town and so joined in carrying him. He could not determine yet what had happened as Thomas had heard no shout or alarm warning of any blasts or sliding of earth.

Two other workers, Thomas Cunningham and Pat Kelly provided the details of the fatal accident. Some men were in a ravine below ground level, digging to prepare for a blast to bore through the earth. Suddenly they heard a blast and a shower of dirt and rock came crashing down on top of them. A late alarm was raised with one man yelling 'Murder!' but it came too late. The men ran in all directions, but Michael Crolly was the closest to the bank and was caught by the mass of earth and buried under it. Immediately all the men began digging to retrieve their fallen co-worker and Dr Henry was called.

The doctor arrived quickly but when he examined Crolly, he found that he was cold, pulseless and unable to speak. Dr Henry determined that neither his back nor spine had been injured, but that his death resulted from the violent concussion caused by the mass of earth falling on him.

The verdict was death from injuries accidentally sustained by a bank of earth falling on him whilst engaged working on the Dundalk and Enniskillen railway.

Each man that provided information to the coroner's jury stated that at all times when a fall was expected, a person was appointed as a look-out man. On this particular occasion, there doesn't appear to have been a look-out man assigned for the day. The jury was outraged and pointed out that there had been great neglect in not having a man specifically appointed to act as a look-out. Whenever danger might be apprehended in the course of the work on the line in question, one person must be appointed as a look-out man, and for no duty other than that.[33]

Building Bridges: Watch Your Step
The Death of Phillip McManus, Clones, November 1861
During the formation of the junction pile bridge, one man fell to his death. John Tully and Phillip McManus were standing on a stage working a jack screw to force an iron girder of the bridge into its bed. Robert Breen, the working foreman, had instructed both the men to be very cautious and watch that nothing shifted in its place and if it did, to call him. They worked away at reinforcing the girder and McManus finished his turn. An engine passed beneath the stage where the men were working, shaking and agitating the displacement of part of the stage without their knowledge. As McManus went to step down off the stage, he missed his step and fell to the ground – a distance of fourteen feet. He landed on his belly across one of the girders being used at ground level for construction.

Immediately he was placed on an engine and driven into Clones. He was placed in the poorhouse under the care of the medical officer, Dr Henry. The doctor attended him and had him put to bed. The external injuries were minor: a cut over the right eye and a contusion across the stomach. Unfortunately, it was his internal injuries that were fatal. Shortly after his arrival, while in the presence of Dr Henry, McManus vomited 'half full of a basin of blood'. By the next morning, Dr Henry knew it was a hopeless case. The verdict was death from injuries sustained on 15 November 1861 whilst working at the junction bridge being made for the railway from Clones to Cavan.[34]

Follow the Rules
Loading and Unloading Wagons
Although the wages for those working railways were considered ex-
cellent, a high price was paid when mistakes were made. While building the Clones to Cavan railway, a man was killed when the horse he
was riding suddenly fell to its knees catapulting him into the path of
a railway wagon. He was killed instantly.[35] Unfortunately, this was
not the only accident of its kind.

James Butcher, a ganger working on the stretch of railway being
constructed near Clones for the Dundalk and Enniskillen railway, made
clear the rules for filling and emptying wagons to avoid accidents. He
provided this information at the inquest of Felix McCabe, a member
of his gang who was killed.

James told the coroner and jury, 'The rule is that a full wagon is
followed out of the cutting on foot by those engaged in filling it, it
being narrow indeed. They then push an empty one to be filled.' He
went on to explain the mistake McCabe made that resulted in his
death. 'The deceased jumped up on the full wagon, lost his balance,
staggered and fell back on the coupling chain of the next wagon. He
then fell to the ground and the succeeding wagon passed over his
body – over his right thigh and down his right arm,' he said.[36]

Killed by his own Wagon: The Death of William Keefe
Monaghan, Monaghan Parish, February 1857
William Keefe had been working for the railway for several months
loading and unloading wagons on the Armagh and Monaghan railway
near Monaghan town. On Wednesday, 11 February 1857, while having
his wagon emptied of earth and rock, he began unhooking his mare.
Suddenly, while in the act of taking her off the line, William stumbl-
ed and fell and his wagon passed over his body. He had fallen on his
face, the rails were between his legs and the wagon crushed his back
parts, his thighs and hinds. A priest was immediately called as death
was anticipated. William died at the Monaghan infirmary a few hours
later that evening.[37]

Spraying the Wagons: The Death of John Linch,
Cladowen, Clones Parish, August 1857
John Linch was in charge of 'spraying the wagons', which involved
stopping wagons by thrusting a stick between the wheel spikes. He
had been carefully attending to his duties all day when, just at the
end of the working day, while attempting to stop some loaded wagons,
he missed his footing. The result was fatal. The wagon passed over the

lower part of his body through his midsection. His father, who was present, cradled John in his arms but he died. The verdict was death from injuries sustained on the Dundalk and Enniskillen railway from a loaded wagon passing over his body.[38]

Opening the Gates to the Train, Closing the Gates of Life
To manage the trains coming and going and to ensure each part of the track was safe, policemen or 'signalmen', and gatekeepers were assign-ed to sections of a route. Safety in the early days was largely in the hands of policemen, who operated along a 'beat' and had their own line-side 'sentry boxes' which are shown on the early Ordnance Survey maps.[39] These men would operate signals at each section along a track and were responsible for the points which changed the tracks the trains ran upon. The signalling system was in place to avoid train collisions and injury to persons. In the early days of steam, signalling was carried out by railway policemen using a form of semaphore with either simple hand and arm signals or with flags, while at night, candle lamps were used.[40]

Gatekeepers were similarly equipped. Expert Mark Kennedy of the Ulster Folk and Transport Museum explains the role of the gate-keeper. 'The gatekeeper was a lesser job than signalman whereby a man was stationed at a small or little used road. Responsibilities in-cluded making sure the gates were closed to the roadside when the train was passing through, to ensure the safety of the public. A gate-keeper was often a retired railway man or even widow who might be given a cottage to live in next to the railway at preferential rates.'

In Co. Monaghan, when a cottage was not provided for the gate-keepers, it appears that they were provided with accommodation with a local family and a small sentry box for them to sit in while they waited to open and close the gates.

Kennedy says that gates were used as a safety measure to avoid public access, particularly at a level crossing. Level crossings meant easy access for persons and animals to cross and extra precautions often needed to be taken to prevent them from being struck by a train. Gate-keepers might be responsible for some forms of signalling such as keep-ing a lamp lit at his station post. The dangers of the job appear to have occurred when the gatekeeper, like many other railway employees, lost track of time or became careless in crossing the tracks as trains were passing, as the following inquests will show.

No Signal at the Crossing: The Gatekeeper is Missing
The Death of William Heartly, Srananny, Donagh Parish, November 1858
The train was travelling at a comfortable eighteen miles per hour on
a particularly dark and foggy morning and was due to arrive at Glaslough station at 8.40a.m. As Charles Aspinell, the driver of the morning train, began to make his approach and reached Scots Crossing,
he could see through the blanket of grey mist that the gate had not
been opened for his passing. Using every ounce of exertion, Aspinell
began to reduce the speed of the train immediately and sounded the
whistle to those ahead. Just moments later, when only fifty feet from
the gate, he could see that a man had opened the gate but was still
quite close to it. As the train passed, its speed had been reduced to
about nine miles per hour, but the buffer of the engine struck the man
standing next to the gate, knocking him down. Aspinell saw that the
train had not passed over him and held out hope that he might survive the collision.

When the train finally stopped, Aspinell and the guard on the
train, Isaac Walker, ran back to the gate. Samuel Eivers, the gatekeeper, was kneeling down next to the injured man, William Heartly,
who lived in the house right across from the station

One woman, Eliza Clarke, was able to explain what had happened before the train arrived. She had walked down the line that morning to bring breakfast to her husband, who worked on the railway,
when she noticed that the gate was closed. About ten perches after
passing it, she heard the whistle of an approaching train. She immediately set down the tins with the breakfast and began running back to
open the gate, fearing an accident would occur. While running, she
saw the gatekeeper, Samuel Eivers, and William Heartly running towards the gate as well. It was clear that Heartly would reach it the
gate first, so she stopped running. After the train had passed the gate
and stopped, she saw Heartly lying doubled-up and raised the alarm.
She did not actually see the accident happen since they were on different sides of the line and the train was between them. After the
crowd gathered around Heartly she turned to Eivers, the gatekeeper,
and asked him why he had not been at his post. He replied that he
had been ill all night. She felt he was telling the truth as he looked
ill when she saw him.

The day before the accident, Samuel Eivers was sent from Belfast
to Glaslough, to report to the station-master, James Laverry. Laverry
told Eivers he would be working at Scots Crossing and would take up
duty immediately. Daniel Donaghue, the porter of the gate, explained

the duties to Eivers and the times that the train would pass. Donaghue advised Eivers that he should leave the gate open a few minutes before the train's approach and that he should take up lodgings at the house of William Heartly. Heartly lived right across the track near Scots Crossing.

On his first shift as the new gatekeeper, Eivers was ill. A little past 6a.m., George Scott was walking past the gateman's box, saw the door open and on looking in, saw him lying across it. Scott put his head in and asked if he was sleeping. Eivers replied no, he wasn't sleeping, but was very sick and had been all night long. Scott offered him a cup of tea but the man insisted that he was too ill to take it. He left the gatekeeper, feeling sorry for him as did not look well at all.

Just a short while later, Eivers arrived at the house of William and Eliza Jane Heartly. He was very sick and had walked back to their home to get warm by the fire. The next train would be arriving in about a half-hour. While there, he spoke with the couple and their friend, Ally Mahony. Unfortunately, as luck would have it, the clock in the Heartly's home was fifteen minutes slow. All parties froze when they heard the first whistle of the train. They'd lost track of time. Eivers jumped to his feet, headed for the door and began running at full speed for the gatehouse. William Heartly, who had just left the house to get some turf for the fire, began racing to the gatehouse with a head start on Eivers. Heartly was the first to arrive at the gatehouse and he began opening the gate.

Heartly's wife watched from the yard of her house as the men began running to the gate. She saw her husband opening the gates for the approaching train and then watched the train pass. After it had gone by, she then saw her husband on the ground with Eivers standing over him.

When Dr McKinstry attended him, he found him 'pulseless and in a dying state'. He remained with his patient for an hour and used restoratives to revive him. They worked but the effect was only temporary. William Heartly died just three hours after the accident.

Samuel Eivers was arrested and an inquest was held by the coroner. Dr McKinstry performed the post-mortem examination and found no marks of injury on the body, except for two small wounds on the top of the head. He concluded that the cause of death was the shock to the nervous system of having been knocked down with great force by some object (the gate) coming violently against him. The verdict of the coroner's jury was that William Heartly came to his death on 10 November 1858 from injuries sustained whilst opening the gate at

Scotts Crossing on the Ulster Railway for an approaching train. He died in consequence of the absence of the gatekeeper, Samuel Eivers. Eivers had been ill the night before and that morning, and had gone to the house of deceased Heartly to warm himself. They also concluded that the clock in Heartly's house was fifteen minutes slow of regular time.

The coroner also recorded an addendum made by the jury. The jury desired to say that some accommodation for the warmth and comfort of the gatekeepers should be provided in their box as the absence of such led to Samuel Eivers leaving his post and the present painful circumstance.[41]

Confusion in Clones: The Gatekeeper is Killed
The Death of Edward Keely, Clones, October 1868
Edward Keely, a gatekeeper with the Irish Northern Railway, was responsible for the gates at the level-crossing in Clones at Pound Hill and Fermanagh Street. On 31 October 1868, he opened a gate to let carts go through towards Pound Hill and then began shutting the gate for the coming train which could be heard in the distance.

A child of about eleven years old, Agnes Ann Rock, was coming from a house on the hill and walking across the railway line as a short-cut. As she approached the Pound Hill railway crossing, she noticed that the lamp at the gate was not lit. Shortly after, she saw the old gatekeeper open a gate to let the horses and carts through. He then shut the Pound Hill gate first, then the other, as he was expecting the train to arrive. He then walked towards the signals with a lamp in his hand, but before he reached them, the train struck him as it was going towards the station house. The whistle then shrieked through the air alerting all of an accident.

Ann Sheenan had also watched the gatekeeper opening and then shutting the gates for the oncoming train. She could see the train approaching and when it grew nearer, she heard a man on the train call out, 'Ned! Stand to one side!' The gatekeeper, with a lit lamp in his hand, was going towards the far side, but before he had jumped off the line, one of the railway cars knocked him down. The entire train passed over his body.

The gatekeeper lay on the ground and Ann Sheenan ran towards the limp and fallen body. She heard him say 'Will no person lift me?' and then the eyes turned in his head. Mary Reilly, another witness who heard the old man calling out for help after the train passed over him, claims to have heard him say, 'Oh! I'm done for! Will no one come to my relief?' He died within moments after the accident.

The authorities were alerted and Dr O'Reilly was called to examine the body of the dead man. He found his left thigh almost torn off and smashed to pieces and the right leg, a little above the ankle, was crushed as well. There was a wound on the left side of the hindquarters where all the skin was torn off and hanging. All these wounds were sufficient to cause his death.

An inquest was held by the coroner and many witnesses were called to give information. Most gave depositions that exposed the great inconvenience and danger arising to the public in consequence of a level-crossing being at the foot of Pound Hill and Fermanagh Street, instead of a bridge. The coroner also concluded from the information provided, that the railway officials were to be exonerated from any blame with respect to Keely's death. It arose from his own imprudence in crossing the rails while the train was in motion. The jury's verdict was that death occurred when the gatekeeper, Edward Keely, was struck accidentally by an Ulster train on the railway while he was discharging his duties of attending to closing the gates of the level-crossing at Pound Hill in Clones. The deceased was sixty-five years of age. The jury further stated that they were of the opinion that no one man could faithfully discharge the duties required at those gates with safety to himself and the public. They strongly recommended that something be done immediately to rid the public of this level-crossing which was a 'perfect nuisance'.[42]

Public Access to the Lines: The Deaths of Pedestrians
An engine-driver was a highly qualified professional who, along with his other responsibilities, worked with a fireman. This driver/fireman team was known as the footplate staff. While one drove, the other fed coal to the engine. Like the driver, the fireman was highly skilled. They had to watch that the engine had the correct steam-pressure for the load, gradient and speed the engine had to travel. Many men started work as cleaners and served long enough to rise to the grade of fireman and then driver. Footplate staff were among the best paid of all railway workers.[43] The driver, besides making sure the engine was working properly, used his experience and knowledge to run the train according to the working timetable, and kept a look out for dangers on the track ahead. Although the driver relied upon the system of signalmen, permanent way gangs and gatekeepers, to ensure the safety of the track, dangers did lurk day and night as people of the countryside would often jump the many fences and gates along the route for their continual convenience in travelling.

Yet, there was danger involved for drivers and firemen. One particular example of these risks is illustrated in the case of John Finegan, a young fireman working on Engine No 12 of the Clones to Cavan railway.[44] Having been supplied with coal and water, the engine was being pushed back into the shed by another engine, where it was to remain until the morning. When the engine had been pushed back far enough, he got between the buffers to unloosen the couplings when his foot slipped and he fell across the rails. Another engine, which was still moving, passed over him and he was killed instantly.[45]

Most accidents involving drivers did not involve injury to the driver himself, but to members of the public and 'pedestrians' illegally walking the railways. It was a continuing problem often captured in the news of the day. There were fatal outcomes for many who took the risk of walking along the lines.

The Respectable Young Countryman
The Death of William Heazlett, Billis, Donagh Parish, July 1866

William Heazlett left Monaghan town at 1 o'clock in the morning, saying goodnight to the night-watchman of the railway and telling him that he would walk home by the railway line. The night-watchman warned Heazlett against walking on the lines as it was dangerous, explaining that he might come in contact with some of the trains passing through. Heazlett reassured the man, telling him that he frequently met trains and there was no danger. Heazlett, a respectable young countryman, went about his way and the watchman felt that he was sufficiently sober to be able to take care of himself.

A short while later, on the approach of the early luggage-train from Belfast to Monaghan, the driver of the train observed the figure of a man lying on the rails at the bridge under the seminary and immediately put on the brake. When he found the body of Heazlett, it appeared to have been dead from some time. The mail-train from Belfast had passed some hours previously and he believed it might have been the cause of the man's death.

Upon reaching Clones, the guard of the luggage-train mentioned the circumstance to the guard and driver of the mail-train, but they both insisted that they did not experience any obstruction at the seminary bridge. They all went to inspect the mail-train and found evidence to prove they were mistaken. Stuck to the front of the engine were blood and fragments of human flesh. It was clear that poor Heazlett was hit and killed upon impact.

Heazlett's body was taken to Monaghan town where the inquest was held. Mr Swain, the general manager of the railway, attended and brought with him the guards and drivers of the two trains. Daniel Rock, a guard on the Ulster Railway, told the jury that he saw nothing on the line nor was he aware of having come in contact with any object whatsoever.

James Brown, a guard on the 11p.m. train from Belfast told the jury, 'We were due at Monaghan at 4.15a.m. and when beneath the seminary, I was signalled to put on the brake, which I did – but 'ere we had passed over the body of a man. I at once got down and diagnosed the body … evidently he had been there for some time as I found clots of blood on the planking bridge.' He continued, 'The train proceeded on to Monaghan whilst I and the assistant brakesman remained with the body till the police came to us. When I got to Clones, I examined the wheels of the train which had preceded mine and on the guard in front of the wheels, I found both flesh and blood.'

Brown told the jury that when he mentioned the occurrence to the driver of the train, he seemed much astonished, being quite ignorant of having come in contact with any person or thing on the line.

The jury returned the verdict of death which occurred at the Blackwater Railway Bridge, near the seminary, by the mail-train due at Monaghan at 2.55a.m. having passed over his body. William Heazlett was aged 35 years.[46] They added that the Ulster Railway Authorities should enforce more stringently the act of parliament prohibiting trespassers on the rail. Further editorial comment was added in an article published in *The Northern Standard*:

> We are informed that it is quite a habit with the peasantry residing between Monaghan and Glaslough and near the railway to use it as their road to and from the town. This is a most dangerous practice and we trust the sad example set in the death of poor Heazlett will prevent a recurrence of what is a trespass on the railway. We think it right to observe that there is but one place on the line where people can get off the high road on to the line – that is the old temporary station, where the line is close to and on a level with the road. A temporary wire fence was put up, but it has been broken down. The Railway Company should make such a fence here – say a strong high wall, which would effectually prevent trespassers going on the line.[47]

Dying to Save a Cow
The Death of Thomas Woods, Drumhirk, Aghabog Parish, May 1869

An accident occurred about two miles away from the Newbliss railway station, on the Dundalk side, on 5 May 1869. A young boy of fourteen years of age, Thomas Woods, was working for Mr James McCleary, a cattle herder, whose land ran on both sides of the Irish North-West-

ern Railway. Thomas and his father, John, had been living and working for Mr McCleary for over a year. On the day in question, the boy
was tending the cows when one got over the railway fence and, being
afraid that she might be killed by the train, he tried to turn her off
the line.[48]

The 4.20p.m. train from Dundalk was heading his way. At the
34-mile post, the driver, Thomas Glover, saw the boy trying to turn
a cow off the line. The boy came from the hedge and, in trying to get
the cow off the rails, he got too close. Glover immediately sounded
the whistle three times which signalled to his guard, Joseph Gille-
land, to put on the brake. Glover told the coroner's jury, 'When the
buffer struck the boy on the back, as quick as possible I stopped the
train and then returned to see about the lad. He was living and I lifted him on the train to bring him to Newbliss station. By the time we
were there, he was dead.'

Matilda Wright was on the railway bridge and saw the entire
accident. She saw the boy struggling to get the cow off the line. After
the train passed, she saw it stop and heard someone say, 'Whomever
owns that child – he is killed.'

Thomas was put in a first-class carriage with immediate medical
aid. Unfortunately, he was too badly injured and died in the six-min-
ute journey to Newbliss station. The verdict was 'death on 5 May
1869, being accidentally killed by a passing railway train whilst turning a cow off the line which had broken over where the fence was
insufficient. Aged 14 years.'[49]

CASUALTIES DURING CONSTRUCTION
Monaghan Cathedral

The construction of St Macartan's cathedral in Monaghan town began in 1862 and many skilled workers in the county were employed
including stonecutters, carpenters and other craftsmen. The cathedral, which still sits high upon the hill overlooking Monaghan town,
symbolised not only the resurgence of Catholicism in the nineteenth
century, but some of the hard-working men from that time, who donated not only their talents but their lives towards its construction.

Failures of the Heart
Death Strikes Workers at the Cathedral
In November 1862, George Alford was a mason employed in the
building of the new cathedral. On 13 November, George was at his

work beside his co-worker, Dan O'Neill, and both were working under the supervision of John Farrell, the overseer of the building of the cathedral. Dan asked George to fetch him some boards. George obliged but when he rose up, he suddenly exclaimed, 'O Dan! O Dan!' and then fell into his arms. Dan O'Neill said that 'after that he was insensible and never spoke again.' The Revd Fr Gillen gave the last rites of the church to the dying man and, by the time Dr Rush arrived, George Alford had died. He was prone to chest pains and was being treated for palpitations of the heart. On his person were found an order of the Royal Bank of Ireland for £1.5.0, a second one for £5, £4 in cash and the key of his trunk. These were taken from him by John Farrell who went to where the deceased lived with a Mr Treanor and found a further £29. Farrell lodged £31.9.0 into the Ulster Bank of Monaghan and used the rest for the funeral and other expenses. He also wrote to Alford's next of kin 'apprising him of the event and requesting his presence'. George Alford died as a result of disease of the heart.[50]

Another man working at the cathedral died as a result of heart disease. John Kane was 32 years of age and married and was working as a stonecutter. A barrowman at the new cathedral, John McKeown, worked with Kane and often observed him change colour from red to blue. Having finished work on 7 February 1867, the two men were in town together and in good spirits, chatting cheerfully. Kane stated he had to go home for dinner. His wife, Margaret Kane, sat down with her husband and poured the evening tea, her husband, apparently, being in good health after his day at work; until half an hour later when he dropped dead on the floor.[51]

Don't Blame the Scaffolding: Death at the Cathedral
The Death of John Mehaffy and John McQuillen, Monaghan, March 1875
Although heart disease took the lives of the mason and the stonecutter, eight years later the scaffolding took the lives of two more. On 19 March 1875, at about 12.45p.m., carpenters John Mehaffy and John McQuillen were working close together on a scaffold near the roof of the church at a height of 70 feet from the ground. Charles Whelan, superintendent of the works at the cathedral, watched from below.

Mahaffy was engaged in driving home a bolt with a sledge-hammer when the 'footlock' (which measured four inches by three inches) broke in the centre and the men began to fall through the air to a pile of rafters on the floor below. Whelan watched as sixteen-year-old McQuillen fell straight onto his head and was killed instantly;[52] John

Mehaffy was not as fortunate. He hit the timber and his body re-bounded, landing about three feet from where he first landed.[53] He appeared to be in extreme pain and was taken instantly to the infirmary. Mehaffy died just five minutes after his admission to the infirmary. He was 46 years old. The two men had fallen from the north side of the cathedral at the nave near the transept.

The inquests that followed were long and detailed as the coroner appeared to be interested in uncovering the state of the scaffolds upon which the two were working, suspended at the top of the cathedral. Another worker, James Byrne, narrowly escaped death by jumping to another plank of timber as the scaffold gave way. There was nothing to the unprofessional eye to show the awful and sudden manner in which they came to their end.[54]

The newspaper stated that the cathedral was at that time eleven years in the building and that was the first 'accident' that had occurred in it. Mahaffy was a native of Keady and left a wife and four children at the time of his death. McQuillan was only 16 years old and was 'the only son of his mother and she is a widow'. The Northern Standard tried to raise a subscription for the affected families of the deceased men and donated £2 to get the fund started. They commented that they 'are certain the people of Monaghan and its vicinity will respond liberally to any appeal made to them under such circumstances.'[55]

The Stonecutter Falls
The Death of Thomas Cunningham, Monaghan, November 1875
Another man, Thomas Cunningham, a stonecutter, fell to his death at the new cathedral just several months after the first accident. James Connolly, a co-worker of the deceased, revealed the details of the accident that occurred on the evening of 22 November 1875: 'We were descending from the roof; I was by the turret stairs, he by the treacle rope. I was lowering him when he called to me to hold hard and again to slack and then that his hand was caught – at which point he immediately fell to the ground (about thirty feet). I ran to him and raised him up and asked him where he was hurt. He said, "My back". Thomas was taken to the infirmary immediately.'[56]

Surgeon Young was present when Thomas was brought into the county infirmary. 'He was suffering from a violent concussion of the brain and spine,' he said. 'He lived till the afternoon of the 30th. His death was a result of the injuries received from the fall.' The verdict was death from injuries accidentally sustained 'which was the result of his own want of caution in attempting to descend by a rope instead of the winding stairs.'[57]

Thomas left behind a wife and one infant child. Money was collected for the family, as stated in the following article which appeared in *The Northern Standard* after his death.

Friday 10 December 1875
Our readers will be glad to observe from the list published in another column that a sum of money is being collected for the Widow of Cunningham who was killed at the new Cathedral. This woman has been left penniless with one infant child; and without any means of support whatever. Any sum that may be raised will go but a short way to make up the irreparable loss she has sustained and the committee hope that those who have not yet contributed towards this fund, will be good enough to forward their subscriptions to the treasurer Mr Peter McCulloch, in time to be acknowledged in next issue of *The Northern Standard*. To the charitably disposed in this town and neighbourhood, it is unnecessary to say more. They are a numerous class and ever ready to contribute where suffering and distress exists.

Beware for whom the Bell Tolls: The Death of James McGaghey, Gortnana, Killeevan Parish, December 1857
On Christmas Eve in 1857, James McGaghey and Mick Boyle were just two of many men working late to raise and hang the bell of the chapel of Cure in Killeevan in time to ring it out on the holidays for the pleasure of all the parishioners and those throughout the countryside. After the bell had been raised and securely fixed to its position about thirty-four feet high, all those participating in its construction began repeatedly ringing the bell. Delighted with the task accomplished, James McGaghey desired everyone there to go to the altar and offer a prayer.

After the prayers, the workers immediately returned to the belfry and recommenced ringing the bell, while James and Mick stayed on the ground enjoying the festive evening and the delight of having finished the task. About ten minutes later, the bell stopped ringing and fell to the ground, landing on the head of James McGaghey.

James was immediately lifted up and attended to by the parish priest and Dr O'Reilly, but the injuries were so serious that he died about seven hours later. His skull was pushed out through to the brain from front to the back of his head. Of those present, only one could offer some explanation of what had gone wrong. James Murphy stated, 'I cannot possibly account for the accident unless the violent ringing of some of the parties caused it to swing over so to get it out of its bed or position and so it came down.'

The coroner's verdict was death from the accidental falling of a large bell on the head of the deceased in the belfry of Cure Chapel.[58]

FALLING FROM A HEIGHT
Roofs, Scaffolding and Trees

Impaled on the Hill
The Death of John Treanor, Monaghan Town, January 1872
People in the neighbourhood of the hill in the town of Monaghan, were much alarmed on Friday morning, 23 January, 1872, as a crowd gathered to watch a man, John Treanor, as he lay asleep on the roof of one of the highest buildings in town – Mr Thomas Wright's office. Treanor, at sixty-eight years of age, was employed to repair the slate roof but he had imbibed an extra quantity of liquor either the evening before or prior to coming to work. While he was attempting to perform his work repairing the tiling of the roof, sleep overcame him and he lay unconscious some sixty feet above the ground. There was a great excitement and intensity amongst the onlookers as they expected him to roll off the roof at every instant. After a considerable amount of time, two men named Carson and Talbot, at imminent risk of their own lives, ventured to take him down. It was reported, 'It was no easy task, but they were successful after some time in saving this man from what in all human probability must have resulted in an untimely death. We hope it will be a lesson not only to him, but to others who habitually make beasts of themselves in this way.'[59] This story was reported in the morning before the rest of the tale unfolded.

After the crowd dispersed, John Treanor, while still unfit to work, climbed back onto the roof. A woman named Leticia Henderson was standing at Mrs Hanna's door across the street observing Treanor on the building above. She watched him tie himself to the roof with a rope. As he moved his position on the ladder, it suddenly came tumbling down and Treanor along with it. William Grimly was also standing in front of Mr Wright's office when he heard a noise as if something were falling. He looked up, saw a ladder coming down and at the same time he saw a man lying across the iron fence – impaled by the railing spikes through the bowels, chest and right arm. Both Grimly and Henderson, shocked by the gruesome accident, immediately ran to assist in lifting Treanor off the spikes. He was still alive. He was taken to the dispensary and treated at the infirmary, where he was seen by the doctor, A. K. Young, Esq., Dr Young stated, 'Upon seeing Treanor,

I'd say he had about the full of a slop bowl of his bowels hanging out. I put them back through a wound between the navel and lower part of the belly that was about five inches long. Higher up on his right side there was a large portion of skin torn from the right arm and elbow and another wound in the chest that evidently entered the lungs, breaking several ribs.' Dr Young, Dr Temple and the Revd E. Gillen, parish priest of Killeevan, visited the man throughout the day. Having lingered for eleven hours, John Treanor died.[60]

Hilton Park Heartbreak: Man Falls to his Death
The Death of William Smith, Hilton Park, Currin Parish, December 1873
William Smith was high up on the scaffolding at Hilton Park, the residence of John Madden, Esq., for the purpose of cutting some branches off a tree that was interfering with some of the work going on. He had cut off one bunch of branches and, when moving to another branch to secure his footing, while simultaneously trying to cut, the branch gave way with his weight and he fell to the ground.

James McDermot, William Walker and John Lamp were working with Smith doing their own jobs nearby. McDermot had been yelling at Smith to be more careful, that he was 'running a great risk in the way he was carrying on with it' but Smith continued. When the branch snapped, all the men looked up to see Smith falling through the air. He landed at the feet of McDermot who at once raised him up, but he was already dead.

The verdict of the inquest was the deceased came to his death on 8 December 1873 from falling accidentally from a scaffold where he had been working at the residence of John Madden, Esq., at Hilton Park. The jury made a point to add a comment: that the said scaffold was built with great attention to the safety of the men at work and that no blame attached to any person whatsoever. William Smith was 30 years of age.[61]

Whose Fault was it? Jonathan Fleming vs the Dead Man –
An Accident at the Monaghan Courthouse
The Death of John Hetherington, Monaghan, March 1862
Thirty-five men employed by the contractors John Hetherington and Jonathan Fleming, were employed in cleaning and painting the outside of the Monaghan courthouse and the ceilings of the Crown and Record Courts within. On 22 March 1862, while all the men were 35 feet above the ground on the scaffolding, performing their duties, there was suddenly a loud crash – the scaffolding had broken and all

debris and bodies came falling to the ground below. Many escaped injury, however several were hurt: George Thompson, aged sixty-two, had his thigh-bone broken and his elbow dislocated; George Farrell escaped with some injury to his spine; a man named Hill had just left the scaffolding and had his feet on the upper steps of a ladder which rested on the gallery. The impact of the crash caused him to lose his hold and he fell on the gallery, but escaped with slight injuries. There was one fatality, John Hetherington, a respected and industrous young man, aged 25, originally from Clones. He was the man in charge of the crew that day and coincidentally, the man being accused of erecting the defunct scaffolding. It appeared that he fell on his back onto the iron railing that separated the outer court from the inner court on the ground below. He was carried to the county hospital and died only a few minutes later from a dislocation of his vertebrae.[62]

Almost immediately following the accident, the responsibility for the poorly-constructed scaffolding was being debated. The story was covered in the The Northern Standard. Along with the details of the accident was the following statement:

> We cannot close our notice of this melancholy accident without expressing our disapprobation of the careless, unsafe and unskilful manner in which the scaffolding, on the stability of which so may lives depended, was erected. The material was evidently too slight, the space over which the transverse planks rested too distant one from the other, and the material of the worst description. We only wonder at the recklessness of the men who ventured upon it.[63]

The coroner held an inquest later on that same day. The testimony of only two men was recorded; the first was the account of George Hill. He had been hired by John Hetherington to assist him in the painting of the Monaghan courthouse for which scaffolding had to be erected in the Crown and Record Courts. When George joined the work, the scaffolding had been erected. He then stated, 'When I saw it, I objected to it as too slight. He considered it sufficient and the workmen ascended to the scaffold, but scarcely were they on it when with a loud crash, it broke and all came down to the flagging below – a height of about 35 feet.'[64]

Jonathan Fleming, Hetherington's partner, explained that the erecting of the scaffolding was left entirely to the deceased as no one was allowed to interfere with him in doing so.

In that week's The Northern Standard, a letter written by Jonathan Fleming was published, in which he defended himself from apparent gossip in town that he alone was responsible for the scaffolding, the injuries to the men working for him and the death of his partner, Hetherington. He gave his deepest sympathies about the death of his partner, as well as the injuries to the men, but stated that he was in Armagh at the time of the accident and that he had nothing to do with the construction of the scaffolding other than buying poles and planks and bringing them to the building site.

> I was grieved to heart to hear, when I came home, that some malicious minded storyteller had circulated that it was I had put up the insufficient scaffolding, and thereby caused his death. It is a grievous thing to be charged with any crime, even though guilty; but how much more so when one is innocent. I think I need scarcely say that I am innocent of the charge ... I was totally exonerated from having anything to do with it ... I got poles and planks at Hetherington's request, and he got some himself. I spoke to two men of experience to assist in putting up the scaffolding but when they came, Mr Hetherington, and the men that were to work on it, had it nearly erected, and it was all done under his own superintendence. These men remarked that the timber for the ledges was light, and I advised him to get more planks, and tie two together and have it strong; he said there was not occasion for them, as it would bear a ton of weight, which unfortunately for him wasn't the case.[65]

Additionally, the foreman of the jury in the coroner's inquest, Thomas Little, wrote in to confirm that Fleming was free from any blame or negligence. He explained that it was the testimony of George Hill which exonerated him; that Hetherington alone was responsible for the erection of the scaffolding.

None of the other workers was asked or came forward with any testimony. According to the local paper, Jonathan Fleming had been cleared in the court of public opinion.

Felling Trees: Crushed by the Giants in the Forest
The Death of John Kerr

The trees that stand at Rossmore Park today are large and impressive. One hundred and twenty-five years ago trees similar in size were removed from Lord Rossmore's estate for the purposes of clearing the land, using the wood either to built other structures or as firewood. The following is a case in which one of the men working for the estate was killed when such a tree was cut down.

John Kerr was employed in the service of Lord Rossmore as the keeper of the gatehouse at the entrance to the farmyard. On 20 November 1875, Kerr was working along with others felling trees on the Rossmore estate. One tree had been cut and, being near falling, several hands were pulling it in the proper direction with a rope, so as to direct its fall. Although the men were pulling the tree in the desired direction, it began falling in a contrary position. The overseer began crying out to leave the way but before John Kerr could move, the tree fell upon him and crushed him beneath its weight.[66] James Sharhen and Peter Murphy were two of the men present who helped in bringing John Kerr to the Monaghan infirmary to be seen by Surgeon Young. Dr Young found Kerr in a dying state; he was suffering from a severe concussion, his left shoulder was dislocated and broken, and there was a slight wound on the forehead. He remained alive for only about an hour after the accident.[67]

There was great public sympathy for the thirty-three-year-old man who left behind a pregnant wife and young child. A letter sent to the editor of the newspaper very clearly explains the impact of Kerr's death on his family:

The Northern Standard, Friday, 17 December 1875
To the Editor
Dear Sir – while I have no wish to depreciate the praiseworthy efforts made to raise some money for the widow of Cunningham who was killed at the cathedral [inquest no.18.1154], I cannot but express the surprise of many of your readers that a collection has not yet been started for the widow of the man killed previously at Rossmore Park. Mrs Kerr is in my opinion by far the greater charity of the two. She is all but blind; has one young child and expects to be shortly confined again. She is totally unable to work and owing to the loss of her eyesight cannot contribute towards her own and her child's support in any way. I am certain that this matter needs only to be mentioned to be responded to with liberality which is so characteristic of the Monaghan people. I contributed towards the Cunningham fund and will be happy to subscribe according to my means towards a fund for the benefit of Mrs Kerr.
Your obedient servant
A sympathiser.[68]

GOING TO MARKET
Fair-days in Monaghan

Fair-days brought people from all over the vicinity and sometimes farther off to trade their wares, sell livestock, pick up supplies as well as socialise. Very often, accidents and fatalities occurred on fair-days primarily owing to the nature of the condensed close space of man and animal or man and machinery, although ignorance contributed to many injuries and deaths. Drink was also a contributing factor to death on fair-days – especially later on in the evening.

No Respect for the Living – or the Dead
The Death of James Duffy, Monaghan Town, January 1873
Patrick Mitchell was in Ballybay on the day of the fair with two
heifers which he sold early in the day. The buyer, James Duffy of Lis-
nashannagh, now wanted to handle them but one of the animals
would not stand for him. The more he tried to the manoeuvre the
animal, the more it shifted and eventually it broke free and began
trotting up the road. Duffy quickly began chasing the heifer. In the
distance, as he ran behind the cow, he could see a man up ahead who
was standing right in the line of the animal. As the cow and Duffy
approached, the man quickly pushed the cow's hips away from him –
the cow's hips swung back, hit Duffy and knocked him to the ground.
Mitchell and another man present, Thomas Meighan, assisted in lifting Duffy and carried him to Dr Adamson to have his leg set. He was
later taken down to Monaghan Infirmary.

Surgeon Young of the Monaghan infirmary found James Duffy
suffering from a compound fracture of the right leg and other wounds
of the same limb caused by the trampling of a bull or heifer. James
Duffy was admitted and was doing well, until a few days later when
his state of mind changed. The infection in his leg caused swelling
and inflammation and he began raving from erysipelas (a contagious
disease of the skin due to strep) and then mortification (gangrene).
Duffy died on the morning of 22 January 1873. Upon the conclusion
of the coroner's inquest, the verdict was 'James Duffy came to his
death from injuries accidentally caused in Ballybay fair from being
thrown down by a young passing heifer. Aged 65 years.'[69]

Unfortunately, the story of James Duffy didn't end here. *The Northern Standard* ran a short story that same week stating the facts of the
case, but with great insensitivity to the death of James Duffy and his
grieving friends and family, they poked fun at the wording used in the
description of the verdict. It appeared as follows:

Fatal Accident
On Saturday last, a man named James Duffy, of Lisnashanna, when going
through the fair of Ballybay, was knocked down and trampled upon by a
heifer, when extricated it was found that the unfortunate man had received
a compound fracture of the right leg and the bones were protruding through
the skin. He was the same evening brought into the County Infirmary where
his injuries were at once attended to by the House Surgeon. He lingered
until the following Wednesday morning when he expired. An inquest was
held on his remains on Thursday when the following peculiar verdict was
returned: 'James Duffy came to his death on Wednesday the 22nd day of
January, 1873 from injuries accidentally caused in Ballybay fair from being

thrown by a young passing heifer aged 65 years.' We do not think a heifer aged 65 years should be designated 'young'.

Clearly upset by the joke made, someone, presumably a juror in the case, took offence at the article, not so much at the disrespect for the dead man, James Duffy, but because of the implication that the jury concluded the verdict in the incorrect terminology. A letter to the editor was published in the newspaper the following week. The disdain on the part of the publisher, as revealed in the response to the following letter, is reflective of the attitudes towards the uneducated at this time in history.

> The Heifer Aged Sixty-Five Years
> To the Editor of *The Northern Standard*
> Dear Sir –
> The verdickt of they Cornerrs gury which you printed last wick you might hev let pas everry one new that it was the age of the pore man was ment and not the kow, and I kan tel you the gurey was not to blaim for it was the Corner drew it up. They Monaghan gureyes is not so ignorrant as you want too mak it apeer. – I remeane sir with all due respekt.
> A GUREYMAN.
> – *The Northern Standard*, 1 February 1873

> [We print the above letter *verbatim et literatim*, from the manuscript as we received it. Comment is useless. – ED.N.S]

Trampled by Horses

Very often the cramped spaces in which the horses were kept during the fair was hazardous to both buyers and sellers. Francis McCarole was trampled by his own horse when it reared up at the Ballybay fair; some men gathered and helped him get back to his home in Killyfuddy in the parish of Killeevan, but the trauma to his chest was too much for his body to bear. He died later that afternoon at the age of seventy-seven years.[70] In another case, Edward Cusack was taken to the Clones workhouse to be treated by Dr Henry for head injuries. While dismounting from Thomas Howe's horse, he lost his balance and fell off the back of the horse directly on his head. He died just two hours later. Cusack was 40 years old.[71]

Hit and Run at the Clones Fair: The Man in the Windsor Trousers
The Death of Thomas Reighall, Clones, May 1873

Thomas Reighall never saw the horse galloping towards him, the shoulder of the horse hit him on the left side of the ribs, and his only memory of the event was the man on top of the large bay horse, a middle-aged man with a long reddish beard, black coat, felt hat and Windsor trousers.

John Reighall, his son, was at the Canal Stores in Clones when he saw a man he knew, Mr White, with two other men, discussing riding a large bay horse. The owner of the horse would not allow Mr White's man to ride him, but decided to ride himself. John continued walking down the Cavan road and upon returning into town a short while later, he heard a shout 'A man is killed!' He rushed to the scene and through the gathering crowd, saw his father lying on the ground. Thomas, a man of about sixty years of age, was rushed to see Dr Henry and Dr O'Reilly; both agreed it was a bad case. They did everything they could, but Thomas Reighall died early the next morning.[72]

CHAPTER SEVEN

WITH INTENT TO KILL
COLD-BLOODED MURDER?

> All histories are really murder stories. Sometimes they are epic and there are generals and battlefields and regiments of cavalry and foot, and sometimes they are just small, domestic, and there are pairs of men and alleyways and pistols in the back pocket.
>
> – *How to Murder a Man*, Carlo Gebler

The murders examined in the coroner's casebook are remarkably violent and show an intense anger, yet the verdicts of these inquests and the conviction rates at the assizes in post-famine Ireland reflect the attitudes of the general population who were unwilling to assume lethal intent on the part of the killer. Justice Charles Robert Barry, a circuit court judge appointed to the Queen's Bench in 1872, once stated, 'In many parts of the country, the people seemed not to consider murder under certain circumstances a crime at all.' These circumstances might be the fatal blow to the head using a large rock during a scuffle between father and son over land, one man chopping off the head of a perceived enemy in a drunken frenzy or one man shooting another man during a riot with political and religious overtones. The Irish were usually willing to assume a lack of intention to murder, and judges, juries and even relatives of victims often accepted that violent homicides were simply 'melancholy accidents'.[1] One hypothesis suggests that the amount of expressive interpersonal violence is inversely proportional to the power of the state; that is to say that, using the jury system, crimes could only be punished severely if the community saw them as truly criminal.[2] Murder was not considered murder unless there was a combination of overwhelming evidence to show intent to kill, motive and premeditation.

Homicides within families often occurred over disputes about property, inheritance and land: fathers and sons feuding over the land, nephews killing elderly relatives motivated by hopes of gaining possession of the land, as well as sibling rivalry due to inheritance practices, are just some of the reasons for murder amongst families that Waddell investigated. Contrary to the society we live in today, depositions and attitudes of witnesses and jurors at inquests and criminal trials in the post-famine years suggest that the rural populace believed that these fatal episodes were private matters and that there should be no open forum for discussion.

Alcohol-related homicide usually resulted from drunken challenges. Violence among men was common and often occurred as a form of entertainment – intoxicated men challenging each other to a fight, confrontations taking place on fair-days and nights, in public houses or wherever people gathered to socialise. These were common and frequent altercations and, when murder resulted, the assizes juries weighed the circumstances surrounding the case differently each time. Using modern-day mores and acceptable codes of behaviour in our contemporary society, one does not struggle between considering such deaths negligible homicide, manslaughter or first- or second-degree murder. However, nineteenth-century juries were more accepting of such 'accidents', as the great variations in the verdicts shows.

Murder that was considered political or sectarian was often distinguished by the use of a gun; contradicting theories have been produced as to whether these homicides represented national or local issues, or were, in many cases, just examples of public disorder owing to the traditional practice of faction-fighting, or the lack of entertainment or amusements. Even in the cases appearing in the coroner's casebook, there is a recreational element to such deaths as many of these killings took place during a celebration of one faction or the other, with alcohol consumed at such times. The punishment for the perpetrators of such homicides depended on the premeditation involved in the planning of the death as well as whether the accused was attempting to defend themselves against an onslaught from the opposing side.

In Waddell's casebook, there were thirty-eight cases in which death arrived by the hands of known or unknown killers. This figure does not include infant deaths or the multitude of suspicious cases where the verdict of the cause of death was concluded as being disease, heart attack, or accident. There were many inquests where the cause of death was more likely murder but, lacking evidence, the coroner and coroner's juries reached a neutral conclusion.[3] Even when a person was named at an inquest for causing the death, they were not always convicted at the assizes. The weapon used in the killing, the state of the body of the deceased and the circumstances surrounding the homicide were often examined, despite the fact that much of the decision about punishment of the murderer weighed upon his/her clear intent to cause lethal harm. Did most people ignore this behaviour? Or were they aware of the reasons for the outbursts of anger and frustration perpetrated by those without the same rights and freedoms within their family unit or within the community they lived in? For example, those without the right to inherit or those unable to marry owing to a lack of property might have gained the sympathy of the jury in a society which was suffering great change and loss. Did they take a lenient view because they were aware of these disparities? Possibly, assizes juries knew of the motives for the many crimes perpetrated in their communities and decided upon lenient sentences for those reasons.

MOTIVATION
Applying Forensic Psychology

Forensic psychology researcher, Cristy Ettenson, in interviews with the author, offered a psychological explanation for the increase in family violence over the land and the increasing levels of violence within rural Irish society during this time in history. 'The diversion from the norms, such as mental illness, suicide and murder are due to the alienation one feels in a society where morals aren't working anymore. A person's belief that being good always led to happiness and a feeling of well-being in the past, wasn't working anymore and now there was nowhere to turn.' The society as a whole was becoming more 'civilised' and restrictions were regularly put in place. Such changes included the civil recording of births, deaths and marriages, and even dog licences were now a necessity;[4] not to mention the temperance movement attempting to restrict the intake of alcohol through religious guidance and rules. Another large change was the thousands of persons, family members, friends and neighbours, emigrating regularly, never to be seen again. Life had changed since the famine and was continuing to do so dramatically.

Ettenson observes that the psychological motives behind the crimes committed appear to be based on the maintenance of one's family or oneself. 'It can be assumed that some felt that there was no other option, no other way to handle their problems. One common trait of these persons is that they all appear to display a lack of an inner guide. Religion was supposed to be their inner guide, but these folks probably couldn't understand why things were so hard for them; if they were churchgoing, hardworking people, why was there no relief?' Ettenson raises an important point. What was the payoff? For some, the idea of eternal salvation was not helping them here on earth. These were people who clearly felt they had nothing else left anyway. Maybe the afterlife offered more. And besides, their rage was getting the best of them.

'You have to look at the big picture and see what was happening at the time. Today we have television and movie violence that are considered contributing factors to murder. In the nineteenth century, these people had only each other, their society and their family life to model their behaviour from,' says Ettenson. 'When a family refuses to allow you freedoms, specifically the land you need to obtain that freedom, it was the family that became the oppressors, not an outside force in society.' Although the societal changes were contributing factors, as is the case in today's world, looking deeper into the personal background of a killer often yields many more clues to an understanding of motive and rage towards the victim.

Homicides within a family were usually wild, impromptu affairs.[5] The weapons used in the murders of family members were most often rocks, sharp farm tools and household instruments such as knives, pitchforks, axes and spades as well as teeth and fists. These were the weapons of intimate mayhem, the objects most likely to be used in mad quarrels and drunken rages. They were picked up quickly and used without much thought. While attempting to profile the frustrations of a 'killer', using modern-day approaches might not always consistently explain this behaviour. In some instances, agrarian murderers were not brutal assassins, but instead persons willing to do battle with, and even kill, loved ones. This type of *recreational violence* was a long-established cultural tradition in rural Ireland.[6] Post-famine Ireland might be defined by the lack of conscious killing or as a society in denial of the deeper feelings of the murderer. Murderers were often excused for alcohol-related homicide and, in many cases, sectarian murder. Again, assizes juries simply refused to convict if they felt the action had been justified or that the issue should have been settled outside the courts (usually where it concerned murder within a family).

Although firearms were used in some cases, they were usually used in disputes between landlords and tenants or for political and religious purposes rather than in domestic quarrels. One study of the instruments used in agrarian homicide showed that the more socially remote the attacker was from his victim, the more likely it was for firearms to be used.[7] This is an important detail in the profiling of these persons when attempting to speculate on unsolved murder cases from the nineteenth century since modern forensic psychological profiles cannot always be applied. When knives were used in murder, judges and juries appeared less tolerant in accepting that the murderer had no malice or intent to kill. One may suppose that, if the general public considered most murders were unintended, it would be difficult to rationalise someone taking a long, sharp and deadly object and plunging it into another's body. In each case where a knife or blade was used in Waddell's casebook, the murderer was sentenced to penal servitude.

Identifying the murderers in some unsolved cases proves difficult almost one hundred and fifty years later. 'Profiling in unsolved crimes requires a lot more information such as details of the crime scene which many of these cases are lacking,' says Ettenson. 'However, it sounds like everyone in the area knew who did it and at the very least, came to their own conclusion based upon the motives of the time – family disputes over land being a primary factor in these agrarian homicides.' In regard to alcohol-related murder, faction fighting and sectarian violence resulting in the deliberate death of the victim, she believes that most of these often unsolved murders, appear very *disorganised*. One can deduce that they were crimes of passion, persons in a heated rage, possibly intoxicated and their motives either reflecting the rage at their unhappiness with their lot in life or passion about what belonged to them – property, land, inheritance and ultimately, personal freedoms.

BLOODSHED OVER THE LAND
Agrarian Homicide

Tenant right was really an immemorial custom prevailing in a great portion of Ireland, but unrecognised in courts of law, or statute books, under which the ordinary tenant at will has acquired the right of selling the succession to his holding.
– From a speech by T. Hughes to the House of Commons,
reported in *The Morning Star*, 13 March 1868

Agrarian murders often began as disputes between tenants within a neighbourhood or between the land-holding farmer and his family members fighting over the rights and uses of the land they lived on.

Many incidences of riots, homicide and attempted murder of land-lords and land agents in Co. Monaghan have also been investigated, yet they have focused largely on the unsympathetic landlord and his dominance over the poor tenant farmers attempting to rise up against his tyranny and high rents. The reality of agrarian outrage in Ireland was that only 24% of all the agrarian homicides were of landlords and their servants (who usually got caught in the cross-fire). Disputes with-in tenants' families accounted for 32%; disputes between tenants ac-counted for 27%; disputes between tenants and sub-tenants account-ed for 5%; and attacks on those who took evicted land accounted for 10%.[8] Therefore, the most likely agrarian murder was *within the family and amongst the tenants themselves* fighting over the property, the in-heritance and the claim to it. It is these disputes – within the neigh-bourhood and kinship ties (the family unit) – and the factors con-tributing to their disharmony which are the focus of this exploration.

The practice of subdividing (isolating individual plots of the family holding to give to children so that they might settle and work the land) came to an end in the post-famine years. The land had become so exhausted and the landholding so reduced that in a bad season there was often a shortage of crops. Land was now given to only one child, usually the eldest son. In response to the cessation of subdivid-ing, families would join together as a unit to make the land profitable. Many families worked very well together, with everyone accepting their role for the greater good of the holding. In fact, in many ways without subdivision of the land, an effective family unit became more disciplined and often intra-family feuding was reduced by de-creasing the number of claimants who might be disappointed by the share of the land they were given.

Yet the same bonds that brought the family together could tear it apart. Ultimately, occupation and control of the land was a chief source of conflict and there were many consequences resulting from the end of subdivision. It was the decision of the landholding parent as to when the land was to be handed over to the inheriting child and in many cases this transfer of possession did not occur within a reasonable timeframe. Tensions developed as children grew older, often into their late thirties and early forties, still working a farm that would come under their control only when their parents died. They were unable to marry without land and unable to make decisions about the use of the land until it was under their control. At a suit-able time (usually for the parents) arranged marriages were organised, matching the son of a farmer with a nearby or equally equitable farmer's daughter to ensure the integrity of the family holding and to keep close alliances among the neighbours.

The precarious time when land was transferred (either one section of land or the entire holding), was a period of change and adjustment, when most grievances arose between father and son, as well as other family members. One case that clearly illustrates this point is 'The Field: The Murder of Michael Mooney'. Tensions turned to homicide as father and son argued over the land that had been recently subdivided. On the surface, their dispute was about one stray heifer wandering out of the pasture and into the crops, yet the real struggle was about ownership of the land. This case was not unusual or rare. Although the family was the natural and primary fundamental group within rural society in the nineteenth century, it was also the origin of social tension and conflict, especially in regard to their primary valuable asset: the property maintained within the family.

The other children and family members were either encouraged to stay to work the farm as labourers or prompted to emigrate. They might stay on the farm their entire lives as labourers, never having their own land and provided only with the opportunity of a place to rest their head. Therefore, the conflict born out of this structure is quite understandable. For those who stayed, there might be resistance to the lack of prospects, the denial of personal ownership and individual freedoms, as well as the limitations of tenant right which created a hostile environment for those who were unable to create opportunities for themselves. For those not able to inherit land, compensation (household or farming property, or money) replaced the gift of land as a new grievance. For example, one murder was committed by the victim's own brother who was frustrated over 'pecuniary matters' (in regard to land the father had sold) as well as the possession of a household item, a clock. Another case, an unsolved murder, illustrates the suspicion surrounding a labouring nephew who was the primary farmer of a holding owned by his grandmother. His uncle was the only person standing between him and the ownership and management of 29 acres of land. The uncle planned to gain ownership of the farm, sell it, offer the nephew compensation for his work over the years and send him about his way. His uncle was found dead on the side of the road.

As well as land, feuding among family and neighbours might extend to broader matters of property, morality and group affiliation. As mentioned in chapter four in the inquest on Phillip Donaghy, it appeared the family had not called for a doctor or a priest as he lay very ill and had essentially allowed him to die. He and some members of his family had fallen out over some 'trifling property' of his late mother who had recently died at the house of her daughter. That daughter had married a Protestant. Warrants had been issued by the Ballybay police against some of the family. Another such case was that of William Foster of Drumbrean whose health had been failing for over a year after his crops had been burned. This incident was considered not only to have contributed to his bad health but poisoning was also suspected. Someone wanted him off the land. While one might never know the exact reasons for vandalism, violence and crime, it is certain that the closer the relationship between the criminal and victim, the greater the potential for inflicting injury or seeking vengeance.[9]

The Passage of Land and Death: The Murder of Michael McEleer, Drumcoofoster, Tedavnet Parish, May 1861

> … Those fields, those hills – what could they less? Had laid
> Strong hold on his affections, were to him
> A pleasurable feeling of blind love,
> The pleasure which there is in life itself
> … But unforeseen misfortunes suddenly
> Had prest upon him; and old Michael now
> Was summoned to discharge the forfeiture.
> — 'Michael, a Pastoral Poem', William Wordsworth

When Dr John William Moratz arrived at the home of Michael Mc-Eleer, he found the old man complaining of severe headaches and vomiting. He told the doctor he'd been bashed in the head with a rock two days earlier at the hands of his nephew, Pat. Dr Moratz examined the back of his head and found a piece of plaster covering some slight cuts and abrasions. Michael's wife, Ann, visited the doctor six days after this visit to say that he was much better having slept well and taken some breakfast. The next day, when the doctor stopped at the McEleer's home in Drumcoofoster, he found his patient had a taken a turn for the worse. Michael McEleer died later that day, 18 May 1861.

The coroner arrived the next day to hold an inquest. Several family members were questioned and Dr Moratz conducted the postmortem examination. He found a large quantity of blood between the brain and the skull and a depression of the bones at the front and back of the head. On removing the skull, he found extensive fractures. One deep fracture was considered the cause of death.

As the coroner began to question both sides of the family, each person offered a 'unique' perspective as to the events of the day in question. It became clear that the families were fighting over a passage of land between their two farms and it was likely the feud had been going on for some time.[10] Michael's farm was adjacent to that of his brother James' farm where each lived with their own families. Ultimately the question was, 'Why did Patrick McEleer want to kill his uncle Michael?'

John McEleer, Michael's son, told the coroner, 'I saw Pat crossing one of our fields. I went to turn him back, but he kept on. My father saw him and went to speak with him. By the time my father neared their house, my uncle, James, and Pat were there. I heard my father exclaim, "James, *it's* not here. You should be at home". On hearing this, I then saw Pat strike my father and I found him lying on the ground. I raised him up when he told me he had been beaten. He complained much of his head, blaming the stroke of the stone given him by Pat.' It appeared that Pat had been looking for something, such as a cow or farming instrument and considered that his uncle Michael had taken it.

John added, 'I took no part whatsoever in the fray.'

Ann McEleer, Michael's wife, also gave testimony. She told the coroner's jury the following story. 'I was at my own door on the 9th of May when I saw James McEleer, his wife and son Pat. At the same time I saw my husband lying on the ground and ran down to him. He was still on the ground and at same time, saw my son John was also down. His head and shoulders were in a furrow and Pat McEleer was kicking him. I pushed Pat away, on which he left the field and ere leaving it, he cheered three times exclaiming, "He was the colig that was worth a feeding".[11] Ann said that her husband told her it was the blows of the stone that were causing his death.

The next to provide testimony at the inquest was Owen McEleer, brother to Mick (Michael) and James, who was sitting in his house when the fight broke out. 'I was there when James' wife went to the door and exclaimed, "They are after Pat" – "they" meaning Mick's family – at which point James left the house to go to them,' he claimed.

Owen said, 'After waiting some time, I went to the door and saw Mick and James struggling and wrestling. They finally let go their hold on each other. I did not see Pat in the field, but saw him coming home later with his father. After they had come into the house, I heard them say that Mick was knocked down and heard James blame Pat for striking him.'

A verdict was reached by the coroner's jury. Mick McEleer came to his death on Saturday, 18 May 1861 from injuries inflicted on him Thursday, 9 May during a scuffle between James and Pat McEleer and the deceased. In the course of which scuffle he received one or more blows of a stone from the hands of said Pat McEleer and which blow or blows caused his death.[12]

James and Patrick McEleer were indicted for the manslaughter of Mick, but, having heard the charges against him, Pat left the country. This delayed the proceedings of the trial until almost a year later in March of 1862. When the trial began, James stood alone facing the charges without his son. The prosecution attempted to introduce new evidence against James McEleer. It was alleged that James, holding his hands behind his back, came up to his brother, Michael, who was then on his own land and struck him with two blows on either side of the head with a loaded whip shaft. At this point in the affray, Patrick McEleer raised a stone and inflicted a blow on the skull of his uncle.

The defence proved that Michael had struck at James and that James had nothing in his hands, as was alleged by the prosecution. The evidence showed that Patrick McEleer, not his father James, struck the blows that proved fatal.

The jury returned a verdict of acquittal and James McEleer was discharged.[13] The families continued to live next to each other in three separate farms for several generations. In 1864, Mick's farm was transferred into the name of his wife, Anne, and, upon her death in 1897, into the name of their son, John.[14] It is unknown if Patrick McEleer ever returned to Ireland.

The Field: The Murder of Michael Mooney,
Carn, Aghabog Parish, June 1872
When James Mulligan married Anne Mooney, his father, Francis, gave him half of his farm at Carn in the parish of Aghabog. On the four acres he was given, James grew crops, allowed his cattle to graze and raised a family. A few months later, a problem arose. His father, Frank, was short of grass and a dispute arose between father and son over a field where the cattle were grazing – a field that both men believed they owned. Although the cows all grazed together, it was alleged that James' cow constantly trespassed on an adjoining field of oats belonging to his father, which annoyed Frank so much that he was determined to drive her from the grazing field altogether. When James protested, Frank said he never gave the field to him. James said

he'd paid the taxes on it for the past five years and, therefore, it was his to do with as he liked.

As the tension over the situation mounted, James and his wife, Ann, decided to ask Father Duffy to come and help resolve the situation. The priest was not at that time aware of any particulars in the dispute but had made inquires among the neighbours and, based upon what they said, he was determined to create peace within the family. The priest arrived at the father's house and was greeted by another son, John, and a servant girl. Frank got out of bed and came downstairs. He seemed to have a black eye and had the appearance of being fatigued or abused. The priest explained that he'd come to make peace between Frank and his son, James. Frank complained bitterly about James. Father Duffy pressed Frank, reminding him of the necessity of giving his son peaceable possession of what he had promised. Frank said he would give his son the portion of the land that was behind his house, but not what was before the door (the field in question).

Father Duffy then went out and told James to come in so that he and his father might shake hands and have peace. James had a stick in his hand behind his back and his father had a sharp instrument on the table. The blade was about nine or ten inches long and was at the end of a stick. The blade was nearly three times as long as the handle. When James entered the house, Father Duffy explained to James that his father would give him the land at the back of the house, but not the disputed field.

James angrily stated, 'I will have that field or death.'

Suddenly, his father went into a passionate rage, grabbed a pitchfork and made a rush towards James. Before they could come to blows, Father Duffy jumped between the two men, pushed James out of the house and locked the door. Francis and John remained inside, raging, yelling and frustrated. As Father Duffy struggled to calm and sort out the situation between the feuding family members, a cow suddenly appeared in the field and the men became very excited inside the house. The priest told them to leave the matter in his hands, that he would turn the cow out of the field and then arrange matters. As soon as he opened the door, the two men rushed out. Frank had a pitchfork which the priest took from him, but the men continued on their way, prepared for a confrontation. Unknown to all parties, Frank had the 'sharp instrument', the knife, in his possession as well.

Frank and John rushed towards James who was there with his father-in-law, seventy-five-year-old Michael Mooney. The priest watched as they violently attacked each other. Father Duffy began shouting,

'Murder! Murder!' and then attempted to get help from the Donagheys, who lived nearby.

Father Duffy began hurrying away down the road, when he heard someone yelling for him. It was James calling for help. When he returned, he saw James cradling the head of old Michael Mooney. He was lying at the foot of the field, bleeding profusely. By the time they carried the old man back to his home, he was dead.

Constable Robert Stanley was working at Newbliss Barracks on 14 June 1872 when James Mulligan arrived stating that earlier that day he'd had a quarrel with his father and his brother, John, and that in the midst of the quarrel, his father-in-law, Michael Mooney, was killed. When Stanley asked who had killed the old man, James stated, 'My father, Frank.'

The constable asked where his father was and James told him he was at Mr Andre Murray Kerr's, a local magistrate and the landlord of their farm. Stanley left to go to Kerr's; on the way he met a man with blood on his face, he asked his name and where he lived.

The man replied, 'Francis Mulligan of Carn.'

Frank was arrested on the spot and taken into custody for the murder of Michael Mooney. Constable Stanley cautioned him against saying anything that might commit himself. When they reached the barracks, he took possession of Frank's bloodstained clothes as they would be entered into evidence when the legal proceedings began.

John Mulligan was arrested the following day in Ballybay by Head Constable Thomas Irwin. He was charged with murder, read the usual cautions and brought back to the barracks as a prisoner.

The inquest took place two days later on 17 June 1872. The jury was called and Mr Kelly, assisted by Mr Robert Hanley, appeared as solicitor for James Mulligan and the Mooney family. Francis and John Mulligan, the two prisoners in custody, were not professionally represented.

The jury viewed the body and the post-mortem evidence was produced. Dr Moore, who performed the autopsy, observed three slight bruises on the left temple, one on the cheekbone, one on the external angle of the frontal bone and one to the head. The brain and membranes were healthy. The wounds on the head would have resulted from blows of an object such as a common walking stick.

'Next I observed an incised or puncture wound in the right armpit – better than half an inch from angle to angle (surface appearance),' stated Dr Moore. 'There is also a cut on the inside of the right arm, evidently caused by the instrument before entering the chest.

The wound in the right armpit passed between the fourth and fifth ribs through the substance of the right lung. The instrument then pass-ed over to the left side in front of the spine, wounding in its course the descending aorta or the chief blood vessel of the body about an inch from the origin of the left major artery. It then entered the left lung passing completely through its substance.' He and Dr Robert H. Reid, his assistant in the examination of the body, concluded that death resulted from the haemorrhage into the cavity of the left lung. From the point of entrance to the external wound in the left lung meas-ured about 10 inches. A blunt instrument likely made the wound on the back of the head.

The jury having viewed the body, James Mulligan was sworn and examined. The coroner asked James, 'Now, detail what you know of this unhappy occurrence.'

'I will,' said James. 'On Thursday, my cow was driven off the field by the servant girl belonging to my father. The cow was put back again by my wife. She was put out of the field a second time.'

'By whom?' asked Mr Kelly, the prosecutor.

'By my brother, John Mulligan, the tailor. I drove her back again.'

'Did anyone interfere with you?'

'– Yes, my brother and father.'

'In what manner?' asked the coroner.

James responded, 'They jostled me and my father lifted a stone and struck me on the mouth.'

'What size was it?'

'It was about the size of my fist. My father pushed me back and in doing so I fell and he fell over me into the dunghill. I rolled him over off me. John got hold of me by the mouth. I got up from them and then they gathered out.'

'Who gathered out?' asked Mr Kelly.

'My own wife, Anne, and Thomas Donaghoe and dragged me from where I was. They fetched me into my own house, where I remained quietly all that day. That all happened on Thursday.'

James continued, 'On Friday, the man was killed. I had sent for the priest, the Revd B. Duffy to try and settle it. He came to my father's house, shut the door and I did not see him for some time. The dispute was renewed again. Father Duffy did all he could to settle, but it was unsuccessful with my father.'

'And with you?'

'Yes,' said James. 'My father said I never got the field and that I'd never turn a sod in it. I said I did and I would have it with the rest.

He then went up to the room and returned with a pitchfork. He did not do anything with it. The Revd Mr Duffy took it from him and pushed me out of the house. At this time I was trying to effect a settlement. The Revd Mr Duffy remained inside for to make peace with my father. My brother John got out. The cow at this time was in the field and he went down to turn her out. He had a stick and pair of scissors in his hands. He told me he would stick me with them.'

'What sort of stick was it?'

'A cane stick,' said James. A stick was then produced in the courtroom for James to examine.

'That's not it,' he said. 'But it is like it. He ran after the cow to turn her, but I kept between them. My father then came down with an old spear-staff and said he would stick me with it. He attempted to do so by making a "prod" at me. I avoided it by stepping back, but it touched my waistcoat. It was the point that touched me. It would have left a mark, only I stepped aside. Both then ran after me – one with the scissors and the other with the spear-staff.'

'Had you a stick then?'

'No, but I was preventing the cow from leaving the field. I had kept them back with a stick until the old man (the deceased Michael Mooney) came out of my house to make peace,' said James. 'I did not let them in on me.'

He continued, 'When the old man came out, John "took" at him. Mooney had not done anything before that. I am married to his daughter. My brother, John, struck the old man with a stick over the top of his head, bruising it. I said no more because at that time my father was attacking me with the spear-staff. He did not get doing me any injury. The blade was bare. I kept him off and when he came "too tight" on me, I ran away. My father then ran up to Michael Mooney, the deceased and stuck him.'

There was a sudden flood of gasps and grumbling in the room.

A juror then asked James, 'How did you see him when you ran away?'

James replied, 'I only ran a short distance. He was stuck in the right breast. I struck my father over the eye with a stick while defending myself. I cut him. My father-in-law was beating the tailor (my brother).'

He then began to explain the altercations between his brother and father towards Michael Mooney. 'My brother first attacked Mooney. Mooney had a stick with which he defended himself. They stopped when my father stuck Mooney.' He then began to describe the position of the fighting parties.

Mr Kelly asked, 'After your father stuck Mooney, what occurred?'

'My father went into the house. My father-in-law ran down the field immediately after getting the stab and fell within a few yards of the field. He never spoke a word. I ran down to lift him and he fell on his face with his hands extended. I lifted his head and the breath was only in him. The Revd Mr Duffy was only a short distance off at the time and I called him. My father-in-law was carried up to my house. He was between seventy and eighty years of age.'

The next to be deposed was Ann Mulligan, James' wife and daughter of the deceased, who gave a very sad, brief description of the events.

'Of my will, I went away to the Revd Mr Duffy to come over and make peace between my husband and his people. When the priest arrived, I went to the back of the hill just to avoid seeing disputing or quarrelling. When I left the house, my father was in it. When I returned, his corpse was there,' she said.

In describing the dispute between the father and son, Ann stated, 'Spring of this year, Frank Mulligan gave to my husband half of his farm and the field in dispute formed part of our half, but as Frank was scarce of grass this year, the cattle were to graze together.'

The inquest concluded with Francis and John Mulligan held responsible for the injuries inflicted upon Mick Mooney during a scuffle arising out of a dispute about some land.[15] The prisoners were then removed to Monaghan Jail.

A charge of wilful murder was brought against Frank Mulligan and common assault against John Mulligan. The Monaghan assizes were held the following month on 20 July 1872 and the trial began. The jury listened to the testimony of all the parties involved. Two witnesses that were not questioned at the inquest appeared at the trial. The first was Anne McDermott, the servant who lived in the house of Frank and John Mulligan. Anne was asked under cross-examination if it was a fact that she had two illegitimate children, to which she answered, 'Yes'. She was also asked if the report was true that in fact she was the person who set the quarrel going between the father and the son, but she denied it. The last question of the prosecutor was if she was going to be married to Frank Mulligan.

She said, 'He never asked me to marry him except in a joke in front of other people.'

Mr Murray Kerr, JP, was called as a character witness for Frank Mulligan. Kerr stated, 'I've known the prisoner for twenty years and never heard a word against him. I'd never known him to be at the bench.'

Kerr was unaware of the sub-division of the farm and, had he known about it, he would not have sanctioned it.

At the end of all testimony, Chief Baron Richard Pigot[16] instructed the jury at considerable length and expressed his conviction that the Crown had very properly withdrawn the charge of murder and that the prisoner, Frank Mulligan, had pleaded guilty to a charge of manslaughter. The jury soon afterwards formally handed down a verdict of guilty against Frank Mulligan who was ordered to stand aside for sentencing. John Mulligan was found guilty of common assault.

Frank was then called forward to receive his sentence.

Baron Pigot spoke to the prisoner and the court: 'You have been found guilty on a charge for which there was no substantial defence – the manslaughter of that unfortunate old man who met his death at your hands on the 14th of June last. My words will not be many.'

The baron then pronounced the following to the hushed crowd in the courtroom. 'The time for admonition to you with any view of reforming your conduct and abating the violence to which you seem from time to time to have given way – the time for all that is passed. You have come to a period of life when punishment must be awarded rather for the purpose of deterring others from similar acts of atrocity than from any prospect of amendment in you. That would, perhaps, be too much to expect during the short remainder of your life. Death has been inflicted on that old man under circumstances of very considerable aggravation. According to the evidence, he was a much older man than you. From him, old age took away the power of either assault or resistance. He was bowed down with the decrepitude of age. He was for all intents and purposes defenceless at the time you used the deadly weapon against him. I have seldom met a case which terminated in manslaughter which so nearly approached the crime of wilful murder. A very small difference would have rendered it impossible to have acquitted you of murder. But I think the Crown properly distinguished under the circumstances of your case as to one or two incidents to which it is needless to refer and withdrew the charge of murder, pressing most rightly against you the charge of manslaughter. Before you got into conflict with any persons in the field you deliberately prepared yourself for conflict with a deadly weapon, for you had on the table beside you in the house an instrument of death. You did, unquestionably, in the first instance, take a less deadly weapon out with you, but when you were aggravated, and when you were determined on inflicting the severest punishment on the old man – perhaps in a moment of sudden passion – you plunged into his body a sharp weapon, inflicting a wound of unusual magnitude and severity, a wound which extended for six inches through three mortal parts of his body. Old as you are – and under other circumstances I should be desirous of mitigating punishment on account of your advanced age – you are not so old as not to bear the punishment due to your crime. If there is anything in your age or health to diminish the punishment, that is to be considered by others. I must let fall a heavy sentence where death has been inflicted and without further comment on this fearful and abominable deed, I must let fall on you a sentence of penal servitude for five years. If you had been a younger man the sentence would probably have been double.'

The court then adjourned until the next day to determine the sentencing of John Mulligan. The next morning, Pigot remarked that on the previous day John's father had received a very heavy punishment. On John, he would pass a mitigated sentence. Whatever interest the father had in the farm had to be attended to by some person in whom he had confidence. John Mulligan's sentence would be two months' imprisonment, dating from 14 June, so that he would be able to look after the harvest work.[17]

Clearly, subdivision of the land had created great disharmony between the father and son. It appears that the land transfer had not been a smooth transition and that the negotiations had not been handled carefully or clearly. One might only imagine how these families continued to live so close to one another following the murder of Michael Mooney.

Just one year after the sentencing of Francis and John Mulligan, the land of Francis Mulligan was transferred to James Mulligan in 1873. It is possible that his father had died after only one year in prison? Or was the land transferred prior to his sentence to secure the family holding? The field where the murder took place was sold to William George Williamson in 1876. Although in later years, John Mulligan did lease several other acres of land in various parts of the townland of Carn, the Mulligan's never again re-purchased or lived on the field where the murder of Michael Mooney occurred.

BROTHERS KILLING BROTHERS
Fratricide

The first murder in the Bible, that of Cain and Abel, has allowed us to examine the nature of the jealousy and rage that occurred between brothers for centuries. There are a few cases in the coroner's case-book in which brothers became angry with their lack of control over land, money or property, while their dear 'brother' inherited that to which another brother felt entitled. What is the trigger that makes a man kill his own brother? Or two brothers?

Double Homicide Over Land, Money and a Kept Woman
The Unsolved Murder of James and Robert Shaw,
Belderg, Donagh Parish, January 1861

On the afternoon of 4 January 1861, Thomas Hamilton walked through the townland of Belderg to the home of James Shaw to pay him back some money he had borrowed. Upon reaching the threshold of the house that James shared with his brother Robert, Hamilton made a shocking discovery. The two brothers lay on the floor in pools of their own blood. James Shaw was lying on his back with his feet outside the house, his head and shoulders inside. His brother, Robert, also lay on the broad of his back, staring ahead, his leg resting underneath James' head and shoulders. They had both been shot in the head, their brains and blood spraying across the lintel and doorpost.

When the authorities arrived, Head Constable Trimble and Acting Constable Henry McMullen evaluated the crime scene. Trimble noticed immediately that the house did not appear to be robbed and was undisturbed. The brothers' watches, money and bank deposit receipt were untouched. It did not appear to be a robbery and was, therefore, highly unlikely to be the work of strangers. The killer or killers knew these men. The bodies were moved from the front door of the home to a room off the kitchen after he arrived. Both had their shoes on without stockings, cord trousers and sleeved waistcoats, their heads uncovered and dreadfully mangled.

The shooting had taken place at the front door of the house. While examining the entrance, both constables evaluated the front of the home outside the door and saw the mark of a bullet on one of the stones on the porch. There was blood and bits of grey matter from the brains of the men spattered on the right side of the door. McMullen found a small piece of bone in the thatch above, which Dr Douglass said was part of one of the deceased men's skulls. It appeared the men were somehow called or lured quickly to the front door of their home where they were then attacked with gunfire.

Trimble, McMullen and several other constables began asking around the neighbourhood, interviewing friends and neighbours. Several pieces of information were furnished. One report described

Robert and James Shaw as unoffending men, holding small farms, yet they were 'pretty well to do'. They were in the habit of lending small sums of money out at interest but it was rumoured they had made enemies for exacting a high rate of interest.[18] It also became clear that the two men lived on bad terms with their brother, William Shaw, and that suspicion in everyone's minds rested on him, as he was the one person who would benefit the most from their death. It was said that the entire population of the district were so indignant about so great a crime being perpetrated in their peaceful circle, that the authorities received every assistance to help them to solve the crime and identify its perpetrators.[19]

Four men were immediately considered suspects. The first man held in police custody was Richard Jackson, a servant of Mrs Ellen Hoey of Billis. He'd been picked up after a neighbour of the Shaw brothers, Peter McGough, told police that he believed he'd heard Jackson's voice calling for the brothers on the night of the murder. 'I live within 100 perches of the Shaw brothers,' said McGough. 'I went to their house at 9 o'clock on the morning of 3 January to borrow a ladder. That same night, myself and my wife, Catherine, were woken by the barking of our dog, which prompted me to find the cause. On going outside, I stopped and listened for two or three minutes when I heard a voice call "Robert Shaw" and "James Shaw" and which voice, at the time, I considered being that of Richard Jackson.' He also said that the voice seemed to be coming from the front of the Shaw's home.

Arthur McEnally, a close friend of the Shaws, indicated to police that there were two other men who should be closely examined in regard to the double homicide. McEnally had known the brothers for nine or ten years and had their confidence in important matters. Over the past several years there had been bad feelings between James and Robert and their brother, William Shaw, over property, money and a woman who William Shaw kept. McEnally said, 'Over the past four months both the brothers were in my house and in conversation about a family dispute between them and William Shaw and Thomas McNiece, nephew of William Shaw.'

'James and Robert both told me that they were in danger of their lives from McNiece both of his robbing and murdering them,' said McEnally. 'The feud had been going on for the past four or five years in consequence of a dispute between themselves and William Shaw. They often made these remarks when they were perfectly sober.'

Constable Scanlon, Constable McRoberts and Inspector McKelvey made a visit to the house of William Shaw of Lisboy. They searched the house and, in a press, found a tin canister with some lead slugs and a canister with gunpowder. Other items included a powder flask and a small case containing some shot. A loaded gun was found, filled with powder and shot but appeared not to have been discharged for some time as it was twisted in the muzzle.

They also found a waistcoat which had stains of blood on it and asked Shaw and McNiece whom it belonged to. William Shaw told them that it was an old coat of his but that it now belonged to McNiece. When they asked McNiece about the coat, he told them, 'I wore it, but it belongs to my uncle.' As the inspector went through the pockets of the coat, he found a musket ball and three percussion caps.

McRoberts, in helping with the search of McNiece, said that he did not find any fowl feathers in the pockets of the coat, despite an insinuation that McNiece had been hunting birds. He remarked that he did not see any blood in the pockets.

Thomas McNiece was then taken into police custody.

William Shaw was still the prime suspect but the police needed more information to bring him in. The issue of the brothers fighting over land became a focus of the investigation. A. H. Murray Kerr, Esq., the land agent to Lord Cremorne, overseeing the matters of land between James and William Shaw had information as to the disputes between the family. 'There was a great deal of bad feeling and much of legal disputing carried on in the family,' he said. It came to a point where he felt called on to interfere and try to settle the matters between them. 'I considered James the most violent brother, but William the most dangerous. During the last three years I have heard little about them in the way of disputes as previous to that period. I had made a judgement between William and James Shaw. There was a farm in William's possession which I would have taken from him and given to James in order to separate them, but from what I knew and from what I heard the neighbours say, I feared there would be lives lost if I did so,' said Kerr. 'I would have done this in consequence of an award (order to pay a fine or a cost) made, by which it said the farm was to go to James but subsequently made another award leaving the farm with William, who now has it.'

On 7 January 1861, just three days after the murders of both his brothers, William Shaw called in to see Mr Kerr at his offices in Monaghan. When the subject of the murders came up in conversation, William Shaw told Kerr that he believed he was blamed in the matter. Kerr answered him honestly, 'William, in my own mind, I do not quite hold you free.' In a very serious and solemn manner, William knelt down on his knees and protested his innocence. His lip quivered and he appeared very agitated.

After this conversation turned, the subject of the possession of the farm of James Shaw was raised by William. He asked Kerr if he was now the owner of James' farm.

Kerr asked him, 'You? Not another brother?' There was another man living on a farm in the townland of Lisboy, John Shaw, most likely the other brother referred to by Kerr.

'Is there not a lease or the promise of one which made the farm mine?'

Kerr replied, 'It remains with Lord Cremorne whether or not you will be allowed to hold James' farm or not.'

That same day, William Shaw was arrested by Head Constable Trimble while in Monaghan town. He was told he was a prisoner in the Queen's name on suspicion of being concerned with the murder of his brothers. He replied, 'Thank God. I'm innocent!' He was warned to say nothing which might incriminate him.

On the way back to the barrack, he told the constable that he'd ought to arrest James Steenson. Constable Trimble also stated that 'he thrice repeated himself'.

The statement was made that Steenson should be arrested on suspicion as he was indebted to the Shaws. James Steenson was investigated by the police, but there was evidence that on the night of the murder, he had not left his house.

When the coroner held his inquest, the suspects, William Shaw, Thomas McNiece and Richard Jackson were present. Depositions from previous witnesses were read aloud and also information from police was again provided.

Some witnesses had heard strange noises of heavy footsteps and their dogs barking loudly on the night of the murders, but Peter McGeough was the only witness able to identify one of the men believed to be at the Shaw's home. Another witness, Jane Little, living in the home of William Crookshank of Drumginey, deposed that on the night of 3 January she was lying in bed with her sister when she heard three shots. Two shots nearly sounded off together and a third shot about a minute after. In discussion, her sister, who did not hear anything, asked where she thought they came from. Jane told her that they sounded as if they had come from Millen Gate or Drumcaw. The townland of Drumcaw lies between Belderg and Drumginney.

There were two witnesses called by the coroner who gave Richard Jackson an alibi. Robert Stewart was staying with his aunt, Ellen

Hoey of Billis, on the night of 3 January. He explained that Richard Jackson, being one of his aunt's servants, was in the house after 9.30p.m. as he closed the door and went to bed. Pat White, a fellow servant in the Hoey household, said he slept with Jackson in the same bed the entire evening. 'On going to bed Jackson was there before me and fast asleep. When I awoke in the morning, he was up and dressing. During the night he could not leave the bed and return to it again without my being aware of doing so,' White stated.

The post-mortem examinations were carried out by Dr A. K. Young and Dr Allen E. Douglass. First the evidence from the autopsy of Robert Shaw was provided. Both deposed to having examined the body of the deceased and found that Robert had received two gunshots to the head. He had a shot or wound on the right side of the head behind the ear with shot and slugs. The other wound on the left side of the head was a gunshot wound, the bullet passing through to the brain and spinal cord and it appeared to have broken his jaw in two places. At the exit wound in the right side of the neck, Dr Douglass found paper which he considered to have been the waddling of the charge. Bullet, shot, pellets and paper were given to Head Constable Trimble. It was this last wound that had caused the death of Robert Shaw.

The autopsy of James Shaw resulted in the discovery of marks of gunpowder and slugs in his face. There was a gunshot wound on the left side of the head above and behind the ear, a wound which came out to the left side of the crown of the head. This was the shot that caused death. It appeared that Jane Little's account of three shots was accurate.

Common firearms in the nineteenth century, such as old blunderbusses, were often loaded with scrap metal that sprayed in different directions. Some of these pistols were loaded from the front through the muzzle as was common at that time. Other types of guns were considered 'percussion' weapons (guns that have a little nipple at the breech end of the barrel over which a percussion cap is placed to ignite the charge inside). Because they were neither accurate nor lethal, a murder with such an instrument would require planning and a closeness to the victim in order to kill. James Shaw's face had marks of gunpowder and the slugs found embedded in his skull indicated that the gun was fired at possibly a distance of six to eight inches away. One fact that is worth remembering – ammunition for each type of weapon was found at the house of William Shaw.

In developing a case for potential suspects, one fact has been pointed out in regard to agrarian murder. It seems that assassins fired less accurately at landlords than at their friends and relations.[20] One obvious reason for this is that family members would be more likely to get closer to their victim than to the landlord. It was the close range of the gunshots that made the attack on the Shaw brothers effective. By evaluating the execution-style killings, which involved being shot behind the ears, a reasonable scenario begins to emerge. They were likely called by a familiar voice to the front of the house, they rose quickly and were ambushed upon opening the door. The assassins were waiting on either side of the entrance and, when James walked through, he was shot first with a single shot to the back of his head behind the left ear. Robert, following right behind him received a shot to the right side of the head, and another shot from the left side which was the shot that killed him. If there were only three shots fired, as was heard by witness Jane Little, the slugs and buckshot taken from the faces of the body and around the sides of the front door could be explained as other scrap metal flying from the barrels of the guns randomly. There must be more than one killer. These murders were well-planned and carried out without fear of being caught.

There was much circumstantial evidence against McNiece and Shaw, but without murder weapons, it was impossible for the jury to name them at the inquest as the killers of the Shaw brothers. Jackson had an alibi and although plenty of materials used with a gun were found in the house of the two primary suspects, along with a coat considered to have blood on it, it was not enough. The verdict of the inquests was that Robert and James Shaw came to their deaths from certain gunshot wounds inflicted on them, but by whom inflicted, the jury had not sufficient evidence to enable them to decide. The three men were discharged.

A year later, still no one was charged with the murder of the Shaw brothers. A letter to the editor appeared in *The Northern Standard* asking why no one had yet been prosecuted for the murder. The single question about the killers in these murders was 'Who had motive?'

Almost two years later, in November 1862, Colonel Leslie, MP for Monaghan was suing William Shaw.[21] Their case was heard in front of the court of the Queen's Bench. Leslie was the owner of the land at Belderg (which Shaw inherited as a result of the murder of his brothers) and he was charging Shaw with not paying the rent. Several irregularities were found in the case showing that Leslie wanted Shaw off the land. When Shaw inherited the land, he did not know it came with a lease. A year later, when Leslie produced the lease, it was discovered that Shaw needed to reside there in order to avoid higher fees. According to the document produced, Shaw now owed £56 to Leslie for back rent and fees. Shaw was also served with a notice of ejectment. When Shaw realised that his back was to the wall, he had his solicitor, Mr Wright, agree that he would sell his tenancy from year to year. However, when tenants approached Leslie's agent, Mr Cunningham, they were cautioned against having anything to do with the matter. He was telling them not to buy. Without selling the rights to the land, Shaw would have to forfeit the land to Leslie and probably pay the heavy rents and fees in addition to the forfeiture. Editorial comment about the lawsuit appeared in several publications defending Leslie – suggesting that he did not want a possible murderer benefiting from the property of those he killed.

It appears the house the Shaw brothers were murdered in was torn down in 1864 and the land eventually taken over by William Shaw in 1870. McNiece never appeared in any of the land records as having occupied his own farm. No one was ever prosecuted for the murder of Robert and James Shaw.

The Clock that made Time Stand Still
The Murder of Patrick Muckian and the Trial of James Muckian,
Castleblayney, August 1870
The town of Castleblayney was thrown into a great confusion upon discovering that James Muckian, a 24-year-old local man, had killed his older brother, Patrick, by stabbing him with a knife during a quarrel. It was said that the father of the deceased and of his murderer, Francis Muckian, resided years before on a small farm of land on the estate of the Marquis of Bath close to the Culloville Station on the Dundalk and Londonderry Railway.[22] Upon leaving the land, which consisted of a little more than six acres in the townlands of Corcullioncrew and Corcullionglish in the parish of Donaghmoyne, he moved himself and his family to Castleblayney. The dispute between the brothers arose respecting some pecuniary matters regarding inheritance and property.

At two o'clock in the afternoon of 16 August 1870, James Muckian went to the home of his brother, Patrick, at Market Square in Castleblayney and began a quarrel that resulted in Patrick lying on the ground in a pool of blood, dying from his wounds. Lucas A. Treston, Esq., the Resident Magistrate (RM), happened to be passing at the time, and heard the cries of 'Murder!' coming from the house. He entered the premises, found the two men grappling and saw the fatal wounds delivered to Patrick Muckian.[23] He took the knife from James Muckian and helped the authorities to take him into custody. The trial was set for the next assizes to be held in February 1871.

James Muckian's trial began on 25 February 1871. The prisoner stood indicted for the wilful murder of Patrick Muckian, his brother. The first witness called was Mary Muckian, wife of the murdered man. She explained to Mr Mullholland, one of the prosecutors, her account of the fatal events:

'I remember 16 August. It was a Tuesday. I remember James (the prisoner) coming to my house from the door leading into the kitchen. It was after one o'clock and my husband was upstairs at the time in a sort of work-room. His brother, Peter, was also present at the time,' she said. 'James asked for my husband. I said he was upstairs. My husband came down before I had time to tell him. When my husband came down I could not tell what the prisoner said. Some words were passed. I heard James say that "this was the last day he (my husband) had to live". James kept both hands in his coat pockets. After the use of that expression, my husband said, "I thought I could make you wise, but I couldn't". My husband passed from one counter to the other. I saw James strike a blow on his shoulder and my husband put out his two hands and pushed him from him.'

Mary continued, 'The blow did not knock James down. It was then that James struck him with the knife. He stabbed him more than once. I called out. My husband did not fall at that time. I then saw Mr Treston come into the shop. I remember Peter coming down. Patrick was wounded before and after the other men were present. My husband was twenty-eight years of age and in good health.'

It was also mentioned to the jury that Mary and Patrick Muckian had three children. She was now a widow and the children fatherless.

She was then cross-examined by Mr Monroe, the attorney for the defence. Only her responses were recorded. 'My husband sold leather as well as made shoes. James purchased leather from my husband. The first time I noticed the knife in James' hand was when he got up after being knocked to the counter. My husband had a finishing machine,' said Mary. 'I heard voices in altercation. Some words I could not hear. I was in the kitchen and the voices were quiet. I heard James say some words, but I could not tell what they were.'

Next, the deceased's and the prisoner's brother, Peter Muckian, was called as a witness. Peter stated, 'I am the brother of the deceased and also of the prisoner. I heard the voice of James before I went downstairs. He was asking was Pat in the house. Immediately after Pat went

downstairs I heard James say, "This is the last day you have to live".
I heard the word "knife" used. I immediately went downstairs and
saw the deceased and the prisoner in "holds". I would know the knife.'
The knife was produced and Peter said, 'Yes. That's it'.

Lucas A. Treston was the next witness. He heard the shouts coming from the house and entered the premises to investigate. Treston told
the court, 'I was near the deceased man's house. I heard the scream
of a woman as I was passing by. I heard her cry "murder!" I went into
the shop and saw a man going out the back door. It was James Muckian. I saw the other man bleeding. He was lying on two sacks. I apprehended the prisoner. I tried to take the knife from the prisoner. I
did and marked it and gave it to the police. I remained with the man
until he died which was thirty-five minutes after my arrival.'

Mr Treston also identified the knife in court as the same one
used to kill Patrick Muckian.

James Quinn was called to testify. Quinn told the court, 'I saw
the prisoner. He was passing our house and he did not have his coat
on him. I saw him a second time and he then had his hands in his
pockets. He appeared to be going to his brother's house. I recollect
James being in our house prior to the incident and he was speaking
about Patrick. I could not give the words.'

Mr Law, the prosecutor instructed him, 'You are not asked to
give precise words.'

The justice additionally ordered him, 'Just give the substance.'

Quinn then admitted, 'Well ... James said he was not pleased
with Patrick about the fortune.'

Upon cross-examination by Mr Monroe, Quinn said, 'I never
heard that James was a man of bad temper.'

James Hanratty was brought forward, sworn in and examined by
Mr Mullholland. 'I remember 16 August. I saw James Muckian. I have
known him for three years. Sometimes he would be in bad temper,'
he said.

Mr Monroe then asked him, 'Do you remember when he threatened to cut your head off?' The courtroom erupted into laughter.

Hanratty replied, 'I do not.'

Several other witnesses were called including Susan Muckian,
Phillip Brennan and Pat McCarroll, whose testimony was in relation
to conversations with either James or Patrick Muckian but the judge
considered that they were unimportant to the case. Another witness,
Head Constable McGivern, gave evidence as to the arrangement and
layout of the house where the murder took place.

Dr Gilmore was the last witness to give testimony. He deposed to finding two wounds on the breast of the deceased. Afterwards he found a total of four and a number of 'scrapes'. There was a wound in the stomach. It was the mortal wound. 'He might have recovered from the wound in the lungs, but the other was mortal,' he stated.

After all the witnesses were called, the jury then deliberated for one hour and came in with their verdict. James Muckian was found guilty of the wilful murder of his brother, Patrick.[24]

The sentencing portion of the trial gave James Muckian his only opportunity to speak to the public to give his explanation of the events of the day his brother died. His story was different than those told previously. James said first that the knife used in the murder was in his possession when cutting a piece of wood a few days before the murder. He'd used the wood to put under a clock in the house to make it level and claimed that the knife was with the clock.

After fixing the clock, he'd proceeded to St Mary's Church for mass with his wife, leaving his mother and father, who lived with them, at the shop. James made it clear that whichever way he walked to the chapel, he could have been seen from his brother's shop. He found when he returned that, in his absence, his brothers, Patrick and Peter, had been there and taken the clock. When he went upstairs he found both the clock and the knife were gone. He explained that his mother went to Patrick's house that same evening. Patrick told her he was going to Dundalk the next day to purchase goods for Wednesday's market and he would take a message to his sister who lived there.

'I told my mother that evening that I would go up on the following day, when my brother would be away and finish repairing a pair of boots for a Mrs Hunter as I had promised,' he said. 'On the next day, the 16th, at one o'clock, I went to my brother's house under the impression he was in Dundalk. I saw his wife, Mary, and asked where he was but she gave me no satisfactory answer, but instead, contempt.'

The crucial part of his story of his encounter with his brother is vastly different from the story produced in the courtroom by the prosecution and the witnesses that came forward. James said he heard his brother coming down the stairs and, when he was within three steps of the bottom, his wife, Mary, who had been washing the dishes in the kitchen, struck him in the face with the dirty towel and Patrick pushed him into the shop. Patrick had the knife in his hand.

With emotion, James continued, 'I did not go to the house with the intention of meeting Patrick and I did not have a knife. If the

Lord Jesus Christ was in the position of his lordship and he was tried by the twelve apostles, I am speaking the truth.'

When Patrick shoved him back into the shop was when James received the wound on his wrist. It was still visible and it was his brother that inflicted the wound. A struggle took place in the shop and he took the knife from his brother, who knocked him down and fell on top of him. He found his brother falling on the knife and he tried to pull it from him. With difficulty they got up again, but Patrick held him down with his knee and it was then that James used the knife. He admitted he had used the knife, but in self-defence and for the preservation of his own life. Mr Treston had admitted in his evidence that James and Patrick were in holds when he came in and that in his presence, the prisoner accused his brother of having inflicted the wounds on his wrist.

James then knelt down in the dock and begged for mercy: 'I am now done and humbly implore your lordship's mercy. I am speaking the truth.' Continuing pleading, James did not rise from his kneeling position until one of the turnkeys was ordered by the justice to raise him up again.

The justice then passed the sentence in the course of a lengthy speech explaining the nature of the crime and justifying the prisoner, James Muckian's fate. He reminded James that he was asking for mercy but that he had shown his brother, Patrick, little mercy and he should not deceive himself with false hopes for his own future. The most intense part of the justice's speech to the prisoner was about to come:

'You have been found guilty of the crime of murder. Murder in its most aggravated form. Murder of a character committed by the first murderer, whose crime the everlasting curse of the Almighty perishes. You thought yourself aggrieved for some real or fancied offence in connection with the taking away of that clock. You went to your brother's house, I am willing to assume that it was by accident you had that knife with you, but for a small thing of that kind, you rushed upon him and inflicted no less than three deadly wounds. Why did you not then stay your head? Why did you not then think of your brother, the companion of youth, the companion of your later years, and the one who showed himself kindly to you in endeavouring to establish you in the world? Why did you then hurl him unprepared before his God?' said the judge emotionally. 'That interesting young woman whose conduct you have now impeached is now his widow. You have made her a widow and turned her upon the world with three helpless orphans.'

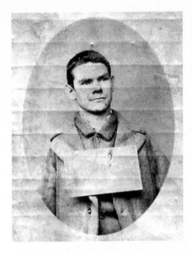

James Muckian on 14 March 1871 upon his reception at Mountjoy Prison. [James McKian, GPB, PEN 1888/49, National Archives, Dublin]

He then addressed the crime and sentence. 'Now it becomes my duty – the most painful duty that can be imposed upon man – to pronounce upon you the dreadful sentence of the law. And that sentence is that you be taken from hence to the prison from whence you came and on Friday, 24 March next, you shall be taken to the place of execution within the walls of that prison, and that you be then and there hanged by the neck until you are dead, and that your body be buried within the prison in which you have been last confined.' He added one last comment. 'I have only again to add that you need not delude yourself with a false hope, and conclude by praying that God may have mercy upon your soul.'[25]

But James was not executed. Since he had never committed an offence before this 'crime of passion' in which he killed his brother, James' sentence was commuted to one of life in prison by the Lord Lieutenant. He was committed to Mountjoy Prison on 14 March 1871.

For many years, James served his time with violent offenders behind the cold confines of prison walls. On his first day in prison, as he was received at Mountjoy, he was written up by the prison guards for having smuggled in monies of 7d and a small bit of tobacco. The first entry of many on his prison record reads:

15 March 1871, Offence: For having retained 7d in money and a small piece of tobacco which were found on him when searched after being cautioned on reception from Co. Gaol on 14th March; Punishment: Specially reported to Director 15/3/71. Money forfeited. Two (2) days bread and water diet. Sgt P.J.M 18/3/71.

James spent the first nine months of his imprisonment in solitary confinement and in December of 1871, he was allowed to enter the general population.[26]

He spent the first eight years of his sentence at Mountjoy working as a shoemaker and keeping in contact with his mother, Anne, in Dundalk, Co. Louth. There does not appear to be any correspondence between him and his wife. In the ninth year of his sentence, his health began to fail. James had developed dyspepsia (a difficulty with digestion). J. W. Young, the medical officer, recommended that he needed a change in environment and, in April 1879, James was sent to Spike Island for four years. He appears to have had several confrontations with other prisoners, as well as breaking the rules by playing prohibited games during dinner, malingering and using improper language. These offences became so prevalent that he was threatened with being put on a 'new marks system', a method by which, with good behaviour and attention to work and duties, a prisoner might be eligible for early parole. Being put on a *new* marks system would mean, essentially, starting over again.

By March of 1886 and back at Mountjoy, James was suffering from rheumatism and still appealing for a licence for parole. When he was released on licence from prison on 1 May 1888, he was forty-one years old. He had served seventeen years in prison for the murder of his brother, Patrick. He began to rebuild his life again in Dundalk.

Coincidentally, the year that James Muckian was released from prison, Patrick's widow, Mary Muckian, cleared out of their shop and residence in Market Square in Castleblayney. The property was leased to Thomas Maguire that same year in 1888.[27]

James Muckian's anger about money and possessions changed his life forever. The clock appears to have represented one possession too many that was snatched from James but it was the sale of the land, and his lack of proceeds from the family holding, that was the spark to the eventual explosion. The justice system came down harder on James Muckian than on the other agrarian outrages in the county over the years. Was it his weapon of choice since knives were considered less than honourable? Were juries more sympathetic when murder was committed in a rage about land rather than property? Or was it the relationship of the victim and his attacker that the jury found so offensive? The most likely reason for the death sentence, and the seventeen years Muckian served in prison, was that the evidence at the trial showed premeditation.

DRUNKEN AND DISORDERLY
Alcohol-Related Crime and Murder

Alleged Assault with a Pitchfork
James and Patrick McKenna, father and son, were summoned at the suit of
Constable Timoney on the charge of assaulting James Gray. Gray was examined and stated that he attended Scotstown fair on Saturday last, and
left that village about half an hour before dark to walk home. At Knocka-
tala, he called at a house called Coulter's and saw James McKenna and Patrick McKenna there. He entered into conversation with them and left the
house in their company and proceeded a considerable distance along the
main road with them. His brother, he was aware, was following him on the
road. He waited for him. The McKennas then passed on. A short time afterwards witness and his brother came up with them. The elder McKenna,
James, had a long stick in his hand and struck witness with it, knocking him
down.
Constable Timoney: I'd say you got a prod with a pitchfork?
Gray: I got a light thrust with something. I could not say it was with a pitchfork. [Is the skin broken?] Yes, in two or three places. The coat I wore on
the occasion is at home and there are two or three tears in a sleeve of it.
Timoney: Did he call you an informer?
Gray: I believed he accused me of being an informer at Coulter's.
Mr Murray: What was the cause of the quarrel?
Gray: Whiskey, your honour (laughter).
John Gray deposed that on the night in question he saw his brother struck
by McKenna, sen. and fall over a ditch. He could not say the assault was
committed with a pitchfork.
Constable Timoney: Did you tell me that night your brother was nearly
killed with a pitchfork?
John Gray: I did not. I was ten perches from him when he was struck. I ran
away as fast as I could.
No evidence was forthcoming to implicate the young man in the matter
and he was therefore discharged.
    James McKenna was detained in custody pending the production of
two men to bail him out with £5 each, that he would be of good behaviour
for twelve months.
                                – *The Northern Standard*, 24 March 1883

Evidence exists suggesting that alcohol-related violence was a lethal
form of entertainment in nineteenth-century Ireland. Characters at
the pub, fairs and markets often instigated fighting by name-calling
and coming to blows as both a display of dominance and especially,
for amusement. Challenging others verbally and physically was how
many such murders occurred. On 27 December 1859, James Farrell
was killed after he drunkenly challenging another man, Pat Smith,
to a fight. While at Robert Goudy's public house on Dublin Street in

Monaghan town, Farrell initiated the altercation by saying to him, 'I could beat a better man than you' to which Smith replied, 'I could beat a better man than *you*'. Farrell was then knocked down and Smith stamped on his belly. Farrell was taken upstairs in the pub to rest and recover. When Dr Temple arrived the next day, he was startled by the symptoms and told his patient that he would not live and that 'he might arrange and prepare for his change'.

The verdict was death on Wednesday 28 December 1859 from injuries inflicted on him by Pat Smith (of the townland of Anna-cramph) on the evening of Monday 26 December 1859.[28] Although Pat Smith was considered to have caused extensive internal inflammation in Farrell's body and killed him, no documentation could be found to suggest he had been sent to trial at the assizes. Being named as a killer at the inquest did not guarantee a trial at the assizes and penal servitude.

Rioting between opposing sides or factions after a race, game or other social gathering such as a dance, was another opportunity for yelling insults, challenges and alcohol-related fighting. On a Thursday evening in the month of January 1857, James Corr and a friend got into a fight with two brothers named Murphy as they all walked home from a dance. The dance was held at Pat Herbert's in the townland of Killykeskeame, in the parish of Killeevan. Corr's master, Thomas McCarvle, heard about the fight and came charging down the road to Corr's defence. As the two parties began to separate, someone began yelling 'derisive cheers and insulting language' that so enraged the Murphys that the fight began again. At the end of the affray, McCarvle had been hit in the head with a stone and lay unconscious on the road. He died the next day. At his inquest, those he'd fought to defend couldn't recall who actually had hit him. In fact, the verdict stated death came on Friday 16 January from injuries sustained on the morning of the 15th, but how sustained or by whom inflicted, the jury had no evidence to show them.[29] A side note was added by Waddell stating, 'James Corr gave evidence that exonerated the Murphys from injuring the deceased.' Often, a coroner and his jury were either unable or unwilling to name a person responsible for the death, especially if conviction of the accused appeared inappropriate if not impossible to prove. The same problems occurred when such cases went to the assizes. One judge is recorded as commenting, 'Perjury in Ireland only refers to giving false evidence to convict an innocent man, no sin in lying to exonerate.'[30]

Excusing Crime and Murder: Blame it on the Drink?
Drink played a big role in the life of the poor throughout the century
and in an 1873 report, government inspectors stated that drunkenness was the main source and cause of crime.[31] It is believed that poverty turned many people towards drink, either the legal stuff or the
illicit poitín, although other sources reveal that people drank less during times of depression and more during times of prosperity.[32] Socio-
logists have pointed to several causes for heavy drinking, such as the
low marriage rate prevailing after the famine, the growing sexual puri-
tanism (the practice of celibacy) and they have suggested that heavy
drinking was most characteristic of middle-aged bachelor farmers and
that the all-male drinking group offered an emotional substitute for
marriage and family.[33] Bachelors make up the largest segment of those
appearing in alcohol-related murder and death in the coroner's casebook.

A drink was often needed before and after committing a crime.
It also brought newcomers into the criminal class as they committed
assaults while drunk, or did a crime to buy drink.[33] The crimes perpetrated while under the influence of alcohol ranged from disorderly
conduct charges (such as loud verbal attacks or public drunkenness,
resulting in a short amount of jail time and a fine) to assault, rape,
manslaughter and murder, with sentences at various prisons. When
crimes were recorded by the police, alcohol was only recorded in relation to the incident if the perpetrator was being charged with drunkenness or as being drunk and disorderly. The problem with recording
statistics in this manner is that it will show only a small portion of
offences that are alcohol-related, when the incident rate is much higher. It is safe to assume that in many of the cases of crime and murder,
drink played a larger part than has been documented.[34]

Disorderly conduct: Several men are arrested for assaulting each other
on the road in the townland of Shanmullagh having been at the public house for a 'harvest bottle' and several rounds of whiskey.
   Larceny: John Goodwin stole £5. 10s. from his acquaintance, Pat
McQuellan, while they shared a room with a quart of whiskey and
two girls.[35]
   Assault and stabbing: Having been drinking for four hours, two
men taunt back and forth about 'pinning' each other down. One no
longer believes it is still a joke, brandishes a knife and stabs the other
in the belly.
   Illegal pawning: An old man lodging with strangers steals their

cow, sells it and later, when found at a pub, offers to buy them a drink with his new money.

Theft: A man steals a purse from his host, who had offered him drink and lodging. He is apprehended later at the pub.

Vagrancy: Two women, both said to be 'of bad character', with no known residence, were found lying in the street in a state of intoxication. A guilty sentence was passed, which gave them the option either of paying £2 in fines or of being transported.

Assault and abduction: A girl's father had refused a potential suitor for an arranged marriage. The man and his friend later drink too much on fair-day, overtake the cart the girl and father are travelling in, beating the father and taking the girl against her will in the hopes of getting better acquainted with her.

Furious driving: A lawsuit was filed by a man injured when another crashed with a horse and cart into his own having drunk *macrone*, a combination of brandy and whiskey.

Using threatening language: After several hours of drinking in a public house, a drunken man threatened to burn down another's house.

These crimes illustrate just how often drunkenness was a factor in criminal acts. Offenders were either fined or punished by short imprisonment. However, in regard to homicide, there is an interesting pattern that emerges in relation to alcohol and the 'class' of victim and killer. When homicide was examined by assizes juries to determine the most appropriate sentence, the state of mind of both the victim and the attacker was evaluated. The following case of crime, prostitution, alcohol and murder and the final verdict of the assizes jury best illustrates how drunken behaviour and the state of mind of the victim and the occupation of the primary witnesses influenced the outcome of justice.

Robbery as the Motive for Murder?
– or did Intemperance and Prostitution Sway the Jury?
The Murder of John McBride, Maghernakill, April 1872

> Robbery was the motive in less than 3 per cent of homicides. Non-fatal robberies were often impulsive acts, committed when a victim left a fair with money in his pocket and as the police reports might note, 'the outrage was possibly suggested by the victim's intoxicated state' ... Drunks were ideal targets for two reasons: they were easy to rob and they were highly unreliable as witnesses.
>
> – Carolyn Conley, *Melancholy Accidents:*
> *The Meaning of Violence in Post-Famine Ireland*

On 6 March 1872, a fair-day in Castleblayney, John McBride, an elderly man from Broomfield, was in town all day enjoying several rounds of drink. At 10.30p.m. McBride walked out of a pub and encountered a woman standing on the street. He asked the woman, Mary McGarvey, if she might 'help him to the livery stables where H. Kernan lived, in order for him to get a ride home'. She took him by the arm and, while they were walking up the road, a man she knew, twenty-year-old Terence McGuigan, came up to the odd couple. McGuigan put his finger to the old man's forehead asking, 'Who is this?' and didn't wait for a response. He began beating the old man in the face with his fist, knocking him down on the ground and kicking him. Mary was screaming, 'Don't kill the old man!'

McGuigan then turned on Mary. He cut her over the eye with a knife, then threw her to the ground and kicked her. While she lay on the ground, he kicked her repeatedly and told her he would 'put her from speaking'. After the attack was over and McGuigan had walked away, Mary went over to the nearest water tank and washed her face. She didn't know what had become of McBride, as he had left the scene. She went to Dr Gilmore's to have her face dressed.

At six o'clock the next morning, Mr Jonathan Whitby was travelling along the Dundalk-Castleblayney road when he found John McBride lying on his back. He was covered in blood, the side of his face was swollen and one shoe was off. McBride was alive, but too weak and sickly to travel. He complained of internal injuries, particularly in his chest. Whitby retrieved a car for him and with the help of Head Constable McGivern, he was removed to Phillip Daly's lodging house in Castleblayney where they decided to take him on to the hospital. At that time, Constable McGivern took a statement from McBride in which he identified his attacker as Terence McGuigan.

Over the next few weeks, McBride's condition worsened. He was discharged from the hospital and sent to his home in Maghernakill, ultimately, to die. McBride was suffering from the beating he had received and gangrene had set into his left lung. Constable McGivern arrived on 30 March to take another statement from the dying man, in which he stated that he believed he was about to die and go before God. He again explained that the injuries he received on the fair-night three weeks earlier had left him in the state that he was in. Once again, he stated clearly that Terence McGuigan had beaten and kicked him, during which attack he'd begged McGuigan not to choke him. It was McGuigan who left him on the side of the road where he was found. Just three days later, on 2 April 1872, John McBride died of gangrene of the left lung. An inquest was held by the coroner which resulted in a verdict which read: John McBride came to his death on 2 April 1872 from injuries wilfully inflicted on him on the night of the 6 March by Terance McGuigan, such injuries having seriously accelerated the death of deceased. Aged 56 years. McGuigan was arrested the same day at Casey's public house in Drumganus in the district of Broomfield. McGuigan was indicted for the murder of John McBride and additional charges were brought against him for feloniously wounding Mary McGarvey.[36]

When the trial began at the Crown Court in Monaghan on 13 July 1872, the Hon. Justice Barry explained the charges to the jury and instructed them how they should decide upon a verdict: 'If a man inflicted violence on another in a delicate condition and it accelerated death, then that violence became of a most serious character. If you have evidence that the intent was to rob him, and that the intent was not to kill him, but that the violence resulted in death, you will find your bill (presumption of guilt) accordingly,' he said.

First it was established that, on 6 March 1872, the deceased, John McBride, had been drinking heavily with a labouring man named Peter Kelly. Patrick Rudden, who ran a public house in Castleblayney, testified that the two men had been in and out of the pub several times throughout the day and night. Rudden said that McBride was drunk when he left, but was able to take care of himself. McBride's son, John, and Peter Kelly were drunk and had left before the old man.

The next witness was Mary McGarvey. She explained that it was on the street, while walking with McBride, that Terence McGuigan approached them, hit and knocked down the old man, then drew a knife and struck her above the eye. She fell and was blinded with blood flowing from the wound, while at the same time McGuigan kicked her as she lay on the ground. Under cross-examination by the defence, she admitted that she was a prostitute and had spent four years in Mountjoy Prison for robbery.

The man who found McBride the next day, Jonathan Whitby, told the jury how he found the beaten man. However, under cross-examination by the defence, he admitted that McBride did smell strongly of whiskey and that long before the attack, McBride walked with a stick and appeared to be paralysed.

The other witnesses testifying as to the physical state of health of John McBride included several doctors and policemen. All the stories were corroborative – McBride had told all of them he was beaten by Terence McGuigan and most of the medical men were in agreement that, although McBride wasn't in the best physical shape before the attack, his death was a result of the injuries received. Dr Robert Morten explained that he had examined McBride the day after the attack and, at that time, he did not have an abscess on his lung. 'I consider his swollen face was caused by the injuries inflicted and, taken in connection with the exposure to which he was subjected that night, hastened his death,' he said. Dr Robert Morten, Dr Arthur McKeown of Crossmaglen and Dr Samuel Gilmore were all in agreement.

One deposition was taken from McBride prior to his death by a Dr McBlaine, but was not allowed into evidence, as it had not been taken down by a magistrate. Another deposition was allowed into evidence: Head Constable McGivern read out the dying words of McBride, although it had not been signed because, at the time the statement was given, McBride could not even move his hands.

The focus of the trial then shifted to the whereabouts of Terence McGuigan on the day of the attack. It was first established that McGuigan was in need of money on the day in question, 6 March 1872. He had taken in a grey flannel shirt to a local pawn shop to attempt to get money (presumably for drink). The woman working at the shop, Anne Hewitt, recognised the shirt as the same one McGuigan's mother had just bought back for him and refused to give him any money for it. He left empty-handed. According to witnesses, the next day, 7 March, he first appeared at Margaret McDonnell's eating house very early in the morning with his father. They were drunk and had something to eat. McGuigan made a point of telling McDonnell upon paying her for the breakfast, 'Mrs McDonnell, take up your money'. They were next seen at Alice McEneaney's public house in Castleblayney at nine o'clock in the morning buying a pint bottle of whiskey. Catherine Rooney of Broomfield, who worked at Francis Casey's public house in Drumganus said McGuigan and his father had come in and bought half a pint of whiskey each and another half-pint bottle. The prosecution was clearly trying to establish that McGuigan had money to spend the day after the attacks and that possibly that money came from robbing McBride.

The most interesting piece of testimony came from Michael Coyle, who kept a public house in Castleblayney. On 7 March, McGuigan, his father and an 'unknown woman' were in his pub. He said the two men came in while the woman or girl waited outside. She would not come in. McGuigan ordered three half-glasses of whiskey and he brought one outside to the woman. She kept her face hidden with a hood and shawl.

'When the woman got a little soft, she came in and said to give them three more,' said Coyle. 'She reached and gave McGuigan some money out of which he paid. After they had finished those drinks, the woman ordered some more, but I refused her. She said, "You might give them more drink for I have whips of money." She then claimed that McGuigan was her husband. She claimed that a man from New-townhamilton gave her twelve sovereigns last Saturday. Then she be-gan to cry for her orphan children that she said she left at Castlebel-lingham. The woman always kept her face covered and I could not see it at all.'

Was this woman Mary McGarvey? Was her face covered because of the injuries received the night before? This woman appears to have been a beggar or prostitute as the testimony suggests. Was the attack on McBride a violent outburst by the jealous boyfriend of a prosti-tute? Or was it staged – he beat up the victim and she took the money?

The jury recessed, deliberated and reached a verdict. On the first charge of feloniously wounding Mary McGarvey at Castleblayney, the defendant was found not guilty.

On the charge of the wilful murder of John McBride, he was again found not guilty.[37]

How could these verdicts have been reached? One reporter cover-ing the case summarised the evidence and provided the following explanation:

> It appears that it was contended for the defence that the intemperate habits of McBride, coupled with the debility of his constitution, had nearly caused his death, which had been accelerated by his exposure all night on the roadside from his being too drunk to get home; that owing to the state of his mind on the day following the alleged attack, the identification was not to be relied on, and that the suggested motive of robbery of a few shillings was insufficient to account for the crime.[38]

How could all the testimony of the witnesses, especially the medical evidence have been ignored? The verdicts suggest that the jury felt it was McBride's own alcohol problem combined with his physical state that prevented him from getting up from the side of the road. In other words, it was the victim's own fault for being drunk. Would he have been able to walk for help if he had not been drunk? Considering that he was bedridden until the day of his death, the answer is likely no. It is shocking that they did not feel that the motive of robbery of a few shillings was sufficient to account for the crime when it had been presented that McGuigan attempted to sell a shirt to get a few shillings for drink earlier on the same day. Possibly it is true that the motive was not robbery. The jury may have made presumptions that were not disclosed in the courtroom. Was McBride soliciting McGarvey for her 'services' when they were interrupted by her 'lover' McGuigan, who, in a jealous fit beat and robbed them? Or is it possible that she was just helping an elderly drunken man to catch a lift home, when she was accosted by a man she admittedly knew? In either scenario, it can be seen that both McBride's association with McGarvey, a known prostitute, and his drunken state, meant that his credibility was in question before the trial even started.

The jury completely disregarded the charges and testimony of Mary McGarvey. Although attitudes and laws against prostitution were somewhat lax, it appears that society at large, as represented by the members of the Monaghan jury, discredited one's character and honesty, based upon the intolerance of intemperance and sexual immorality at this time. Prostitution existed publicly on the streets of many small towns and villages in Ireland and was, on the whole, ignored, until it involved violence, disturbed the peace or became so noticeable that it became an issue of public, and hence of police, concern.[39]

Burying the Hatchet on St Patrick's Day
The Murder of Michael McGale, Killycooly, Donagh Parish, March 1884

> With every day, and from both sides of my intelligence, the moral and the intellectual, I thus drew steadily nearer to the truth by whose partial discovery I have been doomed to such a dreadful shipwreck: that man is not truly one, but truly two.
>
> – *The Strange Case of Dr Jekyll and Mr Hyde*,
> Robert Louis Stevenson (1886)

In the townland of Killycooly, the Kellys and the O'Briens were said to be feuding with each other since the Christmas of 1882. The Kellys had been arrested by police for drinking on licensed premises during prohibited hours. It was rumoured that they believed the O'Briens took some part in their being prosecuted. Since that time, the two families disliked each other, hatred grew and a year and a half later, the Kellys were still angry.

On 17 March 1884, St Patrick's Day, twenty-six-year-old Michael McGale had just arrived at a pub in Emyvale. He'd just been at the funeral of a man named Johnny Boxty and there was probably a lively atmosphere in town that St Patrick's Day. Michael ran into John

O'Brien of Killycooly at the pub. The two men, along with another friend, Frank Donnelly, eventually left for O'Brien's house. Patrick O'Brien, John's brother, was at the house when they arrived and the men remained there for several hours. At 10p.m. McGale and Donnelly decided to go home.

Throughout the evening, their neighbour, Frank Kelly, could be heard shouting different warnings and obscenities from across the fields at the O'Briens. It was night and as Patrick O'Brien later told the coroner's jury, 'God knows how far you could hear him. It was night and you might be able to hear him all the way to Glaslough.' Fearing trouble, John decided to walk with his friends a short while on their journey home. Before they left, Patrick went to see if there was any trouble ahead and make sure the coast was clear. The Kellys were unpredictable.

As John, Michael McGale and Frank Donnelly walked along the road, suddenly through the darkness of the night they heard Frank Kelly scream, 'To hell with the O'Briens, the Indian-meal-fed O'Briens, and black blanket carriers!'[40]

John recognised the voice as Frank Kelly's and then saw his own brother, Patrick, scuffling with Frank Kelly on the road ahead. John then addressed Frank Kelly by saying, 'What do you have to say to me?' At the same time, several members of the Kelly family appeared. In the darkness, Owen Kelly, Frank's brother, was coming up over the fields in a stooping position, looking ready to pounce on the men fighting with his brother. Owen came up behind John and hit him on the back of the head with what looked like a short stick.

As John lay on the ground, Patrick and Frank Kelly were still wrestling. When Patrick looked up, he saw Michael McGale just starting to bend down to try to get Frank Kelly off of him. Suddenly, behind Michael a figure appeared. It was Owen Kelly with a hatchet raised in his hand, arm cocked. The hatchet landed at the base of Michael's neck. He hit him once while he was standing, then again as he was lying face down on the ground.

Donnelly later told the coroner, 'Owen Kelly hit him a chop on the neck and the blood gushed out. I didn't see it because it was dark, but I heard it coming like the steam from the pipe of a kettle and the stream ran down on the road from under him.'

Michael McGale was killed almost instantly. The men put him upon their backs to carry him back to the O'Brien's home, but it was too late. He was dead. Owen Kelly had severed his vertebrae and the spinal cord with the hatchet. He was nearly decapitated.

In the days that followed, the inquest was held at the O'Briens' home. The entire neighbourhood was distressed by the incident, but no one more so than Margaret McQuade, Michael's aunt, who cried through most of the inquest. She told the jury that she raised her nephew from the time he was four years old: 'When my sister, his mother, died, I took him having no family of my own. He was twenty-six years of age, a credit to me and my good luck ... On Monday, he was in his usual good health, in the best of spirits. He was an eleven-stone man,' she said.

Surgeon G. H. Manning told the jury, 'Dr Houston assisted me today in the post-mortem examination which I made of the body. We found a deep incised wound extending a little below the angle of the left jaw to slightly beyond the mediate line at the back of the neck where it terminated an inch above the beginning of the hair of the scalp. The wound penetrated the deep tissues and took a slanting direction downwards from the ear, dividing the second vertebra of the neck. The cut was deeper than the spinal cord on either side of it and in consequence, it must have been crushed by the weapon used. Many of the minor arteries of the neck were severed and haemorrhage must have been very profuse. The wound was evidently caused by a heavy and tolerably sharp instrument and tremendous force must have been used. A weapon such as the hatchet produced could have inflicted these wounds. I believe death resulted from the injury to the spine and must have been almost instantaneous. There was also a trifling discolouration of the skin on the abdomen which was the only other injury to the body.'

The verdict was death from injuries inflicted on Michael Mc-Gale by Owen Kelly.

The assizes commenced in July 1884. Owen Kelly, Francis Kelly, Sally (Sarah) Kelly and Anne Hagan were charged with different offences for inciting and participating in the riot and all pleaded guilty. Owen was charged with murder. Mr Boyd, who represented all the parties, contended that there had been no premeditation whatever and entered a plea of guilty to the lesser crime of manslaughter.

Francis Kelly was charged with assaulting Patrick O'Brien, thereby causing him actual bodily harm. He was ordered to be incarcerated for 18 months with hard labour. He was considered by the justice to have been morally responsible for the murder of Michael McGale. The judge told the court, and Frank, that none of the unfortunate events that happened would have occurred if it had not been for him. It was clear to all in the courtroom that, had Frank Kelly not antago-

nised the O'Briens and their friends, confronted them on the dark
road that night and then been in need of assistance when he was not
able to handle the altercation he had started, his brother Owen and
the others would not have needed to come to his rescue.

As for Owen Kelly, the judge said he was sorry that he would have
to inflict a very heavy punishment upon him. He believed that Francis Kelly was the author of all the disturbances and that the death of
McGale was attributable to his conduct. He felt that Owen Kelly was
of high character and that if this wasn't so from the evidence, he
would have passed a much heavier sentence. The prisoner was sentenced to penal servitude for a period of ten years.

Many explanations can be offered for this brutal murder, but none
makes more sense than the simple fact that alcohol was involved. The
Kellys were probably drinking through the evening and the entire clan
incited to violence by Frank, who spent the whole evening yelling
obscenities at the O'Briens. When Owen took a hatchet and buried
it into the back of Michael McGale's head, it was in a passionate moment that was unlikely to have occurred if not mixed with drink, bad
temper and the instinctive need to protect his brother. Again, these
drunken altercations and challenges between men were commonplace
and a test of masculinity and strength.

Owen Kelly served his sentence at Mountjoy prison. When he
arrived, he was a single man of fifty-three years of age. Like most prisoners, he spent time picking oakum and at trades such as carpentry.
According to Owen's Mountjoy records, his brother, Francis, wrote to
the governor of prisons on his behalf on several occasions and was able
to help Owen get released a few years before the end of his sentence.
After only five years, he was released on 19 July 1889. He returned to
live once again at the family home in Killycooly amongst the neighbours in his townland, who included the O'Briens and the McQuaids.

FIGHTING ABOUT RELIGION ON ST PATRICK'S DAY?
The Price of Fun, Fighting and Freedom

Several deaths and murders appearing in Waddell's casebook were believed to have resulted from sectarian feeling stirred during religious
holidays and social events. St Patrick's Day, Orange Order marches in
July and election days in November were often triggers for such out-
breaks of violence among both Catholics and Protestants. Yet most
of these killings were not motivated solely by politics and religion.

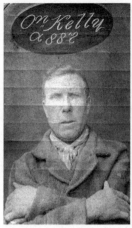 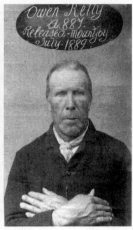

Prisoner Owen Kelly
when he was received
at Mountjoy Prison
and upon his release
five years later.
[Owen Kelly,
GPB, PEN 1889/79,
National Archives,
Dublin]

Fighting fuelled by alcohol was often the primary form of entertainment and, during such affrays, defining sides of 'us' and 'them' served the social function. This labelling offered ease and identification as well as justification for recreational violence very similar to other types of faction fights.[41] The distinction however, is not easily identified and not likely to be isolated in many of the cases believed to be sectarian.

Men challenging one another, wrestling, fighting and rioting was a common occurrence during the celebration of St Patrick's Day. Newspaper reports of sectarian homicides supported party lines and political agendas and once all the facts were revealed, many of these murders appeared to be a result of drink, erratic behaviour and random outrage. Such was the case when the murder of the Protestant, Owen Fox, was reported, but fear and partisan journalism quickly abounded. In the case of Fox however, the newspaper quickly retracted their original claims of sectarian violence and corrected itself by publishing the facts.

Murder on St Patrick's Night
The Murder of Owen Fox, Lisgillan, Aghnamullen Parish, March 1866

> It is feared that the death of Fox is only the beginning of the bitter fruits of the lying reports of agitating journalists.
>
> – *The Northern Standard*, 24 March 1866

In March of 1866, the headline in the newspaper read, 'Murder on St Patrick's Night'. The victim, Owen Fox, was described as a Protestant labouring man working for a respectable farmer in the parish of

Aghnamullen, who while walking with two Roman Catholics was assaulted by them. The report claimed there had been a dispute between the parties when discussing the late trials in Monaghan. They were referring to the trial of the infamous Warren Gray, a Protestant man with a notorious reputation who had recently been acquitted on charges of murder. Fox's employer was one of the jury in Gray's case and it was alleged that he was justifying his master when the final blow to the head, with a loaded butt, fractured his skull. The article implied that more Roman Catholics would be striking out against Protestants as a result of the trial of Warren Gray.[42] Edward Warren Gray, a Protestant from Ballybay, had been acquitted of shooting and killing two Catholic men during a party fight on election night in 1855.[43] Warren's father, Sam Gray, was a notorious figure in Co. Monaghan for abusing justice and had also been charged with the murder of a Catholic – and acquitted – years earlier.

No evidence was produced at Fox's inquest to support the newspaper's claims. Waddell's inquiry revealed that the story was pure sensationalism, used to allow journalists and editors to publicise their own political agenda. Owen Fox had been drinking at a public house in Ballybay with his brother Pat, their sister, Susan Fox, his wife, Ann, and their family friend, John McGough. When walking home they met three men. Both parties had been drinking, some words passed and Fox's party, including his sister, Susan, were knocked down. John McGough clarified the content of the conversation during the altercation, as well as identified the men who attacked them:

'I was in company with the Fox family when, near Mr Dunbar's Gate, we were overtaken by three men, two of whom were John and Thomas Lattimer. Some trifling words as to the weather were passed, and when Thomas Lattimer gave the lee [leeway] he then knocked Pat Fox down, struck Susan and then knocked Owen down. I saw no more, but fearing my turn would be next, made off for home.'

Pat Fox described the hours before Owen died. 'Owen was bleeding. We all hurried to Nancy Hand's near Drumskett. After washing up Owen, we then hurried on to Mr Thomas Rowland's, the deceased's master. Owen was put to bed and he died in the morning. From the time he was knocked down till his death, he never spoke or answered when spoken to, although sensible of what was said to him.' The verdict was death from injuries caused by Thomas Lattimer on the night of 17 March 1866. Owen Fox was aged twenty-seven years.[44]

The following week, a retraction of the story was published explaining that the newspaper had received letters from a local magistrate. These letters stated 'not a single word had been uttered between the two parties or in any way identified either party with religion or politics.' Additionally, the Revd Mr Clifford wrote that 'There is not in the whole world a more peaceable, sober, loyal, well-conducted people than the Catholics of this neighbourhood, and I can appeal to every gentleman in this and the surrounding parishes to bear testimony to this truth.' The editor of *The Northern Standard* continued saying that they had published the story from *The Daily Express* and that 'we regret giving it [the story] publicity as the circumstances there stated, were not by any means correct. Correspondents in writing to journals should be careful in giving the true statements, not colouring them by their own prejudices or feelings.' If not for the facts gathered by the local authorities, specifically the coroner's inquest, it may be possible that the truth would have continued to elude the general public and to incite fear amongst the populace.

SECTARIAN AFFRAY
Murder and Death at the Orange Marches

Within the twenty-year time-frame of Waddell's casebook, many deaths and murders took place during or as a result of the marches of the Loyal Orange Order in July. The marches brought such frenzy of participation that, each year within the crowds themselves, men were accidentally trampled in the multitudes. The Orange march of July 1872 at Bessmount was one in which two men were killed by their own party members as a result of horse and cart crashes. On the afternoon of 12 July, several witnesses saw a young boy at the head of a horse harnessed to pull a carriage and passengers, trying to fix the horse's winkers as it rested on the side of the road. The boy made every attempt to keep the horse steady, but it broke free and the runaway carriage swung side to side through the crowd. Coming down the crest of a hill just a short way off, the horse and carriage knocked two men to the ground as they walked with fellow Orangemen in the march. The Revd Mr Ash was in attendance, brought the men spring water and wine and took both injured men, David Gorman and James Shaw, to his home in his own cart. Gorman died soon after the impact.

Dr William Woods later examined Gorman's body and found that death resulted from a fracture of the lower part of the sternum and a fracture of one of his ribs. There were serious contusions on the left side of his body and on the face and head. Gorman was forty-eight years old.[45] Shaw was taken to the county infirmary and upon death was considered to have died as a result of a concussion of the brain and the contusion to his head from coming in contact with the horse and cart. Shaw was forty years of age.[46] The owner of the horse and carriage, Edward William Story, was chastised by the coroner's jury for his negligence. They noted that he should not have used that particular horse on that busy day as it was proved that Story knew it to have a bad temperament. It was recommended that Story offer some monies to the families of the men his runaway horse had killed.[47]

Other deaths occurring at the marches did not appear to be accidents. Marches were anticipated well in advance not only by Orangemen, but also by members of such groups as the Irish Republican Brotherhood (IRB), also referred to as Fenians. Deaths and murders surrounding such events stirred huge emotion when they occurred and, years later, those participating were identified as local heroes, rebels and outlaws for each cause.

Creating Heroes, Rebels and Outlaws

The history between the IRB and the Orangemen is a long, tangled and intricate web of battles and uprisings as well as plateaux and peaks in legislation for both sides. One may regard the agendas and movements of each faction at national and local levels as often triggering other events at those same levels (ie national to local or local to national), actions within a network that might be best thought of as a single body's nervous system. Feelings of pain or perceived pain might result in a variety of actions and reactions targeted at the alleged source of that pain. However, there is debate amongst historians about the validity of connecting outrage at local and national levels.

'Fenian fear' was a constant topic of news and information as the movement grew throughout the nineteenth century. The newspaper was the primary source used to spread news, but it also bred fear and terror amongst the predominantly Protestant readership. Any violent event, riot, death or murder that appeared in the newspaper, if at all within the realm of possibility, was attributed to the growing 'revolution' of the Catholics and kept the other factions fearful and ready to act. The editor of *The Northern Standard,* as well as other culprits in the country, would associate any aggression between two parties – Catholic and Protestant – to Ribbonism, the Irish Republican Brotherhood or growing sectarian 'partyism'. (Ribbonism has been gradually refined within the academic community, so that the term is now used in both a wide and narrow sense. Originally, the expression covered the gamut of manifestations of Irish agrarian social upheaval, and was used as a 'convenient generic label for peasant disturbance in general'.[48] The term is now used more specifically to denote those clandestine organisations which used quasi-Masonic secret signs and symbols to discern their initiates and which were determined to overthrow British rule in Ireland by means which were never particularly well defined.[49]) Although the majority of newspapers were Protestant-owned, Catholic and Liberal newspapers around the country used the events of the time to support their own causes as well. It is from the actual events around the county, local gossip and partisan journalism that folk heroes and *outlaws* were born. By their mere association with either party line, or as martyrs for the cause, the murdered men and their murderers became local heroes and villains. Regardless of the principles, values and moral foundations, or the lack thereof, in each story, a hero was born to each faction out of the womb of violence.

When murder was considered political, religion was used as the group identity for the accused and the corpse. During such investigations, witnesses lied, newspaper reports were biased, fuelling larger political agendas, and the motives of the accused were unclear. The result of a criminal investigation or trial was perceived as a victory or loss not only for the accused, but for all those of the same religious and political beliefs. Corruption and false information were commonplace. Although murder could be carried out with fists and weapons, in premediatated murder, assassins used guns. They were the primary weapon of choice and used to define sectarian murder.

Several inquests capture the events surrounding political murders in Co. Monaghan, detailing eye-witness accounts of political affray. Many of those mentioned are still a part of contemporary memory. Some are remembered in folk songs, while others have been forgotten during the transition from generation to generation and the blurring of actual events over time. Unless the death or murder was heralded as having changed a way of life, encouraged a revolution or was recorded on a plaque or monument *in memoriam*, many of these persons have been forgotten. They have been resting in the coroner's casebook or in the microfilm of old newspapers. In the stories that follow, each man regains his 'humanness' as a distinct individual and is reborn into history and folklore. The reality that faced these men illustrates the sacrifice they made for their cause – at the expense of their families and their freedom. Through their actions and the circumstances surrounding their deaths, they are remembered as a morbid yet vibrant part of Irish culture and heritage.

Murder at the July Marches
The Death of Thomas Hughes and the Trial of David Baird,
Monaghan, July 1868

> And when they saw their man was fall their agents falsely swore
> That David Baird a man had shot out of his father's door.
> Our hero then was taken and placed in prison strong
> For seven months and better he suffered in the wrong.
> — 'The Conquering David Baird', Folk Song

The year was 1868. Irish Protestants became fearful that the English government was turning its back on them and the proposal of disestablishment of the Church of Ireland became a real possibility. As a measure of support and in an attempt to maintain their power and demonstrate their strength at a local level, Orangemen gathered over 1,900 supporters in small groups around Co. Monaghan to show their support for their cause and to commemorate their heritage. On 13 July there was a gathering of supporters at the house of John Lindsay, who allowed the Orangemen to hold their celebrations of the Boyne victory at his home in Brandrum, located just two miles from Monaghan town. It was on their way back into town that men from the Bellanagall L.O.L. 1142, ran into an angry mob of Catholic and Fenian supporters.

Fourteen Orangemen were ambushed by a large mob of close to one hundred persons as they walked back into Monaghan town. They were forced to fight their way back towards their lodge on Dublin Street under a shower of insults, fists and stones. Having retreated to the lodge on the second floor, just above Baird's pub, while the mob threw stones at the windows, shots rang out and all those on the street began running for cover. Several people were wounded by the gunfire and were either left there or helped to retreat up the street. As the street cleared, the body of Thomas Hughes, a young man from Tyholland parish and a suspected Fenian supporter, lay dead amongst the rubble of stones. His body lay for two hours before anyone dared retrieve it as it was believed the shooters might still be lying in wait. They were believed to be hiding at Baird's pub, the spot from where witnesses later claimed the shots were coming.

Waddell conducted the inquest the next day on 14 July 1868. A jury was assembled and many witnesses were called to provide evidence as to what actually had occurred during the riot that evening. However, while this case is being researched years later, a contradiction arises between Waddell's notes and the court records. Waddell recorded that he interviewed one witness, namely James Hughes, brother of the murdered man. James Hughes stated that the deceased was his brother and explained that Thomas was a small farmer and butcher from Crumlin, Tyholland parish. That was the only information Waddell recorded for that day. He also wrote that the inquest was adjourned and then resumed two days later on 16 July 1868 at 9a.m. This information conflicts with newspaper reports and entries in Bishop Donnelly's diary. It appears that the inquest resumed later on the same day it had been adjourned. Donnelly recorded that fourteen Catholics and nine Protestants were on the jury, and that they had, earlier that day, wished to bring a verdict of wilful murder but that Waddell had refused it.[50] He then dismissed them and, later, he and some of the jury reassembled to record the following verdict: 'The verdict of death was wilful murder by David Baird of deceased, Thomas Hughes on 13 July 1868.'[51]

Why did this irregularity take place? It appears that the Catholics on the jury, eager to name David Baird and gain justice for the murdered man, insisted upon concluding the inquest and expediting the criminal process. The killing of Thomas Hughes was no ordinary murder. It created another martyr for the Fenian cause, while at the same time it challenged those sympathetic to the Crown and Protestant interests to stand up and support their brethren who attempted to defend their right to march. David Baird was becoming a local hero to the Protestant population. They felt an injustice had been done to him and his defence for the assizes was already being constructed. If it could be found that Baird shot in self-defence, in this instance that he was firing because he had been fired upon, then a jury at the assizes could not find him guilty of murder.

Reviewing the depositions of witnesses at the inquest, it was clear why David Baird was found to have committed murder. There were several eyewitnesses stating that shots were fired only from Baird's pub. Constable William Murdock told the coroner's jury that he heard no firing from anywhere except Baird's house. In fact, he'd been trying to control the crowd on the opposite side of the street from Baird's, a mob of about 100 angry rioters throwing stones at the building, and to encourage them to move out of the line of fire. Sub-constable Gilligan also saw shots fired from Baird's window and made a note that he did see bullet holes in the houses across the street from Baird's (McCabe and McKean's homes), but none in Baird's. There were also witnesses stating that Baird, and his brother and cousins (the Clarkes) had run up to the second floor with guns in their hands. Shots were then heard from the second-floor window. The most damning deposition came from an eyewitness, Anthony Meighan, a shoemaker and resident of Dublin Street. Meighan was also a Catholic. He claimed that he saw shots fired by David Baird and John Clarke from the door and the window above. 'I saw Hughes shot. He was standing beside me and was shot by David Baird. As myself and Hughes were standing on the street, balls were coming from upstairs and downstairs. The bullets were coming thick. At the time, Baird was firing from the door downstairs, there were two or three firing from above the windows. I swear it was the ball from David Baird's pistol that killed Hughes,' he said. 'I saw Baird open the door and fire but could not say which half of the door that he opened. He fired six shots. My friend, young Hughes, fell with the second shot.'

There was contradictory information provided by several witnesses depicting the circumstances on the evening of the murder. Dr William Temple examined the body and determined that the gunshot wound on the left side of the chest fractured Hughes' ribs and passed through the left lung, then out the chest on the right side between the fourth and sixth ribs. He added, 'I consider the shot that caused the wound was fired from above.' In addition to the deposition of Dr Temple, three constables from the Manchester police force happened to be inside Baird's pub on the evening of riot as they were travelling home from Dublin. Andrew Drysdale, an inspector of the Manchester police told the coroner's jury that he was in the company of Sergeant George Morris and Constable John Morris at Baird's pub at approximately 5.15p.m. when they heard the noise of a commotion outside. 'We looked out the windows when one of the Morrises said to move away from the window and sit down. As soon as I sat down, two or three bullets came through the window of the room where we sat. They seemed to have been fired from the opposite side of the street at a 'dead level'. The inspector had a bullet hole in the collar of his coat, proving that in fact a bullet had been fired into the room in Baird's pub where they sat. David Baird and his men were not the only persons that day with guns. Someone else from the crowd had been shooting into Baird's pub.

The inquest verdict stating that David Baird had wilfully killed Thomas Hughes, aroused passion for both Catholics and Protestants. The Catholic funeral of Hughes was an event used to arouse conflict. The coffin containing Hughes' body was carried by six men in a crowd of 3,000 marching down Dublin Street, displaying their grief and contempt for the murder. They stopped at the door of Baird's pub, put the coffin in the middle of the street in front of the house and yelled out, 'Murder!' They said prayers aloud and cursed the Baird family, asking the Virgin Mary to have vengeance poured down on their [the Bairds'] heads.[52] On the other hand, David Baird came from a well-known Protestant family, dedicated to such causes as the Orange Order and, as a result, a David Baird Defence Fund was organised to help support his legal costs. There was a surprising donation to the fund of £30 by a Bro. J. Waddell of Australia.[53] Is it possible that even Waddell's family had a personal interest in the outcome?

Mr John Rea, the famous Belfast lawyer, was hired to represent Baird. The first action Rea took was to make an application on behalf of David Baird that the coroner's warrant (the warrant issued for David Baird's arrest) was illegal. Rea also opposed the coroner's proceedings as it was maintained that the jury had remained some time in deliberation, were unable to agree on a verdict and were discharged – yet some jurors returned and signed a verdict of wilful murder. Although, throughout the casebook, adjournments did occur, it is difficult to determine from this coroner's casebook when the inquest reconvened. In the end, Rea's request was denied.

John Baird and John Clarke were also charged with wilful murder. John Baird was charged with having aided and abetted the murder and it would be proved that he handed his son the pistols that his son fired into the crowded street. Clarke would also be proved to have been present and to have aided and abetted the murder as charged in the indictment.

After seven months of imprisonment and a long drawn-out trial, David Baird and the others were acquitted on all charges. As in many other cases of sectarian affray and murder, if a person was proved to have acted in self-defence against an unwarranted attack, they were not held responsible for murder. Although a subject of debate amongst historians, it would appear that the small group of Orangemen were taken aback by the large crowd opposing their march. Having been chased back to their lodge and rocks having been hurled at the building, it appears David Baird and the others decided to keep the crowd at bay with the use of their guns. The entire incident suggests that although there was sectarian feeling amongst the opposing parties, there was an element of recreational violence that went very wrong – especially for the victim, Thomas Hughes. But even before the criminal proceedings to decide the fate of David Baird took place, another murder shared the spotlight in an already tense political climate.

Election Night Murder
The Murder of James Clarke, Monaghan, November 1868

> On the 23rd of this present month, a ruffian found his way at or after eleven
> o'clock at night into one of our Hotels and deliberately shot one of the men
> so brutally and wantonly attacked on the 13th of July (previous). The funeral
> of this murdered man took place yesterday and was attended by at least
> 3,000 of his brethren, as well as a large number of the gentry of the town.
> Fifty Masters of the Orange Lodges wearing scarves and hatbands headed
> the procession. No maledictions were uttered ... The immense crowd ac-
> companied by the body to the Presbyterian burial ground and separated in
> perfect quiet and good order. The contrast of the two funerals [Thomas
> Hughes and James Clarke] is suggestive and needs no comment. There is
> however a quiet determination on every face which it would be well not to
> try too far.
>
> – The Two Funerals, *The Northern Standard*, November 1868

On election night November 1868, only four months since the murder of Thomas Hughes and while David Baird sat in a jail cell waiting
for the outcome of his trial at the assizes, Baird's first cousin, James
Clarke of Corness, was shot dead in Campbell's Hotel in Monaghan
town. The man charged with the murder, John McKenna, was believed to be a Fenian supporter and rumoured to have been fighting
with Clarke on the day of the riot on 13 July earlier in the year. Vigi-
lante justice for the murder of the Catholic Hughes was believed to
have been the motive.

The inquest on the body of James Clarke was held at the courthouse in Monaghan town in front of a large crowd. Twenty witnesses
were subpoenaed to provide evidence on the events of the night of
23 November 1868. Dr William Temple's deposition regarding the
wounds on the head of the deceased was dramatic. 'I saw a deep incised wound on his forehead that a knuckle might do. I have not seen
so severe a wound inflicted by a man's fists; it was more likely done
by the barrel of a stick,' he said. 'I examined the wound of the deceased and it is of my opinion it was inflicted by the discharge of the
two barrels simultaneously.'

What brought about such a violent death for James Clarke? Witnesses were called to explain the sequence of events. McKenna was
greeted at the door of the hotel by Mary Catherine Tailor, a servant
at Campbell's Hotel. She told the coroner's jury, 'I heard a knock at
the front door about 10.15p.m., opened the door and saw a stranger.
I told the man at the door that Mr Campbell would admit no one
that night.' Tailor stated that she identified the prisoner in the dock,

John McKenna, as the man she'd seen that night. 'He made no answer but pushed me aside and went into the hall, then into the commercial room, which is on the left-hand side. I followed him in and told him there was no one there for him. He (McKenna) went in, saw the deceased in the room and said the boy was here that he wanted. I then left the room and went upstairs. I returned on hearing the shot.'

John Baird, Jr., brother of David Baird, deposed that he saw McKenna come into the door. He said, 'I heard a bustle in the hall and went out to look. I got on the third step of the stairs and saw McKenna strike Clarke, who then returned the blow. At that moment, McKenna fired a pistol. I saw it plainly. When the pistol 'twas fired, Clarke put his hands on his belly and ran into the commercial room of the hotel, then came back out into the hall and fell going into the kitchen. McKenna ran into the kitchen.' It is not surprising that this witness claimed he saw McKenna strike his cousin first.

Other guests in the hotel had seen the scuffle and more came immediately upon hearing the shot. Some attended to Clarke while others locked McKenna in one of the rooms of the hotel until help arrived. Sub-inspector of Police, David Harrell, Esq., arrived to arrest the prisoner as well as to take possession of the pistol believed to have been used in the shooting. The verdict was James Clarke met his death on the night of 23 November 1868 in Campbell's Hotel, Monaghan from a wound inflicted by a pistol shot fired wilfully by John McKenna. The deceased was 26 years of age.[54] The newspaper reported that the jury in the case handed the coroner a document signed by the minority of the jury stating that McKenna fired the shot in self-defence. The coroner declined to receive it.[55]

There could be little doubt that Clarke had been a victim of a foul conspiracy. Was the murder of Clarke a retaliatory act for the murder of Hughes and if so, were both Hughes and McKenna members of the Fenian Brotherhood?[56] Christopher McGimpsey in his article, 'Border Ballads and Sectarian Affray', asks this same question. McGimpsey's in-depth look at the murders of Hughes and Clarke via Orange folk-songs and research into the backgrounds of those involved reveals that, indeed, both Hughes and McKenna belonged to the Fenian organisation. There was still motive for the murder, even if not committed in retaliation for Hughes. McKenna had been an active participant in the riot in July and it was rumoured that he and Clarke had been fighting on the day. Also, John Clarke, James' brother, had brought McKenna up on charges of possession of a pitchfork.

Sam Clarke, father of the deceased man, claimed that it was a premeditated murder. He told the coroner's jury that early on the day of the election, McKenna, Daniel Fowley and Frank Smith were standing in Church Square while his son, James, stood across the street by himself. James had been engaged in bringing in voters to be polled. Sam was startled when Frank Smith came up to him and said, 'Your son is a great man now, but he will be shot tonight.' Sam later told his son and made James promise that he would stay at Campbell's Hotel for the night.

One thing is clear: if the murder was planned, it was poorly planned. When Clarke did not leave Campbell's Hotel, McKenna decided to just go in. It is uncharacteristic of an assassin to go in and shoot in front of a hotel full of witnesses. Is it possible that this was an angry man whose temper got away from him? What if McKenna only wished to resume his fight with the Clarkes from back in July but when he began to get beaten, he fired without much thought?

When the trial of John McKenna finally took place, his defence charged that the homicide was justifiable. The fight was rumoured to have started when Clarke, sitting with his friends, thought they might get some sport out of McKenna and a short jostling match occurred; shortly after that the shot was fired.[57] McKenna claimed that he had shot Clarke in self-defence as he'd received serious injury when the two began scuffling in the hallway. Even those present in the hotel after the shooting testified that McKenna was beaten up pretty badly. Mr Alexander Montgomery said he saw Clarke hit McKenna first and McKenna hit him back. Then Clarke began pummelling McKenna, in particular with 'two ringing blows'. It was after this he heard a muffled shot and saw smoke. At this point in time, Montgomery believed McKenna fired the shot.[58]

The jury returned a verdict which the authority presiding over the case, Baron Deasey, did not understand. They handed him a verdict of not guilty of murder, but guilty of justifiable homicide. Shortly after, Deasey said to them, 'Gentlemen, if you come to the conclusion that the homicide was justified by reason of self-defence, it is your duty to acquit the prisoner. If you come to the conclusion that the act was done in self-defence or under reasonable apprehension that his life was in danger and that he felt it necessary, the verdict should be acquittal.'[59]

Mr Butt who was defending McKenna asked to have a word. He stated that he sincerely trusted that the result of an acquittal through the law, would show them that their true protection was in the laws

of the country and that he who violated them took away the best
protection to men such as the prisoner at the bar. He hoped that the
prisoner, his friends, or party in Monaghan, would not look upon the
verdict as a triumph over their opponents but as a triumph of law and
justice and that they would exercise it so as to put an end to the ridi-
culous, absurd and mischievous party feeling in that country.[60]

McKenna was found not guilty.

James Clarke was buried at the First Monaghan Presbyterian
Church on Dublin Street, Monaghan. His gravestone reads:

Erected
By the Orangemen of Monaghan
In memory of James Clarke of Corness
Who was shot by a Fenian
Campbell's Hotel Monaghan

CONSPIRACY AND ASSASSINATION
Killing for the Cause

Fear binds people together. And fear disperses them. Courage inspires com-
munities: the courage of an example – for courage is as contagious as fear.
But certain kinds of courage can also isolate the brave.
 – Susan Sontag, from her essay 'The Power of Principle'

The most popular stories appear to have been conspiracy plots to kill
men who were leaders or in a position to continue executing the laws
and practices opposed by the growing faction of Fenian supporters.
Fenian conspiracy was the most publicised and most feared form of
violence found to threaten the institutions established in the country. When a man named Patrick Burns came back to Ireland from
America and changed the name of the secret society referred to as
Ribbonmen, Bogmen or Rednecks to the Republican Brotherhood,
many took up the cause. They met in abandoned barns, along the
edges of fields and sat along the river under small stone bridges where
they developed their plans to combat those who oppressed them. They
fought the land agents, the landlords, the government, the English
and the Orangemen, attempting to develop a regime to change a way
of life.

When an assassination took place there was not much need for
determining motive. The motive was clear. The accused had intentionally taken the life of his intended victim. The outcome of such

homicides was almost always death for the convicted murderer. What has emerged through the various murder cases that were tried at the assizes is that juries gave the accused the benefit of the doubt that they did not intentionally kill their victim. However, in cases of political assassination, the only outcome to be determined was the punishment.

In contrast to the heroes and martyrs immortalised in song and tale from the Orange Order, many of those involved in secret societies, such as the Irish Republican Brotherhood or Fenians, were so given to secrecy that it prevented many from knowing enough about them or having enough information to immortalise their memory in folk tales. One example of such a participant in the covert operations of the Irish Republican Brotherhood was Joseph Daly of Kilmurry in the Donaghmoyne parish. Although not an inquest in the casebook, Daly's story is one, which illustrates the background of a failed opportunity, an unsuccessful attempt at murder. The consequences of his attempts were punished based on motive.

Convicted of Conspiracy: A Man from Donaghmoyne
The Conviction of Joseph Daly, Kilmurry, Donaghmoyne Parish
Joseph Daly lived on a small farm with his wife, Bridget, and ten children. He had resided at Kilmurry in the parish of Donaghmoyne since the year of his birth in 1826. One can only surmise from the background of the Daly family from previous generations why he joined the Irish Republican Brotherhood. Oral tradition states that the family, referred to as the O'Dalys, owned large tracts of land in Co. Monaghan before the confiscations. A patriot of the same name, Joseph Daly, also of Kilmurry was documented as a leader of his family group. He was exiled to Van Diemen's Land for his activities against British landlordism in the early 1800s.[61] Now another man of the same name and one generation later was fighting for the same cause.

In the 1880s, Joseph, along with several others had been meeting in the fields and abandoned cottages as part of the revolution attempting to subvert the laws and practices of the British government in Ireland. He'd joined forces with Denis Nugent and Thomas Kelly (both tenants of the Ball estate), Michael Watters (schoolteacher), Patrick Finnegan (labourer) and small farmers, James Hanratty,[62] Patrick Geoghegan, Peter Devlin, John Donnelly, John McBride, and blacksmith, James Duffy. The men had secret meetings throughout the area of Culloville and even at the mill of local resident, Patrick Trainor. They set fire to the mill of John McCullagh of Cornally as well as sent local

Protestants, landlords and agents threatening letters. One of their primary goals was to kill the agent of the Ball estate, Henry Gustavus Brooke, JP, of Glenburne, Rockcorry. He had been evicting people who could not pay their rent as well as taking them to court through 'ejectment proceedings.' One man, Pat Duffy, who was aiding the ejectments was sent the following letter by the group:

> Notice – Take warning that if you go on behalf of that Protestant pup of a policeman, you may first of all make your coffin, and if you prove to one of the ejectments that you served you will not prove any more. You are spared a little too long, and have nothing more to do with Orange Brooke. Let him do his own business while he gets leave – that will not be long. Death is your doom if you disobey and death to Brooke without any delay. – Pat Duffy, traitor to justice and assister of tyrants.

Brooke was also sent a letter:

> To Orange Harry Brooks. Take notice if you do not repair the damage you have done and that at once, you will not get more time to consider the matter. You may choose the best to your pleasure to be a Christian or choose the model picture below and after.' [A drawing of a coffin with the word 'hell' and also 'so repent in time, Tyrant Brooks, Blayney.']

When their demands were not met, they began to act upon their attempt to assassinate Brooks. Instructions were given to James Duffy, the blacksmith who had a forge at Culloville, to carry out the murder. When the assassination plot failed, they kicked James Duffy out of their group, accusing him of being a paid informant of the government and of tipping off their target. Unfortunately for them, they were right. Joseph Daly and the men were arrested and accused of treason and conspiracy to murder. It was James Duffy who appeared in court to testify against them as well as providing one of the most damning pieces of evidence. It was a book of minute notes found in an abandoned house (formerly owned by a man named Conlon) in the townland of Killybane in the Cullyhanna district. The book was written in by the schoolteacher, Michael Watters, and his handwriting was verified as it was matched up with the threatening letters. Several books were found hidden in places built in special compartments in the wall. One contained an oath and many names. There was also a minute book recording a collection of £10 for the purpose of blowing up Dublin Castle.[63]

Duffy went on to detail that the Patriotic Brotherhood branches were headed out of Crossmaglen, Culloville and Cullyhanna and that the officers were called 'Bs' and 'Cs'. He stated that prisoner Daly was a B. Their connection with the more nationally-known figures was explained. They had indeed been founded by Patrick Burns and they received letters from O'Donovan Rossa to encourage them to continue fighting for the cause.

The prisoners were found guilty.

Joseph Daly, aged fifty-four years, began his ten-year sentence at Mountjoy in March 1883. He left behind his wife, Bridget, and ten children. Joseph spent his first nine months in solitary confinement removed from the rest of the prison population. Unbeknownst to the prisoner, two weeks after he began his sentence his family had suffered another great tragedy. His daughter, Mary, had died. Bridget waited until after her husband was out of solitary confinement, almost a year after her daughter's death to tell him. She communicated this news in a letter composed to the warden:

Kilmurry, 26 March 1884
M. Murphy Esq.,

Sir, In reply to your letter of the 23rd beg to state hoping you will convey the same to my husband that Mary died on the 9th April a fortnight after his conviction. Her disease was unknown unless a broken heart. I would have sent him word about it at the time but he being a delicate man before his confinement, I thought it better not to mention it for fear it might have a bad effect. Hoping he will get over it better now.

Yours faithfully,
Bridget Daly,
Kilmurry.[64]

Over the years he spent in prison, he was visited by his sons Arthur, Joseph and Thomas, his daughter, Ann, and his sister, Catherine Far-

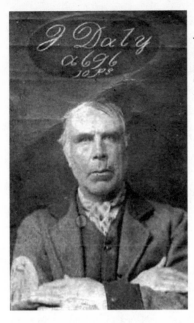

Joseph Daly, member of the Irish Republican Brotherhood on reception at Mountjoy Prison, Dublin, on 3 April 1883. [Joseph Daly, GPB, PEN 1890/2, National Archives, Dublin]

rell. His son, James, wrote to him towards the end of his sentence:

Kilmurry, Culloville via Dundalk
10 September 1889
My Dear Father,
If you would send forward another memorial [appeal to leave prison on licence patrol] right now it might be successful as your sentence is drawing to a close.
Your loving son,
James Daly[65]

Joseph Daly spent seven years in prison, most of it at Mountjoy. He was released from Downpatrick Prison on 21 January 1890 and returned to Kilmurry where he lived with his family for the rest of his days. After his release from prison, he continued to fight against the government until his death in 1903 at the age of eighty.

POLITICAL HOMICIDE
Compensation for Widows and Orphans

The widows and children left behind when their husbands or fathers were killed as a result of political riot or assembly or political assassination could apply for compensation to the grand jury. The Crime and Outrage Act of 1848 was created to suppress offences and was perceived by the government to have worked. The 1850s and 1860s were documented as the periods of lowest crime recorded in Ireland in decades. When the act was renewed in 1870, it was renamed the Peace Preservation Act and designed to provide compensation in cases of 'agrarian offences' such as Whiteboyism, Ribbonism and Fenianism. Section 39 of the act empowered grand juries to grant compensation in cases where a crime of murder arose out of any illegal combination or conspiracy. In two of the cases in Waddell's casebook, widows did appeal for money for themselves and their newly-fatherless children. With no other means of support, these families found themselves at the mercy of the grand jury at the Co. Monaghan assizes.

The Shanco Murder: The Taxpayers Must Cover the Loss
The Murder of William McMahon, Orangeman, July 1870
William McMahon was gunned down during the Orange marching season on 12 July 1870. As he and a group of men marched from Fort Singleton to their lodge near the Shanco schoolhouse, they were attacked by gunfire. He was shot and after many attempts to save his life over the next four weeks, including an operation conducted by several doctors in consultation, McMahon died. Although there were several suspects surrounding the murder investigation, no one was ever convicted.

In the wake of his death, Mary McMahon, wife of the deceased, entered an appeal for £1,000 for loss and damage sustained by her and her three minor children. She first presented her claim at the Presentment Sessions for Truagh, held in Glaslough in November 1870. She was up against strong opposition since if her claim was approved by the grand jury at the next assizes, the fees would be levied off the barony of Truagh. Her claim was passed at the Truagh Presentments and she next proceeded to the Monaghan assizes in February 1871. With her solicitor, Mr George Wright, to guide her through the proceedings, Mary told the court what she knew. On the day of the shooting she knew about the meeting of the Orangemen at Shanco schoolhouse. 'It was well known. My husband was deputy-master. He left home at nine o'clock while the parties were dining at Mr Moutray's. I saw about a hundred with guns, they were unknown, they assembled at Knockakerwin Hill. I heard a volley of shots and my husband was not dead when I saw him. It was from the effects of the ball that he died. He survived four weeks,' she said. 'His average income was £4. I have three children, the oldest is ten years, and the two girls are nine and seven years old.'

Based on the conditions of the act, Mary needed to show the jury that her husband had been killed as part of a conspiracy or illegal group organised for premeditated violence. What did emerge was that the Shanco lodge members had met at Mr Moutray's home, Fort Singleton, for dinner. During their march they were attacked by a large group of men, many of whom were armed and opened fire on the Orangemen. They were said to have been strangers and no one claimed to recognise them. There could be no doubt that these persons had prearranged their meeting to attack the marching men. A rumour had also spread through the neighbourhood earlier in the week. A man whose name was Moore told the grand jury that he worked at Mr Smith's mill and had overheard some of the men say that if the Orangemen met at Mr Moutray's they would be attacked. It was well known through the district.

Mr McDonnell represented those opposing Mrs McMahon's claim. He argued that the fees should be levied against the entire county, not just the barony of Truagh. However, the judge presiding over the case told the solicitor that he could not shut his eyes to the fact that a premeditated attack had been made on the school house and Orange lodge in that location. The justice also stated that 'the Orangemen were vain to continue to subscribe to this "stupid mummery" and utterly childish marching with dirty yellow handkerchiefs ... and when they could not persuade the other party to abstain from interfering with their idle and childish processions, the only thing they could do was to appeal to the pockets of the parties and therefore, possibly this presentment would teach them that if they would continue this work – they must pay for it.'

Having considered her claim, the grand jury awarded Mrs McMahon £200 and £100 to each of her children. The justice ensured that the £500 would be levied off the barony of Truagh.

Murder after the Races: Compensation for a Widow and Seven Children
The Murder of Patrick McKenna,
Dernasell East, Tedavnet Parish, March 1873
Patrick McKenna from the parish of Tedavnet was hit in the head with a rock when he and several friends were walking home from the Monaghan races. They were caught in the middle of a riot when mobs from Tedavnet and Aghabog began throwing stones at each other. McKenna had his head wrapped by a neighbour upon returning home, but

no one imagined that the skull was broken.[66] Within a week, he was delirious. Dr Irwin was called, and at once pronounced the case hopeless. The verdict at his inquest was that Patrick McKenna came to his death on the Sabbath, 9 March 1873 from the effects of a wound inflicted on the evening of 20 February from a stone, but by whom it was thrown or inflicted there had been no evidence to show.[67] He left a wife and seven children ranging in age from twenty years down to the youngest, aged three. Three arrests were made and over thirty persons summoned by police from been identified as having taken part in the riot.

At the Monaghan assizes later that year in July, the three men arrested were acquitted by the jury. It was clear their blame for the death of Patrick McKenna could not be proved, regardless of the eye-witnesses. Mary Anne McKenna, the deceased man's widow, applied for a sum of £1000 to compensate her for the loss sustained by her and her seven minor children. The act empowered the grand juries to grant compensation in cases where a crime of murder arose out of any illegal combination or conspiracy. Men had gathered illegally, began rioting and as a result killed a father of seven children. The grand jury gave the widow £30 and each of the children £10 each, £100 in all.[68]

CHAPTER EIGHT

MATTERS OF LIFE AND DEATH:
CURES AND REMEDIES AND LAST MOMENTS ON EARTH

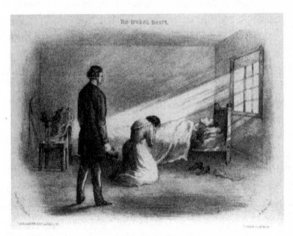

The Broken Heart
[Trench, The Realities of Irish Life (London, 1868)]

Although death came in various 'natural' forms such as disease or heart attack, because of its sudden nature an inquest was often conducted based on the existence of unanswered questions. Extenuating, suspicious or unusual circumstances surrounding such deaths required a more conclusive answer; self-medication, home remedies and treatments performed by the family prior to the death which left physical marks on the body also raised issues. At times a doctor or another official was required to give a more conclusive answer to the death of the deceased.

DEATH BY DISEASE
Why was it investigated?

In 1860, a Select Committee on Coroners Report recommended 'an inquest should be held in cases of sudden death where the cause of death is unknown, and also where, though the death is apparently natural, reasonable suspicion of criminality exists.'[1] An inquest into a seemingly obvious death is illustrated through that of Robert Shannon, who had been living in America for fourteen years, arrived in Monaghan and resumed his residence with his wife, Jane. Just ten days after his return, he was dead. The circumstances of the death caused concern given his brief return to Ireland and the likelihood of an estranged relationship between him and his wife. It emerged in the evidence that he had suffered from consumption in America, but it cleared up during the passage home. However, upon his return, his chronic cough resumed. Dr Rush was called to examine the body and concluded that Shannon had died from consumption. The verdict was death on 24 October 1864 from consumption accelerated by the fatigue of the voyage and journey home.[2] Many other inquests carried similarly reasonable suspicions until the evidence produced cleared and calmed the public's mind as to the cause of death.

The location in which a person was found, contributed towards the decision to hold an inquest. One found living at home alone or a dying person on the side of the road, unable to explain the circumstances prior to death would require an inquest. For example, when Mary McAlier was walking through a field and heard moaning, she looked down and found her grandmother on the ground. The priest and Dr Charles Coote were immediately sent for and attended to the seventy-year-old Ellen McLoughlin. She died shortly after. Dr Coote concluded the old woman fell as result of impeded circulation of the brain, the result of great debility natural to one of the deceased's advanced time of life. The verdict was death from causes natural to one of her time of life.[3]

The State of the Body: Eaten by the Cat
The Death of Robert Connolly, Corragore, Ematris Parish, January 1867
In the townland of Corragore in the parish of Ematris, lived the eighty-year-old Robert Connolly described as having very penurious habits and living the life of a recluse. Although he was reputed to have saved money, the house he lived in was wretched and he lacked either the ability or means to properly care for himself. He was reported to be suffering from convulsions on occasion, and one attack occurred just a few weeks before his death. On the morning of 18 January 1867, Connolly visited his neighbour, Mary Wright. She offered him some breakfast, but he refused and left later that afternoon. It was the last time anyone saw him alive.

Two weeks later, a neighbour, Sarah McHaffy, heard that one of Connolly's windows was lying open. She entered the house, saw him lying on his bed and confirmed her suspicions. Connolly was dead. This was apparent when examining the right side of his face. It had been mutilated and gnawed as if by rats or a cat. Considering his age, the wretched house he lived in, the extreme cold during the previous two weeks and his attack of convulsions, it was concluded that Robert Connolly's death occurred as a result of natural causes.[4]

For some, the reason their deaths were investigated was possibly owing to their occupation or unknown circumstances surrounding the death. For example, a policeman, Charles McCue, brother-in-law of Mr William Johnston of Fort Johnston, died from a heart attack on a July morning. Although Surgeon Rush and Mr Johnston both told the coroner that the deceased had suffered from heart disease for at least twelve months, an inquest was held.[5] It is interesting that an inquest was held on McCue, given that very often the well-known and affluent persons in the community avoided such public inspection of their loved one's death and very often pleaded with the coroner to hold merely an inquiry. In the case of McCue, possibly because of his position as a police officer and the fact that the circumstances were not laid out in the details of the inquest, the death was investigated.

The age of the deceased was also a contributing factor in holding an inquest. Eighteen-year-old Margaret Maguire was working with her father, Thomas, in the bog wheeling turf. After dinner, she complained of not feeling well, and the moment the words passed her lips, she dropped to the ground. Thomas took his daughter in his arms, laid her over his knee to give her some fresh air hoping to revive her, but she never spoke another word. The only explanation offered for her death was that she occasionally complained of pains around her heart. Dr McKinstry was called to examine the body but did not perform an autopsy: 'The body presents no marks of injury but from its appearance and the evidence of previous symptoms, I consider her death to have resulted from disease of the heart.'[6] Although the evidence was inconclusive, more information was sought, possibly in an attempt to clarify how such a young girl might be taken so early in life.

CALLING FOR HELP IN THE LAST MOMENTS OF LIFE
Remedies, Cures and Physicians

Many of the doctors in the coroner's casebook are described as attending to the sick (soon to be deceased) as quickly as possible and providing their utmost care to their patients. Dr Henry and his son, also a physician, were documented time after time as having arrived as soon as they could, providing every necessary treatment in an attempt to save the patient's life. Many other fine physicians were described in the same manner. However, some descriptions are not as flattering. Many people had reservations about calling a physician. One reason for this was the lack of money to pay for his services. Also, a general attitude of scepticism prevailed towards doctors in the nineteenth century, as many felt that these were men that could take advantage by making a profit from helping the sick and dying.

As mentioned previously, Dr William Gillespie had reportedly refused to treat a man whose legs had been severed on the railway tracks and who was lying there in pain and agony. Gillespie complained that the Ulster Railway had not paid him in the past and he would no longer do any work for them. The man bled to death.[7] Poor attendance by practitioners was also recorded when they had been called upon but were not able or willing to help the dying patient. Dr Reid of Slieveroe dispensary was documented as having poor attendance in the case of William Gibson, a one-year-old child who was suffering from burns after he pulled a bowl of boiling water on himself. The boy's mother, Anne Gibson, told the coroner that she'd gone to the dispensary where she saw Dr Reid and he gave her a salve for the child but it did little good. Upon returning to him after a few days, she found Dr Reid intoxicated and he told her he could not attend the child at that time but would see him in the morning. He never arrived. Dr Reid never attended the child again and ten days later, young William died as a result of his injuries.[8]

Due to the lack of confidence in physicians and the medical profession, many persons were more apt to self-medicate than to call a physician. Samuel Benson was one such man. For three months he was in delicate health and complained of pains in his sides and kidneys. His companion, John Slowey, told the coroner that Benson was more disposed to treat himself than to employ doctors. He was taking sarsaparilla, a sweetened, carbonated beverage flavoured with sassafras and oil, distilled from a European birch (it also came in tonic or syrup form) which was often used in the nineteenth century as a herbal medicine, advertised as a cure-all, for rheumatism, skin diseases, a hair restorer, anti-inflammatory, liver-protector and blood purifier. When Benson's health took a turn for the worse, John Slowey asked Dr O'Reilly of Clones to come and see him. Dr O'Reilly had known Benson for a long time and was aware of his forcefulness as to his own health, that he was disposed to treat the case on his own and knew him to also use 'instruments' if necessary.

When the physician arrived at the residence of the sick and dying man, he found him in a 'heavy stupid condition like one after taking a narcotic'. When spoken to, Benson responded gruffly and dropped over again. O'Reilly ordered 'mustard' to arouse him, a pungent yellow powder used in medicine as a stimulant and diuretic, an emetic, or a counter-irritant and then offered him some tea. Benson went into convulsions, recovered, but fell back into the same inanimate state. Dr O'Reilly next gave him some brandy but received no response. Shortly after leaving his patient, the physician got word of his death. The verdict was death on Thursday 24 April 1862 from congestion and bleeding of the brain.[9] Based upon the practices and remedies of the practitioner at this time, it is not surprising that many persons used similar treatments within their own home to try to cure the dying.

Gentian Root: Improving Appetite?
The Death of Alice McDonald,
Smithborough, Clones Parish, October 1874
Alice McDonald was a twenty-one-year-old woman in good health, until the beginning of October 1874 when she began complaining of pains in her stomach and sides. She described them as acute of which the severity was increasing. Her appetite remained good (she did not have heartburn and was fond of fruit) throughout the time of her stomach pain; however, it began to wane. On October 24 she took some milk and whey but vomited it up at 2p.m. She was then given a dose of castor oil by her mistress, Ann Jane Moorhead, but it had no effect. Castor oil was taken to cure a variety of problems such as abdominal disorders, colic, enlarged liver and spleen, nervous diseases, fever, headache, etc. It was used as a purgative in the treatment of acute constipation, intestinal inflammation, and worms.

It was stated that she also took gentian root for the purpose of improving her appetite. Gentian root (Gentiana macrophylla) is a bitter herb popularly used as an anti-diarrhetic and a remedy for anaemia. Gentian can be brewed into a tea or taken in extract form. Other anti-diarrhetics of the time were blackberry, black pepper and ginger. The remedy was used to no avail. Alice died the next day on 25 October 1874. Dr Reid deposed that her death came from inflammation of the bowels.[10]

Bleeding the Patient
Opening Veins and Using Leeches
Many cases document the use of home treatments and cures performed on the dying as a last attempt to save their lives. The practice of bleeding (or bloodletting) was used frequently in the mid-nineteenth century and examples of such treatments exist in the casebook. Bleeding was used for every ailment imaginable including pneumonia, fevers, back pain, rheumatism, melancholia and other types of injuries. In the casebook, however, it was recorded as being used as a technique for restoring animation to drowning victims and other unresponsive persons. An incision was made on the body of the person in distress using an instrument called a lancet, a vein was opened and blood allowed to flow from the patient. It was believed to relieve tension in the arteries, thereby reviving and regaining animation in an unconscious victim. Physicians, as well as relatives desperate to keep their loved ones alive, performed the treatment. Drowning was the leading cause of accidental death according to Waddell's records and in an age before cardio-pulmonary resuscitation was used to attempt to revive the recently drowning victim, bleeding was the common form of treatment. Although the procedure was believed to have restored some back to life, most often, as shown below, such attempts were futile.

Trying to Restore Animation
The Death of Matthew McCabe, Cortober, Ematris Parish, August 1856
One Saturday afternoon in August 1856, James McCabe was walking home when he met two of his three nephews. He chatted with the young boys for a while, inquiring where their youngest brother, Matthew, was. They told him they had been playing with him and he had wandered off just a short while before. None of the parties were concerned as they assumed he was just a short way off. James parted company with the boys and continued down the road, when suddenly he heard the boys screaming to him for his assistance. He ran back to witness his two nephews standing around a bog hole and their little brother, Matthew, face down, floating in the water.

As quickly as possible, James retrieved the boy, but he was dead.

The Rockcorry police investigated the death and recommended to the coroner that an inquest be held. The boy's face had a dark appearance and there was a large wound in his neck. The jugular vein had been cut.

Dr Moore performed the post-mortem examination and explained the state of the corpse. 'I found the face very dark and livid. There

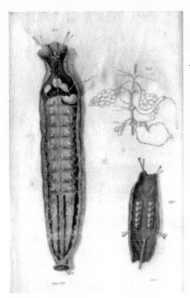

The Underbelly of the Leech
A Treatise on the Medicinal Leech
Johnson, James Rawlins,
(London, 1816)

was an incised wound in the left jugular vein, but the appearance of the face is natural to that of one who was suffocated by drowning. The wound in the neck was made by those endeavouring to restore animation by bleeding.'

The verdict was death from suffocation by accidental drowning.[11]

Bleeding and Spirits: The Death of Thomas Crawford
Clonnagore, Drummully Parish, April 1857

David Crawford and his wife were engaged in trenching corn in their garden and their fine, lively, five-year-old boy, Thomas, was amusing himself beside them. About 6p.m. he wandered a short way off. A little later, when they couldn't see him, they assumed he'd gone back to the house and took no further notice. When they returned home and enquired as to his whereabouts, they then realised he had not been in the house. The mother ran out of the house with the father right behind her frantically searching for their son. She had not gone far when, on seeing his cap floating on a pool of water, she screamed out. His tiny body was floating in the water. David lifted Thomas out of the water and brought him back to the house. Every means was used to restore him to animation – including 'bleeding' him and 'rubbing him with spirits before the fire' – but with no results. The child was dead as a result of drowning.[12]

Bleeding the sick was also believed to relieve the body and rid it of the bad blood, disease and poisons in the system. Leeches were also used. These blood-sucking worms, used to drain blood from the wound, were commonly affixed by inverting a wine-glass containing as many as were required upon the part affected.[13] The leech, when full, contained about half an ounce of blood and, if the blood continued to flow after they were removed, the application of a slight compress restrained it or brandy or spirits of wine were poured over it to seal the wound.[14]

Rubbing spirits on a sick child before the fire was another method believed to restore animation into the unresponsive body, as mentioned previously in the inquest of the child, Thomas Crawford. It was well-documented that rubbing a person with spirits or alcohol of any description, such as whiskey, was believed to put heat into a cold body and had indeed in some cases, brought persons back from the dead. A century earlier, a Mr Glover, a surgeon in Doctors Commons, London, discussed a case of a person who was restored to life after twenty-nine minutes hanging by the neck. The principal means used to restore this man to life were opening the temporal artery and external jugular, rubbing the back, mouth and neck with a quantity of volatile spirits and oil and covering them with warm ashes of salt, administering a tobacco enema by means of lighted pipes and strong frictions of the arms and legs. This was continued for four hours and then an incision was made into the windpipe and air blown into the lungs. It was then that a pulse was detected. The man made a full recovery.[15] This treatment was used for stillborn children and anyone who was no longer responding to life.

A poultice (also called a plaster), a soft, usually heated and sometimes medicated mass/paste enclosed in muslin or linen, applied to sores or other lesions, was often used to reduce inflammation, to induce warmth or, when mixed with mustard, as a counter-irritant. It was believed to be good for arthritic joins, congestion, asthma, coughs, ridding colds and any condition requiring circulation. The two types of poultices mentioned in the coroner's casebook were mustard and warm turnips. Mustard poultices and warm turnips were often used for persons who died from epilepsy, rupture of blood vessels, effects of electricity (struck by lightning), congestion of the lungs and more.

Warm Turnips for Comfort before Death
The Death of Robert Campbell, Crumlin, Tyholland Parish, February 1859
On 21 February 1859, Robert Campbell was working with his uncle and namesake thatching the roof of their house. The old man took many breaks, complaining of not feeling well. He had been a healthy

man until the last few months and the family was concerned. On this day, he stopped early to rest. Later that evening, his nephew applied a poultice of warm turnips on his uncle's chest but unfortunately the old man felt no relief. By bedtime, they found him standing roasting his chest over the fire 'from the great coldness he felt there'. His bed was moved to the fireside to keep him warm, but within an hour, Robert Campbell was dead. The verdict was death from an attack of cramps to which for several months he had been subject.[16]

Turpentine used as a Remedy

Turpentine oil (*Pinus palustris*) ingested with alcohol or tea, was used for a variety of different ailments including gout, rheumatism, typhus, curing wounds and, mixed with other ingredients, to prevent gangrene. It has even been used in the treatment of worms. In several inquests it was revealed that turpentine was used to attempt to soothe those feeling ill, usually complaining of a swelling of the belly and abdominal pain. One sad inquest explains the desperate attempts of Peter Coyle who tried to soothe the severe abdominal pains of his brother, Michael, by preparing some turpentine and caraway for him and sitting him by the fire. Caraway is a herb that can be grown in the garden, an aromatic antispasmodic.[17] It was used for digestion problems, flatulence, nausea, anxiety and to flavour mixtures. The seeds were added to water to make a tea; however, the drink did not have the desired effect. Peter soon had to call the priest as Michael stated he was going to die. By the next morning, he was dead. The verdict was death from a severe attack of acute peritonitis (internal inflammation). Michael Coyle was forty-nine years old.[18]

Treating Burns
Butter and Oils Bring No Relief

> For a Burn: There is a pretty secret to cure a burn without a scar; Take a sheep's suet and the rind of the elder tree, boil both together, and the ointment will cure a burn without leaving a mark.
> – Lady Wilde, *Quaint Irish Customs and Superstitions*, 1896

Usually, burns were treated with linseed oil, castor oil, cream or butter on the wound. They were also wrapped with bandages or homemade salves. In the case of one woman, Margaret McElmeel, when it was discovered that her clothes had caught fire, she was doused with water and the injured parts of her body were 'smeared with sweet cream'. She died just five hours later.[19] These products are known today as some of the worst possible treatments for burns as they trap in the heat, not allowing the skin to breathe. Burns treated with such products and wraps would have been intensely painful.

Rub Butter on the Wound
The Death of Susan Keely, Coolkill, Ematris Parish, August 1857
A mother was working in her home attending to her chores with her young child, Susan, beside her, when she heard a shout of alarm coming from outside. She ran from the house leaving Susan behind, to discover there was a cow in the corn. After about ten minutes, the cow was turned out and she went back to the house. Upon entering the kitchen, she got a terrible shock. Susan's clothes had caught fire and had burst into flames. With the utmost speed, the mother extinguished the blaze, retrieved some fresh butter and smeared the child's body with it. Linseed oil was then applied to anoint the most wounded areas. Susan lingered from about 2p.m. when the accident happened until 7 o'clock the next morning when she died.[20]

Bathing Feet: Soothing but Ineffective
Very often persons suffering from illnesses such as bowel complaint, chest pain, congestion of the lungs and many other aches and pains had their feet bathed in a tub of warm water, usually to attempt to relax them and warm the body to provide some relief from the pain. It was done in combination with a variety of other treatments and, while it did not serve a medical purpose, it was a common practice to calm and comfort the sick.

A Newlywed Dies
The Death of Philip McKiernan, Clonfad, Killeevan Parish, March 1864
Ellen McKiernan told the coroner and his jury that she and her husband, Philip, had been married for about a year. He had good health but was subject to attacks of cholic. He'd had two since the marriage and the last was six weeks previously. The usual remedies had been used and produced a good effect. During the past two days, Philip had been harrowing and sowing oats. On the second day, he'd come home, eaten an egg and some bread and retired to rest. He slept soundly, but at 6a.m. he woke up with an attack of cholic. His sister prepared some warm milk with ginger in it. Ginger was often used for hangovers, to settle the stomach, relieve anxiety and calm the nerves. Unfortunately, when her brother drank it, he quickly vomited. Again it was prepared, and again he threw it off.

Concerned, Ellen prepared a mixture of whiskey and an ounce of castor oil, but his stomach rejected this also. She wanted to send for Dr Taylor of Drum, but Philip refused, saying it was unnecessary. She then gave him some castor oil with tea and, having drunk it, he appeared to be doing well and said he felt better. After a short time, he wished for another drink, at which time Ellen prepared cream of tartar with some boiling water. He continued to feel well. To offer her husband some more comfort, she then bathed his feet. Several hours later, a change for the worse set in. He was in great pain for about a half-hour, until suddenly, he stopped breathing. Philip was dead. The verdict was death on the evening of 23 March 1864 from an attack of cholic.[21]

When Treatments are the Cause of Death
Procedures and Medications

In several instances the treatments and medicines used in an attempt to remedy and cure disease and ailments contributed to the cause of death, although they were not always proved as having done so.

Lanced to Death?
The Death of Emily H. Scott, Skeagh, Drumsnat Parish, April 1865
Margaret Began was a servant of the Scott family of Skeagh in the parish of Drumsnat responsible for tending to the home and their young child, Emily Scott, a small girl three years of age. On 11 April she walked to the residence of Dr Moorhead of Smithborough to have him treat the boil on the back of Emily's head as she had been instructed by Emily's father, William, to do so. When the doctor examined the young girl, he stated that Margaret should take the child home as she would not be alive for long. The child was sick, possibly from the effects of the lump, which, although considered a boil, was in fact described as being the size of a large plum. He examined the lump, took his lance and opened it. A considerable amount of 'matter' came from it. Margaret then left Smithborough with the child, Emily, and headed for Skeagh.

William Scott told the coroner the rest of the sad tale. He had instructed the servant girl to take his child to have the boil lanced. A while after they had left the house, a messenger was sent to tell him that his daughter was dying and he was instructed to go and meet the servant. 'At once I went meeting the girl about half a mile from

MELANCHOLY MADNESS

my own house. By the time I reached them, my child was dead.' Dr Reid examined the body of the deceased child and considered that the death, though very sudden, arose from natural causes. The verdict was death by natural causes.[22]

The 'boil' on the back of Emily Scott's head was possibly not that, but instead a tumorous mass which may have contained enlarged veins and arteries and which, being opened, encouraged too much bleeding resulting in the child's death. Dr Moorehead had diagnosed the child as dying before he opened the 'boil'. However, is it possible that it was the lancing of the tumour and the haemorrhage that followed which actually caused the death? There was no comment from the child's father or the servant that the child had not been well or that her life was in danger prior to the visit to the physician.

How were they Treating the Worms?
The Death of the son of James McCabe,
Magheross, Magheross Parish, January 1861
An inquiry was held on 26 January 1861 after Waddell received a report from the head constable of Carrickmacross that the six-year-old son of James McCabe of Magheross had died suddenly. Accompanied by the head constable, Waddell went to McCabe's home. He learned from the father that the boy had been sick for three weeks and was under medical treatment for worms. James had taken his son out for a little fresh air, but he continued to get worse and died about an hour after their last journey outdoors together. Waddell did not hold an inquest, feeling that the cause of death was most likely from the boy's battle with worms. Although there is no description as to the state of the body of the deceased boy, it can be assumed his poor belly was hard and swollen, that he had sour bad breath, a great thirst, an involuntary discharge of saliva, pains in his sides, a dry cough, drowsiness, cold sweats and possibly epileptic fits. Dying from worms in the intestines was a painful death.

Treatments and cures for worms included rituals and practices that often caused death – although not intentionally. There was a belief among the country people that worms were an evil spirit that had taken over the body, and therefore a myriad of strange and harmful practices were conducted on children. Chanting incantations was likely only the start before bringing the child's body closer to the fire (a practice similar to ridding the home of changelings, as discussed in chapter four). Upon investigating the cures, remedies and treatments for worms, it seems that one or more of the following methods may have been implemented: starvation, serving them raisins soaked in whiskey, ingesting turpentine oils which, in certain doses, are poisonous and prove fatal, bitters and wine, saltwater, as well as herbs and plants such as grains of powdered rhubarb, garlic and rue. Rhubarb (Rheum Palmatum) appears to have been most commonly applied as it was a purgative, laxative, digestive remedy and has antibacterial properties used to allow the body to rid itself of the poisons inside and begin to heal again.

Accidental Overdose of Love
Medication and Children

Nineteenth-century medicines often did not cure disease, unknown to those administering such drugs, but they did have a calming effect by helping the patient sleep or by serving as painkillers. Opium and morphine, although not used often, were narcotics used for numbing pain. Drugs such as laudanum were used to help the sick sleep during their illness. In some cases, however, it was these same drugs that when used without care or not administered properly, caused death.

Listening for a Monaghan Accent: 'Robarb' v Opium

The Death of John Mooney, Castleshane, Monaghan Parish, October 1868
John Mooney was very concerned for his eight-month-old son, his namesake, John. The baby was sick with swinepox (smallpox) and his father was being advised to give him rhubarb pills. Upon running out of the medication, he quickly went to Thomas Henry's of Monaghan where he asked the shop boy, George Alderdice, to give him a pennyworth of rhubarb, which was done. The next day, he gave the child two of the pills as was the routine. Three hours later, the child was severely ill. John picked his son up out of the cradle but the child went limp and fainted. He rushed to the window to get him some fresh air which, fortunately, revived him a little. Knowing something was very wrong, he sent for Dr Donaldson.

Dr Donaldson arrived and examined John. The doctor prescribed warm, watered-down punch for the stomach after being told that the child had ingested Rhubarb. He returned later that evening and examined the child again. It appears what happened next was that the doctor, likely not understanding why the child's symptoms had not changed, examined the medicine. Whether by taste or by smell, he suddenly realised that the medicine was not Rhubarb at all – it was opium. Dr Donaldson immediately prescribed very strong coffee. But the baby would not take the coffee and the parent began rubbing his chest with turpentine to keep him awake. The opium had made the child tired and they feared if he lost consciousness, he would certainly die. The child, John Mooney, died at 2a.m. on the morning of 5 October 1868 from an opium overdose.[23]

The jury verdict was that death came from George Alderdice, the assistant to Thomas Henry, giving the father of the deceased the wrong medicine. Because of his negligence they wished to call the attention of the authorities to see whether Thomas Henry took the necessary precautions required by law to keep dangerous medicines properly separated from others of a more innocent character; and to verify whether they were properly labelled when given out. When the Monaghan spring assizes commenced on 6 March 1869, George Alderdice was indicted for having caused the death of John Mooney. Mr Law QC was the Crown prosecutor and Mr Porter, the defence attorney in the case.[24]

John Mooney told his story of asking and receiving the pills and of the fatal outcome to his infant child. He stated that when he spoke to Alderdice after the child's death, that 'He said I asked him for opium. There was no label on the bottle that I got.'

Mr Porter then addressed the jury for the prisoner and said the occurrence simply arose out of a mistake and was, no doubt, a very painful case that this child came by his death from a drug administered at the hands of his own parents. He pointed out that when at the chemist, Mr Mooney pronounced the word rhubarb 'robarb', as he was not a native of Monaghan, although a local policeman. The young man mistakenly considered that opium was being asked for. Mr Porter argued that the jury, in order to convict the accused, had to believe that the drug was given out of the shop in a culpably careless manner and that the prisoner was guilty of something other than a mistake.

It is important to note that it was common at the time to treat swinepox with rhubarb, followed up with an opiate as the final cure.[25] Is it possible that Alderdice gave the opium willingly or confused the two drugs as both were used to treat the illness?

Mr Thomas Henry, grocer and chemist, Monaghan, was examined and said that the prisoner was in his employment. He said that the prisoner was in the habit of selling drugs and understood his business. It was also made clear to the judge that 'a druggist is not bound to have a licence to deal in drugs'.

The judge charged the jury, and they returned a verdict of not guilty.

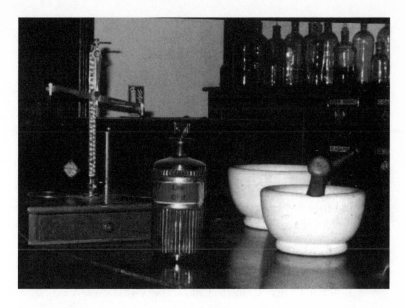

Opium at the Chemist.
[Taken at the Ulster-American Folk Park in Omagh, at the apothecary/chemist shop]

Just a Little More Medicine …
The Death of Thomas McAlier, Monaghan, Monaghan Parish, May 1858
Thomas McAlier had been a delicate child since he was three months old. His mother, Ann, had been receiving medicine and ointment for him for six months past for eruptions on his skin. Dr Temple from the Monaghan dispensary had prescribed a bottle of medicine for the child and gave verbal instructions to the baby's sister, fourteen-year-old Theresa, to give him five drops each night. The baby was attended to very closely.

A few days later, the mother was engaged in washing and the child was very restless. She decided to give him a full teaspoon to settle him down. After the dosage was given, little Thomas sat very quietly and after a while was laid down in the cradle. About 45 minutes later, he was moaning heavily. Ann was alarmed and sent to the apothecary, Mr Robinson, who sent some new medicine for the baby. No change took place and at midnight he was brought to the infirmary and admitted. Mr Young, the surgeon on staff, was sent for to see the child. He saw him repeatedly throughout the night, but Thomas died at noon the next day. Dr Young told the coroner at the inquest, 'I cannot say what was the nature of the medicine given, but if the quantity ordered – namely 5 drops – was a sufficient dose, 60 drops (a teaspoonful) or 12 times that quantity might be sufficient to cause its death, assuming the medicine to be a narcotic.'

As Ann McAlier was most attentive to the child and greatly distressed at his death, no charges were pressed against her. The verdict at the inquest was death on Sabbath 23 May 1858 in consequence of Ann McAlier, mother of deceased, having given the deceased a dose of medicine equal to about 12 times more than that ordered by Dr Temple for deceased through the ignorance and inadvertence of said Ann McAlier.[26]

Eruptions on the skin were often treated by swallowing turpentine and other volatile substances that served as a poison and were often lethal in large doses.

SUDDEN DEATH

When an Angel Came to Call – The Visitation of God

Of the thirty-three deaths recorded with a verdict stating 'death came by a visitation of God', most were elderly people over the age of sixty-five who appear to have experienced chest pain, shortness of breath, instant weakness or paralysis or became speechless prior to their death. In modern terms, these persons likely died as a result of heart attack, the rupture of an aneurysm or massive fatal stroke. Death by a visitation of God does not vary in any technical manner from inquests in the coroner's casebook which result in a verdict of 'death from heart disease' or 'death by apoplexy'. The one shared characteristic of the deaths recorded under this verdict is that a doctor was not called to their inquests to provide his official opinion or certification as to the cause of death. They can quite clearly be distinguished by their sudden and unexpected nature and the reaction of the survivors. Most of the deceased persons were classified as having literally just 'dropped dead' … and God was named as responsible.

Visited by the Almighty
The Death of Owen McCarvle, Corravilla, Killeevan Parish, April 1874
Catherine McCarvle had risen early to make breakfast for herself and her husband, Owen, a strong, healthy man, twenty-eight years old, who had always been free from sickness. Having eaten and chatted, Owen walked over to the fire to sit on the stool to warm himself. He leaned over, slowly putting on each shoe in preparation for the day's

work. Suddenly, without a moan or exclamation, he fell off his seat. Catherine rushed over and picked up her husband's head – only to find that he was dead. Thomas Martin, a boarder at the McCarvle's home, heard her scream and cry, 'My husband is dead!' He jumped up and ran to her. When Thomas found her in the kitchen, Owen was dead, cradled in her arms. The verdict was death by visitation of the Almighty.[27]

From Time to Eternity: The Death of Elizabeth Irwin
Corraghduff, Donagh Parish, September 1859
William and Elizabeth Irwin were married for forty-two years and had reared a family of seven children together. Over the years, Eliza had always enjoyed uninterrupted good health until the past month during which she had occasionally experienced a pain or smothering about her stomach. The pain came on after exertion, but it soon passed.

On the Sabbath, Eliza rose early as usual, took her meals and appeared in good health. At nine or ten o'clock that night, she retired to bed and William joined her soon after. At three o'clock in the morning, William happened to wake and put his hand over on his wife as she felt cold. He spoke to her but receiving no answer he again touched her and realised she was dead. He jumped up and alarmed the family. William told the coroner, 'On striking a light I remarked that she was just in the position on which she had fallen asleep, so much so as to make it evident she had passed from time to eternity without a struggle or the slightest pain during her sleep.' The verdict was death on the night of 4 September 1859 by the visitation of God.[28]

A Short Chat by the Fire
The Death of Pat McEntee, Sandhills, Currin Parish, December 1859
While walking on the road to his stables to see about his young horse, William Noble of Sandhills happened to stop in conversation with one of his tenants. The old tailor, seventy-year-old Pat McEntee was walking up the road towards him, hand in hand with his young child out for a stroll. Noble continued on to the stables, while McEntee stopped in Noble's residence to warm himself. While there, Ellen Judge offered Pat and the child seats by the fire as Pat had complained of the cold in his feet and he took off his shoes to warm them. Another member of the Noble family sat down and engaged Pat in conversation. Pat chatted away, but then stopped suddenly. Ellen turned around to look towards him and saw him in the act of falling off his seat. She caught him in her arms and immediately realised he was dead. The

word was still unfinished on his lips when he fell to the floor. Mrs Carr, who was in the hall, was called in to try to revive him, but to no avail. Life was quite extinct. William Noble later told the coroner, 'I scarcely believed the truth of it and hurried home. When I arrived at my house, I saw the deceased lying with a pillow under his head. Members of the household were all around him. I felt his pulse and found that life was departed.' Pat died by the visitation of God.[29]

*

Great men are not always those who are recorded in history. Because of the nature of Waddell's occupation as coroner, he set down the history of the nineteenth-century common man: a people who lived in extraordinarily harsh and uncompromising times and who must have had great strength to overcome them. These unknown people, destined for obscurity, lost in the memory of a troubled landscape, are now remembered.

APPENDIX ONE

Coroner's Reports held at the National Archives, Bishop Street, Dublin.[1]

Carlow:	1886–1915 (excl 1909 and 1913)
	Coroner's Depositions 1920–25
Cavan:	1914, 1917–19, 1922–23, 1925–39
Clare:	1851, 1864, 1880, 1885–1902 (some gaps), 1911–27
Cork:	None[2]
Donegal:	1865 (abstracts), 1892–94, 1902, 1905–25, 1929–69
Dublin:	1900–1917, 1922–36, 1937–71
Galway:	1907–14, 1920–23
Kerry:	None
Kildare:	1863–85, 1887–95, 1897–1900, c.1959–71 (not yet fully sorted)
Kilkenny:	1874–76, 1925–74
Laois:	1879, 1884, 1888–1911 (excl 1909), 1923–42
Leitrim:	1888–1941 (excl 1939)
Longford:	1888, 1890, 1894, 1897–1900, 1916–26
Limerick:	1919, 1923
Louth:	1908–49
Mayo:	1888–94, 1901–20, 1922–36, 1938, 1940–48, 1950, 1954
Monaghan:	1910–12, 1914, 1920, 1925
Meath:	1900–1915 (fragmentary and damaged)
Offaly:	1922–27
Roscommon:	1884, 1897–08
Sligo:	1877, 1888–1912, 1932–60
Tipperary:	1852, 1863, 1905–06, 1909–29 (excl 1918)
Waterford:	None
Westmeath:	1892–99, 1917, 1930–60
Wexford:	1898–1912 (excl 1905)
Wicklow:	1887–1922, 1926

The papers at the Chief Secretary's Office cover the years 1832–80 and contain coroners' inquest papers and reports for various years and counties. Additionally, the Chief Secretary's Office Reports covering the years 1818–1922 contain a number of reports about individual inquests and matters relating to personnel and organisational issues relating to coroners.

APPENDIX TWO
Recording Death During the Famine
Inquests from Volume One (1846–1855)

It is estimated that Co. Monaghan suffered a death rate of 18,000 between the years of 1846–1850.[1] The coroner documented only a fraction of the deaths that took place during the famine, but the inquests
that were held capture conditions of destitution, starvation and painful death. The conditions under which the deceased were found were
unique in comparison to the inquests which followed in later years
and were not repeated in the second volume of the casebook. Only
two inquests in volume two refer to death by destitution or starvation
and in each case they are easily explained. One dealt with elderly
neglect; the other an apparent stroke victim.

Brian Ó Mórdha, in his *Clogher Record* article 'The Great Famine in Monaghan' states that 'there are quite a number of inquests on
people who died from excessive drinking, or from a combination of
excessive drinking, lack of proper food and exposure to cold.' The bits
of food that were available consisted of Indian meal or grains used to
make a stirabout. Potatoes are only briefly mentioned and turnips to
varying degrees. Any food mentioned in the inquests referred to thin
soups made from water and boiling a bit of turnip or greens for some
variant of nutrition or flavour. Ultimately, these inquests record destitution, persons with no hope for living other than attempts to emigrate or else attempting to find food by begging. Of course, those unfortunate souls appearing in the coroner's casebook found no sanc-
tuary. They died as a result of exposure, starvation and fever.

The first volume of Waddell's casebook is still missing, so the
cases below are taken from the inquests which were reported in the
Clogher Record.

Fear Amongst the People
The following story addresses the fear of the general populace during
the time of the Great Famine. Prior to 1846, the people of the countryside were known for their hospitality and welcoming strangers and
beggars into their homes. During this time of disease and death there
was a great fear of fevers. Beggars and strangers were now seen as spreading these plagues from place to place along their journeys and they
were no longer welcomed into the homes of the countryside. One
inquest depicts a man named Lynch who was refused shelter time and
time again in October 1847. He was found dead the next day with

no food in his stomach or his intestines. The verdict was death from destitution and exposure due to the severity of the weather.[2]

Swarming with Vermin
The Death of Bernard Kelly, Aghalisk, Kilmore Parish, June 1847
Bernard Kelly was starving and homeless. He had no money and no means to support himself. It was June 1847 during the Great Famine when starvation, homelessness and disease was killing hundreds of thousands of his countrymen. He wanted to survive and desperate times required desperate measures.

Jail was the one place where Berny knew he would be given clothes, shelter and at least one meal a day. With nothing to lose, he decided to break the law in a last effort to save himself. Berny went to the house of James Walsh and threw some rocks through the windows, smashing the glass. Walsh, possibly feeling sorry for Berny or just unconcerned about the incident, decided not to prosecute. Adam Clarke, the acting constable, told Berny to go back to his homeplace in Coolnacarte, near Clones. With nowhere left to turn, the sick and dying man decided to try to make his way back to his home. On the way there, he collapsed by the side of the road. He could walk no further.

On Saturday night, Pat Tierney of Anagola heard that there was a man on the road that was very ill. It was late and Tierney decided to wait and see if the man was still around by morning. When Tierney rose, early on Sunday morning, he went out to look for the sick man. He found Berny lying by the side of the road. Tierney made Berny a bed of straw right where he lay and another neighbour, Mr Carson, sent him food. He remained in the same spot for the next day or two receiving food and care from the neighbourhood until Monday evening when they found him dead. The poor man was 'extremely filthy' and his body was 'swarming with vermin'. The neighbours believed that Berny was ill from yellow fever and that was the reason none of them took him into their homes. According to the coroner and jury, they were wrong. The verdict was death from filth and extreme destitution.[3]

Dying to Get into the Poorhouse
Edward McGovern, CC, Parish of Magheross in 1847 told the coroner's jury that many persons were dying suddenly in the parish owing to want and destitution, or starvation and exposure. The coroner recorded Fr McGovern as stating that he 'knows that the number of deaths in this parish on average at present are between seven and

eight each day.' With so many people without homes and food, there was a huge burden put on the local poorhouses around the county who were unable to meet the demands of the public. The following story illustrates just how desperate conditions were during this dark time in history.

Politics of the Poorhouse Kill a Husband and Father
The Death of Pat McCabe, Magheross Parish, March 1847
During the breakfast hour on the morning of 8 March 1847, Thomas Keelan of Greaghletterkepple in the parish of Magheross, near Carrickmacross, had a visitor come to his door. It was Pat McCabe, a neighbour who lived nearby and worked as a cottier. Pat was a husband and father to several children and was now at Thomas' door asking if he might have any food to help feed himself and his family. Keelan gave Pat some bread and milk and Pat went on his way.

As the day continued, Pat went about the district begging with no luck and trying to find help for his daughter who was suffering from fever. But he had to stop, likely from weakness and fatigue, and found shelter in a ditch.

The next day, Pat's son arrived at the residence of the Revd Thomas McEnally to ask for his help. His father was speechless and the family had left their home. They had taken up residence in the ditch, building a fire to keep warm. Fr McEnally recalled meeting Pat just a day earlier. He had found him 'in a state of appearance boarding on idiotism'. The priest was now so concerned that he contacted Fr Edward McGovern and the two men went immediately to the boardroom of the poorhouse to see if they could get the man and some of his family admitted. They were told by the guardians of the poorhouse that they could not admit anyone without the warders of the division being informed first. The men then went away to sort out the situation.

Meanwhile, Pat, hearing that he might have admission into the poorhouse, arrived only to find that he could not get in. He was seen by his neighbour, Thomas Hanlon, walking from the fire near the ditch in the morning and back towards it that night.

About midday on Tuesday 9 March 1847, Fr McGovern caught up with Pat and his family. He had secured admission tickets for Pat and some of the members of his family, but it was too late. As the priest arrived with a horse and cart to take the family to the poorhouse, he found the body of Pat McCabe, lying in an open field, with no covering except his usual tattered clothing. Sitting a short distance away was Pat's wife and her child, exposed to the inclemency of the weather, having no other covering but the clothes on their back which were 'of the worst description'. They had a little milk, but no food. He discovered that the family had been living in the open air for three days and nights and that Pat had starved to death trying to secure food and a means to support his family.

Fr McGovern then ordered a fire to be lit and the neighbours to keep watch over the body until a coffin could be procured and the body removed to a safe place. He then took Pat's wife and child, placed them in the cart, and took them to the Carrickmacross poorhouse.

The coroner was informed and an inquest took place. John McEffer, Esq., MB examined the body of the deceased. Mr McEffer was of the opinion that Pat McCabe died from the effects of cold and destitution. He found his body 'without any appearance of food, but the intestines contained a considerable quantity of digested food. There were no marks of external violence on the body. The verdict was death in consequence of the combined effects of want of a sufficiency of food and exposure to the inclemency of the weather.[4]

No Admittance to the Poorhouse for Suspicion of Having Money
The Death of Bernard Rudden, Killark, Currin Parish, February 1848
Bernard Rudden was a beggar who made regular stops at the house of the Mulhollands of Killark. It was February 1848 and Bernard was again at the door for the second time in about twelve hours. He'd stopped the previous evening with a little bit of meal and had Anne Mulholland make a supper for him with it. For breakfast, he received some light gruel and was again on his way. A short while later, Anne walked out the door to run some errands when she came across Bernard lying face down in a small river just next to the house.

Anne began screaming for help and those in the house came running to her aid. They raised Bernard up and laid him on a bank near the water. It was too late – he was dead.

The coroner arrived to investigate the death and interviewed Anne Mulholland and another neighbour, Ellen Reilly. Both women told the same tale. The beggar had often tried to gain admittance to the Clones poorhouse but could not get in since the guardians suspected that he had some money. During the summer he had got some relief at a soup kitchen but made no other application for relief that they were aware of, save for receiving charity. Bernard had no food, bedclothes, nor shoes or stockings. Dr Taylor said that the poor man died as a result of destitution from want of sufficient food and expo-

sure to the cold of the season. The verdict was death from destitution.[5]

The Food came too Late: A Mother's Sacrifice
The Death of Mary Ann McDermott, Cladone, Clones Parish, March 1847
Mary Ann McDermott had lived in the village of Killeevan since
December 1846, getting by as a beggar to support herself and her two
children. She went collecting each day, walking around the county,
coming home at night with the proceeds of what she'd collected.
Often she would have received some meal and at night could make
a gruel of it for herself and the children. She also got a few pence by
begging and with that she paid the rent of 2d for her house and gave
herself and the children two meals on Sunday.

On 12 March 1847 Mary Ann walked from Killeevan to Clones
on an errand for which she would receive a cupful of meal. The children were left in Clones to go to the soup kitchen for a bowl of soup.
While there, they saved one cupful for their mother for her return.
As Anne made her way back from Clones with the meal to feed her
children, she became very weak. About two miles from Killeevan she
collapsed in front of the house of Bernard Greenan in the townland
of Cladone.

Mary Greenan was told there was a woman at the gate who was
very weak. Mary went to investigate and found Mary Ann lying on
the roadside. The woman quickly went to get some stirabout and
handed it to the weak and trembling creature. Mary Ann was so fra-
gile that she could not hold the spoon to feed herself. Mary Greenan
held the spoon and attempted to feed Mary Ann, but even as her
mouth was open for the food, once in her mouth she could not eat it
as she could not swallow. The stirabout continued to fall from the
sick woman's mouth onto her chest. Mary Ann began struggling very
hard to gain control of her hands and managed to do so for twenty
minutes – and then she died.

Catherine McDermott, Mary Ann's daughter, spoke at the inquest explaining the events of the months, weeks and days prior to
her mother's death. For the past four months, they had been living in
Killeevan with no other way of support except by begging and random acts of charity. About a month previously her mother had a
severe attack of a bowel complaint but within the last fortnight she
had been feeling better. During that time she had no food whatsoever
for herself. She was giving the little bits of meal she was able to scrape
together to her children, making them a bit of gruel each night. It

was only in the past two days that the three of them were able to secure a quart of soup at the soup kitchen in Ballinure.

Dr Hurst of Clones examined the body of the deceased. The appearance of the stomach and bowels was healthy. The contents of the stomach contained some greens of bad quality (likely grass or rotten plants) as well as pieces of raw turnip, most probably only the rinds of the turnips. None of this food was sufficient to sustain life and Dr Hurst considered this to be the cause of the deceased's death. The jury found her death resulted from the want of proper food and nourishing.[6]

APPENDIX THREE
Listing of the Doctors Referred to in the Inquests

There are almost seventy doctors, over the twenty years between 1856 and 1876, referred to in the inquests in the coroner's casebook. Their attendance, remedies, cures and practices (including autopsies) are recorded. The doctors are listed below in alphabetical order along with the area in which they practised.

Adamson (Monaghan Infirmary)
Bayley (Monaghan Parish)
Blakely, Samuel (Aughnacloy, Co. Tyrone)
Carnston, William (Aughnamullen)
Clark, Samuel (Drum)
Coote, Charles (Monaghan)
Corbett, Charles (Monaghan Infirmary)
Coulter, Robert (Donagh Parish)
Davis (Monaghan)
Donaldson (Ballybay, Tyholland, Tullycorbet, Castleshane)
Douglass, Allen Edmond (Glaslough)
Duffy Francis (Carrickmacross)
Fleming (Carrickmacross)
Gillespie, William Henry (Clones, Clones Workhouse)
Gillespie, James (Clones)
Gilmore (Donaghmoyne Parish)
Graydon, Samuel Johnston (Scotstown, Tedavnet Parish)
Hamill, D. (Clones)
Harris (Tedavnet Parish)
Henry, Alexander, Jr (Clones)
Henry, Richard, Sr (Clones)
Hodges, John F. (Prof. Medical Jurisprudence, Belfast)
Hoskins, Thomas Joshua (Clones)
Irwin, Fitzjohn Robert (Mon. Parish)
Johnston (Newbliss)
Joyce, Lancaster (Ballybay)
Knight, Alexander (Clones)
Loughran (Middletown, Co. Armagh)
Mansfield, Robert (Carrickmacross)
Manwhinny (Newbliss)
Martin, Brownlow (Ballybay)
McClure Ross, Daniel (Monaghan Workhouse)
McDowell (Medical Attendant, Monaghan Jail)

McKenna,[1] Bernard (Emyvale)
McKeon, Arthur (Crossmaglen)
McKinstry (Glaslough)
Mooney (Monaghan Parish)
Moore, Robert (Rockcorry)
Moorehead, John, Jr (Smithborough)
Moorehead, John, Sr (Smithborough)
Moratz, John William (Tedavnet)
Morten, Robert (Crossmaglen, Co. Armagh)
Mulligan, John (Aughnacloy, Co. Tyrone)
O'Reilly, Surgeon William (Clones)
Reid, Robert H. (Slieveroe)
Robertson, JC (Medical Attendant, Monaghan Asylum)
Robinson, Andrew (Newbliss)
Ross, D. M. (Monaghan Town)
Rush, Matthew G. (Monaghan)
Scott (Aughnacloy, Co. Tyrone)
Sharp (Coothill)
Sherry, Richard (Currin)
Short, John (Scotstown Dispensary)
Stewart, Robert Wilson (Glaslough)
Taggert, Robert (Carrickmacross Workhouse)
Taylor, John (Drum, Currin Parish)
Temple, John (Governor of the Monaghan Jail)
Temple, Thomas (Monaghan Parish)
Temple, William (Monaghan Parish)
Wall (Aghabog Parish)
Watters (Middletown, Co. Armagh)
Weatty (Monaghan Parish)
Wheeler, R. J. (Carrickmacross)
Woods, William (Tedavnet Parish)
Young, A. K. (Monaghan Parish and Monaghan Infirmary)
Young, James William (Ballybay Parish)

APPENDIX FOUR
A List of the Dead: The Deceased Persons in
the Coroner's Casebook (1856–1876)

The names of the deceased that appear in the coroner's casebook are arranged here in alphabetical order. It is important to note that the names are recorded as they were transcribed by Waddell and then recorded by the author. These names may have been misspelled by Waddell and further research may be required in order to link them to other ancestors. The townland names are recorded in the same fashion. For example, Arablekirk, a townland in the parish of Monaghan, is properly spelled Urbalkirk; however, leaving the names spelled according to the transcription of the coroner allows for individual researchers to make their own assessment of the correct spelling and location. The parishes recorded are the civil parishes. Verdicts of death are categorised for simple review and understanding of how death came. The coroner's verdicts can be found in the original casebook.

For the researcher interested in finding gravestones for the persons listed in the casebook, it may be wise not to conduct an extensive search as this researcher discovered – most simply do not exist. Many of those listed in the coroner's casebook appear to have either been buried in unmarked graves; interred in an existing family plot with no record of their death; or their gravestone is no longer standing. For more information, visit www.melancholymadness.com

Abbreviations

Mon:	Monaghan	Workhse:	Workhouse
Poorhse:	Poorhouse	Infirm.:	Infirmary
Unkn:	Unknown		

Inquest	Name	Year	Townland	Parish	Verdict of Death
2.516	Adams, Francis	1858	Drumgrone	Currin	Visitation of God
15.1077	Airds, Robert	1873	Monaghan	Monaghan	Drowning in a boat
12.677	Alford, George	1862	Monaghan	Monaghan	Heart disease
20.1054	Allwell, John	1872	Clones	Clones	Apoplexy
12.603	Anderson, Christopher	1860	Cornapaste	Currin	Run over by railway wagon
5.580	Andrews, James	1860	Clones	Clones	Drowning
15.1122	Andrews, John	1874	Lisoarty	Clones	Old age and exposure to poor weather
13.1014	Andrews, Leticia	1871	Clones	Clones	Natural causes
	Anketell (young man)	1872	Truagh Lodge	Drumsnat	Violent fall off his horse
16.681	Armstrong, James Jo	1863	Clonkirk	Clones	Burned by boiling water
2.577	Armstrong, William	1860	Lisareark	Currin	Apoplexy
27.771	Armstrong, William	1865	Dunsrim	Currin	Cart and horse accident
10.963	Arnock, William	1870	Kilcorran	Clones	Visitation of God; heart attack
11.964	Bailie, William	1870	Dunraymond	Kilmore	Mill accident; arm ripped off
	Bannon, James	1875	Mon. Asylum	Monaghan	Consumption
5.795	Barker, Michael	1865	Arablekirk	Monaghan	Apoplexy
9.1136	Barker, Michael	1875	Coolshannagh	Ematris	Drowning

Inquest	Name	Year	Townland	Parish	Verdict of Death
	Barker, Robert	1856	Urbalkirk	Monaghan	Sudden death
6.457	Barkey, Susan	1857	Carnbane	Drumsnat	Burning
11.941	Barnwell, James	1869	Clones Poorhse	Clones	Burning
2.773	Beags (Boags), Thomas	1865	Monaghan	Monaghan	Shock and effusion of blood
5.636	Beaty, Nathanial	1861	Kilmore West	Ematris	Suicide; gunshot wound
7.598	Began, Felix	1860	Calliagh	Aghabog	Falling from a haycock
25.989	Bell, William	1871	Emyvale	Donagh	Visitation of God
26.720	Benner, Mary	1864	Sieveah	Tyholland	Mill accident
11.1073	Benson, Robert	1873	Corvally	Tyholland	Drowning
9.659	Benson, Samuel	1862	Garren	Clones	Congestion of the brain
9.523	Berny, Thomas	1858	Three Mile Chapel		Heart disease
	Bethel, William	1871	Drumkeen	Aghabog	Burning by hot water
1.1126	Betty, William, Esq.	1875	Kilcorran	Clones	Heart disease
	Birch, Robert	1874	Carrabrack	Donagh	Retention of urine
3.956	Black, Elisa	1870	Cortober	Ematris	Burning
9.780	Boylan(d), Michael	1865	Emyvale	Errigal Truagh	Drowning
7.521	Boyland, Jane	1858	Monaghan	Monaghan	Suicide; drowning, depression
	Boyle (1st name unkn)	1873	Mon. Infirm.	Monaghan	Accident at Moutries Mill; Emyvale; bled to death
	Boyle, Margaret	1874	Mon. Asylum	Monaghan	Scarlet fever
1.590	Bradly, Edward	1860	Clonickny	Donagh	Head trauma; drunk and head caught in cartwheel
	Brady, Catherine	1876	Mon. Asylum	Monaghan	Debility and old age
15.529	Breaden, George	1858	Monaghan	Monaghan	Crushed by a falling tree
19.1155	Bready, Ellen	1875	Listillen	Killeevan	Apoplexy
6.816	Bready, Hugh	1866	Monaghan	Monaghan	Crushed by cart; accident
13.437	Bready, Hugh	1856	Magherany	Clones	Inflammation of the stomach and bowels
18.609	Bready, James	1860	Tullaghalusk	Clones	Exposure from state of dotage
17.531	Bready, John	1858	Mullnahinshago	Tedavnet	Visitation of God
2.1024	Bready, Robert	1872	Clones	Clones	Falling; head trauma; Runaway horse
16.980	Bready, Thomas	1870	Clones	Clones	Heart disease
13.588	Brides, Ellen	1860	Knockwest	Currin	Drowning
16.875	Brown, John	1868	Monaghan	Monaghan	Heart disease
6.1009	Brown, John	1871	Glassdrummond	Clontibret	Suicide; drowning; fever
7.922	Brown, Martha	1869	Lissimanon	Clones	Burning
15.479	Brown, Mathew	1857	Termadown	Kilmore	Drowning
10.887	Brown, Samuel	1868	Drumullan	Kilmore	Heart disease
1.1108	Brown, William	1874	Glenlough	Drumsnat	Heart disease
14.873	Burk, James	1868	Carronroe	Currin	Natural causes
3.933	Burk, John	1869	Tullyard	Killeevan	Natural causes; heart disease
8.658	Burk, William	1862	Creeran	Currin	Apoplexy
13.715	Burns, Patrick	1863			Drowning
20.484	Byers, John	1857	Creggins	Donagh	Run over by a mail coach while drunk
16.1078	Calaghan, Hugh	1873	Crieve	Monaghan	Drowning
11.422	Caldwell, Sophia	1856	Stranduff	Donagh	Drowning
14.664	Callaghan, Sophia	1862	Clonedrigal	Clones	Effusion on the brain
	Callan, Bridget	1875	Mon. Asylum	Monaghan	Phthisis
9.740	Cambell, George Killen	1864	Glaslough	Donagh	Effusion on the brain
	Cambell, James	1870			Sudden death
4.1111	Cambell, Patrick	1874	Drumnacain	Tedavnet	Effects of a bad stomach
1.533	Cambell, Robert	1859	Crumlin	Tyholland	Attack of cramps
	Carr, Alice	1875	Mon. Asylum	Monaghan	Debility and old age
	Carroll, Michael	1868	Clones	Clones	Old age
18.549	Carson, Jane	1859	Milltown	Monaghan	Struck by electric fluid
19.550	Carson, William	1859	Milltown	Monaghan	Struck by electric fluid
4.748	Caruth, Samuel	1864	Skineharigan	Errigal Truagh	Flax mill accident
19.983	Cassidy, Bridget	1870	Derrycarrett	Clones	Natural exhaustion
6.1134	Cassidy, Catherine	1875	Drummaree	Killeevan	Heart disease

Inquest	Name	Year	Townland	Parish	Verdict of Death
3.894	Caulfield, Ann	1868	Monaghan	Monaghan	Debility of constitution
1.810	Caulfield, John	1866	Killynenagh	Currin	Hanging; strangulation; accidental
9.900	Cavenagh, Ann	1868	Askneskew	Currin	Haemorrhage; childbirth
	Child	1873	Emyvale	Donagh	Unknown
23.953	Christy, John	1870	Golanmurphy	Killeevan	Burning
17.1051	Churchill, Thomas Cotton	1872	Clones	Clones	Apoplexy
17.900	Clark, James	1868	Monaghan	Monaghan	Murder; gunshot wound
22.1128	Clark, Joseph	1875	Confinlough	Tedavnet	Apoplexy
3.862	Clark, Margaret	1867	Mon. Infirm.	Monaghan	Heart disease
11.1005	Clark, Mary	1874	Billis	Donagh	Burning
3.668	Clark, Mary	1862	Carracahan	Drummully	Falling into bog
	Clark, Mrs. Robert	1857	Cadagh (Dromore)		Died in childbirth
25.489	Clark, Peter	1858	Mon. Jail	Monaghan	Starvation
14.528	Clark, Thomas	1858	Rackwallace	Monaghan	Exposure, old age
	Clarke, Mary	1875	Mon. Asylum	Monaghan	Congestion of the lungs
18.808	Clarken, Agnes	1866	Mon. Jail	Monaghan	Chronic bronchitis
2.426	Clarken, Bernard	1856	Mullaloghan	Donagh	Railway work accident
4.934	Clarken, Margaret	1869	Drumbrain	Aghabog	Drowning
2.893	Clarken, Mary	1868	Mon. Jail	Monaghan	Fever
12.423	Clarken, Owen	1856	Kilntibret	Clones	Hit by horse and cart
	Clarken, Pat	1860	Annybane	Ematris	In bad health prior to death
5.500	Clerkin, Hugh	1858	Cooldaragh	Drumsnat	Bursting of blood vessel
16.946	Clifford, Margaret	1869	Liscabrick	Tedavnet	Burning
	Coil, Winifred	1875	Mon. Asylum	Monaghan	Failure of the nervous system's energy
12.436	Colgan, Ann	1856	Lisgow	Donagh	Burning
7.558	Condon, Ann	1859	Tirrevera	Tyholland	Cart accident; head trauma
14.804	Conlon, James	1865	Bowelk	Aghnamullen	[depositions sent to Swanzy]
12.462	Connolly, John	1857	Tullavogue	Tedavnet	Excessive drinking
12.697	Connolly, Mary Ann	1863	Newbliss	Killeevan	Burning
13.1047	Connolly, Pat	1872	Killycohert	Clones	Old age and infirmity
11.1045	Connolly, Patrick	1872	Clones	Clones	Inflammation of the lungs
1.452	Connolly, Thomas	1857	Tilleden	Tedavnet	Falling from scaffolding
7.1041	Connoly, John	1872	Kilnahatter	Kilmore	Struck and killed by train
5.776	Connoly, Owen	1865	Emyvale	Donagh	Cart and horse accident
22.841	Connoly, Robert	1867	Corragoar	Ematris	Natural causes
3.594	Connor, Jane	1860	Creveleagh	Clones	Drowning in canal, accidentally fell in
21.485	Connor, Thomas	1857	Leitrim	Tyholland	Visitation of God
4.881	Conolly, Miles	1868	Carsons	Ematris	Heart disease; stomach cancer
13.890	Conolly, Sally	1868	Lisnagoe	Killeevan	Infirmity and weakness;
18.1124	Conoly, Mary	1875	Monaghan	Monaghan	Crushed by a cart and horse
15.1049	Coogan, Edward	1872	Corranure	Tullycorbet	Natural Causes
13.943	Coogan, James	1869	Drumnacrutten	Monaghan	Drowning
	Cook, Anne	1875	Mon. Asylum	Monaghan	Consumption
9.420	Corbitt, Thomas	1856	Corrinshigoe	Currin	Punctured by stick when jumping over fence
9.560	Corcorhan, Ann	1859	Monaghan	Monaghan	Rupture of blood vessel
16.1050	Corigan, Andrew	1872	Mon. Poorhse	Monaghan	Rupture of blood vessel in the abdomen
	Corly, Female Child	1857	Rushnaglough		Burning
6.708	Corr, Owen	1863	Dundrummond	Clones	Epilepsy
2.1084	Corrigan, Edward	1873	Mullaloghlan	Donagh	Natural causes
3.623	Cosgrove, Bridget	1861	Liscrave	Monaghan	Exposure of the night
1.1129	Cotes, Henry	1875	Clones	Clones	Heart disease
1.1101	Coulson, George	1874	Rockcorry	Ematris	Suicide; drowning
14.978	Cox, Jane	1870	Bagher	Ematris	Burning
12.1034	Coyle, Michael	1872	Maghill	Drumsnat	Acute peritonitis (internal inflammation of intestinal canal)
20.984	Coyle, Owen	1870	Mon. Asylum	Monaghan	Paralysis

Inquest	Name	Year	Townland	Parish	Verdict of Death
24.575	Coyle, Patrick	1860	Cooldorragh	Drumsnat	Drowning; epileptic attack
27.491	Coyle, Phillip	1858	Cooldaragh	Drumsnat	Apoplexy accelerated by repeated intoxication
	Crawford, Billy	1873	Ardaghey	Monaghan	Sudden death
4.455	Crawford, Thomas	1857	Clinagore	Drummully	Drowning
8.867	Crawley, Elisabeth	1867	Carrickmacross	Magheross	Natural causes
	Creighton, James	1876	Mon. Asylum	Monaghan	Debility and paralysis
4.669	Croarken, Hugh	1862	Drummonda	Clones	Internal disease
13.477	Croarken, Hugh	1857	Shanroe	Clones	Natural causes
10.541	Croarken, Infant Child	1859	Kilcorran	Clones	Death at birth
9.460	Crolly, Michael	1857	Clones	Clones	Crushed by falling earth; railway accident
18.789	Crossen, Henry	1865	Drumbrean	Aghabog	Suicide; hanging
8.522	Crow, Joseph	1858	Aughnaskew	Currin	Exposure while under the influence of drink
13.508	Cumiskey, Francis	1858	Pogents	Kilmore	Drowning; fell into canal
19.838	Cunniery, Margaret	1867	Doogarry	Tedavnet	Natural causes
7.884	Cunningham, John	1868	Curraghey	Clones	Heart disease
18.1154	Cunningham, Thomas	1875	Mon. Infirm.	Monaghan	Falling from cathedral roof
13.1075	Curren, Robert	1873	Corrinshigoe	Currin	Fatty degeneration of heart
10.855	Currens, Thomas	1867	Corrinshigoe	Currin	Drowning
7.1010	Cusack, Edward	1871	Clones Workhse	Clones	Injuries sustained from falling off a pony
10.421	Cushla, Mary	1856	Arublekirk	Monaghan	Burning
11.782	Daily, Bernard	1865	Mon. Jail	Monaghan	Suicide; hanging
8.923	Daily, John	1869	Killymuddy	Clones	Inflammation of the bowels
	Daly, Peter	1875	Mon. Asylum	Monaghan	Failure of the nervous system's energy
12.714	Darby, William	1863	Tanmaenally	Ematris	Apoplexy
4.863	Darcy, Thomas	1867	Clones	Clones	Congestion of the lungs
6.626	Davis, William	1861	Cornacrieve	Donagh	Scrofulous disease of the ear
	Dawson, Daughter	1859	Tattygar (e)	Ematris	Scalding by water
14.785	Dawson, Mary	1865	Drumcall	Ematris	Burning
2.533	Dawson, Mary	1859	Tullyard	Killeevan	Heart disease
18.482	Dinny, Elinor	1857	Aughnacloy	Drumsnat	Accidental gunshot wound
11.1033	Divine, Jane	1872	Hollywood	Tedavnet	Suicide; drowning; depression – Melancholy Madness
	Dobson, Catherine	1875	Mon. Asylum	Monaghan	Disease of kidneys and heart
16.760	Dodson, James	1864	Clones Poorhse	Clones	Old age; infirmity; want of care
20.551	Dodson, John	1859	Clones	Clones	Death from effects of electricity
5.896	Dogherty, Michael	1868	Corlat	Tedavnet	Epileptic attack
	Donaghy, Phillip	1857	Edenfirkin		Fever and neglect
8.559	Donaghy, Susan	1859	Corduff	Aghabog	Drowning in a pot of milk
11.435	Donally, Bridget	1856	Carrowkeel	Tyholland	Drowning
1.651	Donally, Edward	1862	Dawson's Grove	Ematris	Heart disease
9.753	Donally, Mary Ann	1864	Annycatty	Donagh	Burning
9.999	Donally, Nancy	1871	Monaghan	Monaghan	Natural causes
18.532	Donally, Pat	1858	Lignacrieve		Murder
8.1135	Donally, Thomas	1875	Corianagh	Tullycorbet	Drowning
12.783	Donnelly (-olly), John	1865	Cremoyle	Ematris	Heart disease
14.1150	Dooley, John	1875	Clones	Clones	Exhaustion
11.661	Doran, William	1862	Cornawell	Ematris	Gunshot wound; accidental
	Dorly, James	1866	Tappa	Monaghan	Falling from horse; accident
11.926	Dowdell, Patrick	1869	Mon. Jail	Monaghan	Visitation of God
11.631	Dowley, Elizabeth	1861	Monaghan	Monaghan	Falling down a deep cutting on the railway
6.959	Drysdale, Henry	1870	Dawson's Grove Farmyard	Ematris	Angina pectoris or breast pang
12.802	Duffy, Bernard	1865	Tetoppa	Kilmore	Visitation of God
27.1061	Duffy, James	1873	Mon. Infirm.	Monaghan	Falling; trauma resulting from collision with heifer

Inquest	Name	Year	Townland	Parish	Verdict of Death
8.419	Duffy, James	1856	Annagoes	Aghabog	Manslaughter; stuck and killed by man riding a horse
5.1133	Duffy, James	1875	Cornacrew	Tullycorbet	Natural causes
12.871	Duffy, Margaret	1867	Tamlet	Monaghan	Burning
	Duffy, Mary	1864	Drummakenna		Natural causes; bronchitis
14.891	Duffy, Michael	1868	Monaghan	Monaghan	Suicide
12.587	Duffy, Nancy (or Mary)	1860	Terrycaff	Tyholland	Natural causes
3.554	Duffy, Owen	1859	Mon. Poorhse	Monaghan	Consumption
24.726	Duffy, Patrick	1863	Eden Island	Donagh	Heart disease
20.611	Duffy, Patrick	1860	Mullanaknock	Monaghan	Suicide; drowning
	Dunbar, Richard	1857	Mulnagore		Complications from a fall
	Dunlop	1862	Killegraggy	Aghabog	Most likely heart disease
	Dunlop, Mary	1869	Killegragy	Aghabog	Burning
14.605	Dunn, William	1860	Smithborough	Clones	Falling off a horse
15.874	Dunwoody, Foster	1868	Tully	Monaghan	Accidental gunshot wound
1.860	Elliott, William	1867	Moy	Donagh	Drowning
20.730	Fannen (Farmer), Francis	1864	Aughnacloone	Monaghan	Cart crash
20.1156	Farley, John	1875	Drumgreeny	Kilmore	Paralysis
2.966	Farley, Mary	1870	Drumarutt	Kilmore	Drowning
1.1063	Farmer, Patrick	1873	Drumdisco	Tedavnet	Heart Disease
15.566	Farrell, James	1859	Monaghan	Monaghan	Murder; kicked in lower belly – internal injuries
31.495	Fields, John	1858	Smithborough	Clones	Exposure
21.840	Finegan, John	1867	Clones	Clones	Railway accident; hit by train
22.766	Finigan, Mary	1865	Mullaghmore	Tyholland	Bursting of blood vessel
24.1058	Finley, Mary	1873	Drumbeen	Tedavnet	Scalding; falling into a pot of boiling hot food
	Fitzgerald, James, Esq.	1858	Clones	Clones	Falling on his head
	Fitzimons, William	1875	Mon. Asylum	Monaghan	Consumption
4.518	Fitzpatrick, Ann	1858	Monaghan	Monaghan	Exhaustion
5.969	Fitzpatrick, Francis	1870	Cremoil	Ematris	Epilepsy attack
6.1088	Fitzpatrick, Hugh	1873	Monaghan	Monaghan	Drowning
24.768	Fitzpatrick, Patrick	1865	Scotstown	Currin	Bursting of blood vessel
2.955	Flanagan, Ellen	1870	Clones	Clones	Haemorrhage
2.992	Flanagan, John	1871	Clones	Clones	Railway accident
	Flanegan, Margaret	1875	Mon. Asylum	Monaghan	Consumption
6.883	Floody, Thomas	1868	Anny	Aghnamullen	Drowning
	Foresythe, James	1875	Mon. Asylum	Monaghan	Consumption and disease of the heart
19.610	Foster, Jane	1860	Clones	Clones	Choked on piece of meat
16.907	Foster, William	1868	Drumbrain	Aghabog	Inflammation of the stomach and bowels
23.411	Fowley, Hugh	1856	Carcrely	Kilmore	Drowning
11.542	Fowley, Patrick	1859	Monaghan	Monaghan	Falling off a horse
15.590	Fox (or Foy), Judith	1860	Lattarossin	Currin	Drowning
2.811	Fox, Owen	1866	Lisguillen	Aghnamullen	Beating; violence; murder
	Frazer, Mrs John	1856	Drurryarving		Weakness
3.774	Fulton, Ann	1865	Rockcorry	Ematris	Epilepsy
12.563	Gallagher, Bridget	1859	Scotstown	Tedavnet	Visitation of God
23.987	Gallighar, James	1871	Mon. Infirm.	Monaghan	Congestion of the brain
13.1107	Gallogher, Joseph	1874	Conaghey	Killeevan	Drowning
	Gartland, M.	1868	Toora	Aghnamullen	Childbirth
6.936	Gartland, Margaret	1869	Ardragh	Magheross	Bowel complaint
11.461	Gavan, James	1857	Dysart (Nart)	Kilmore	Visitation of God
	Gaven, Betty	1873	Stranooden	Kilmore	No cause of death; Ill
13.1094	Gaven, Michael	1873	Clones Poorhse	Clones	Falling; congestion and shock to the system
5.655	Gibson, William	1862	Cornasoo	Kilmore	Burned by boiling water; poor attendance by Dr Reed
3.1139	Gillelan, Catherine	1875	Magherarney	Ematris	Heart disease
	Gillespie, David	1875	Carrafarry		Not enough info

Inquest	Name	Year	Townland	Parish	Verdict of Death
11.902	Gillespie, Michael	1868	Mudley	Clontibret	Trampled by a horse
3.535	Gillis, Jane	1859	Drumginny	Donagh	Old age and infirmity
	Ginely, Margaret	1876	Mon. Asylum	Monaghan	Paralysis
12.1002	Ginely, Rose	1871	Kilnacloy	Drumsnat	Fever; exposure
5.536	Ginley, Joseph	1859	Clenavarne	Kilmore	Exposure and weakness
11.870	Glass, Jane	1867	Tirnamona	Tedavnet	Drowning
7.751	Glen, Michael	1864	Newbliss	Killeevan	Internal disease
15.786	Glyne (Glynn), Mary	1865	Aghabog	Aghabog	Burning
12.1074	Goodfellow, Infant Boy	1873	Kilmore East	Ematris	Murder; strangulation
17.648	Goodwin, Alice	1862	Carneys-Island	Clones	Crushed by falling oats; mill ceiling collapse
16.647	Goodwin, Patrick	1862	Carneys-Island	Clones	Crushed by falling oats; mill ceiling collapse
	Gordan, Jane	1867	Dundrennan	Ematris	Beaten; spousal abuse
28.619	Gorman, Bridget	1861	Donagh	Donagh	Burning
3.1037	Gorman, David	1872	Derryvane	Donagh	Trampled by a horse
8.1042	Gormly, John	1872	Monaghan	Monaghan	Struck and killed by train
19.570	Gormly, Mary	1860	Corravally	Tullycorbet	Natural causes
1.496	Graham, Francis	1858	Monaghan	Monaghan	Effects of drink and debilitated constitution
24.915	Graham, James	1869	Smithborough	Clones	Drowning
9.540	Graham, Jane	1859	Killycoyhill	Clones	Drowning
	Gray, James	1865	Feragh	Monaghan	Natural causes
2.1005	Greydon, Susan	1871	Gartnawhiney	Clones	Cancer; haemorrhage
10.641	Greydon, William	1861	Clones	Clones	Apoplexy
2.733	Griffith, Joseph	1864	Monaghan	Monaghan	Burning
6.737	Grimes, Charles	1864	Templetate	Tyholland	Drowning
9.962	Grogan, Bessy	1870	Clones Poorhse	Clones	Heart disease; water on the chest
4.579	Hagan, Henry	1860	Monaghan	Monaghan	Burning
10.561	Halfpenny, Francis	1859	Gibraltar	Tyholland	Drowned in bog-hole
	Hall, Ann Jane	1875	Mon. Asylum	Monaghan	Chronic diarrhoea
2.667	Hamilton, Elizabeth	1862	Deraneary	Aghabog	Natural causes
9.819	Hare, James	1866	Roosky	Drumsnat	Disease of liver; peritonitis;
	Harper, James	1858	Menintens		Brain fever
15.1095	Hart, Sally	1874	Tully	Donagh	Drowning
26.845	Harvison, William	1867	Monaghan	Monaghan	Natural causes
6.1113	Hazlet, Mrs. Jane	1874	Killgaven	Tedavnet	Car accident
15.834	Hearse, James	1866	Kilcreen	Clones	Burning; lamp with oil
6.637	Hearty, Mary	1861	Monaghan	Monaghan	Epilepsy
16.1019	Heasly, Elizabeth	1871	Monaghan	Monaghan	Suicide
6.656	Heatherington, John	1862	Monaghan	Monaghan	Falling from scaffold
13.527	Heatly, William	1858	Strenany	Donagh	Hit by train
6.1142	Henderson, Eliza	1875	Tullycoragh	Muckno	Heart disease
7.738	Henderson, Thomas	1864	Monaghan	Monaghan	Cart accident
10.909	Hernowin, Michael	1868			Natural causes; exposure
2.821	Hewlett, William	1866	Monaghan	Monaghan	Killed by train
2.879	Higgins, John	1868	Clones	Clones	Crushed by cars at railroad
4.775	Hill, David	1865	Cordoolough	Tullycorbet	Suicide
1.632	Hinigin, James	1861	Lisnagonway	Aghabog	Kidney problems
12.857	Holdcroft, Joseph	1867	Derryleedigan	Clones	Drowning
13.977	Holdsworth, John	1870	Carrickmore	Clones	Concussion of the brain and spinal marrow; fell from cart
12.976	Holmes, Jane	1870	Monaghan	Monaghan	Effusion on the brain
2.917	Howe, Catherine	1869	Drumakelly	Aghabog	Natural causes; heart disease
6.796	Hughes, Ellen (aka Mary)	1865	Dundonagh	Donagh	Drowning
3.705	Hughes, James	1863	Mullaghabog	Donagh	Natural causes; drink
7.627	Hughes, John James	1861	Garren	Tyholland	Drowning
18.948	Hughes, Mary	1869	Monaghan	Monaghan	Effusion of serum on the brain; apoplectic fit
13.784	Hughes, Patrick	1865	Monaghan Jail	Monaghan	Natural causes; epilepsy

Inquest	Name	Year	Townland	Parish	Verdict of Death
1.412	Hughes, Thomas	1856	Sillis	Tynan, Co. Armagh	Accidental drowning, possible murder
22.41	Hughes, Thomas	1856	Lillis	Donagh	Drowning
1.892	Hughes, Thomas	1868	Monaghan	Monaghan	Murder
7.852	Infant Child	1867	Drum	Currin	Drowning
4.849	Infant Child	1867	Faulkland	Donagh	Drowning
7.582	Infant Child	1860	Killegrallen	Tedavnet	Drowning
14.545	Infant Child	1859	Monaghan	Monaghan	Drowning
16.511	Infant Child	1858	Kilnaclan	Tullycorbet	Exposure to open air
9.584	Infant Child	1860	Aughnamulla	Drumsnat	Fractures of the skull
20.839	Infant Child	1867	Annagalln	Tedavnet	Infant death
24.843	Infant Child	1867	Donagh	Donagh	Infant death
5.920	Infant Child	1869	Rockcorry	Ematris	Murder
18.1080	Infant Child	1873	Cornaclue	Errigal Truagh	Murder; exposure
3.918	Infant Child	1869	Monaghan	Monaghan	Murder; Neglect at time of birth; found in canal
11.856	Infant Child	1867	Drum	Currin	Murder; strangulation
9.1090	Infant Child	1873	Drum	Currin	Natural causes
11.1001	Infant Child	1871	Drumsloe	Drummully	Natural causes
23.767	Infant Child	1865	Killeevan	Killeevan	Natural causes
14.589	Infant Child	1860	Knockwest	Currin	Natural causes
3.498	Infant Child	1858	Monaghan	Monaghan	Natural causes
10.741	Infant Child	1864	Roosky	Monaghan	Natural causes
5.749	Infant Child	1864	Stranervy	Donagh	Natural causes
15.646	Infant Child	1861	Monaghan	Monaghan	Natural causes
12.662	Infant Child	1862	Ternahiseo	Tedavnet	Natural causes; corpse buried and abandoned
11.525	Infant Child	1858	Monaghan	Monaghan	Neglect
10.800	Infant Child	1865	Monaghan	Monaghan	Neglect at time of birth; drowning; canal
12.526	Infant Child	1858	Monaghan	Monaghan	Premature birth
10.601	Infant Child	1860	Maghery	Clones	Stillborn
8.503	Infant Child	1858	Nawderpark	Killeevan	Stillborn
24.615	Infant Child (Kells)	1861	Derrrins	Currin	Stillborn or murdered by mental imbecility of mother
19.949	Infant Child	1870	Clones	Clones	Unknown
15.546	Infant Child	1859	Killykespin	Killeevan	Unknown
19.483	Infant Child	1857	Monaghan	Monaghan	Unknown
5.556	Infant Child	1859	Monaghan	Monaghan	Unknown
5.578	Infant Child	1860	Clenamully	Tedavnet	Unknown; found dead on the side of the road
16.665	Infant Child	1862	Clones	Clones	Unknown; found floating in the canal
7.997	Infant Child	1871	Cloncaw	Donagh	Unknown; possible drowning
13.463	Infant Child	1857	Dundrummond	Clones	Unknown; badly decomposed
18.683	Infant Child	1863	Clones	Clones	Murder; persons unknown
6.690	Infant Child (female)	1863	Monaghan	Monaghan	Drowned; strangled
20.571	Infant Child (female)	1860	Monaghan	Monaghan	Exposure
26.770	Infant Child (female)	1865	Dromore	Ematris	Murder
1.1096	Infant Child (female)	1874	Rockcorry	Ematris	Murder; drowning
19.443	Infant Child (female)	1856	Rockcorry	Ematris	Murder; drowning
3.454	Infant Child (female)	1857	Newbliss	Killeevan	Murder; strangulation
9.1012	Infant Child (female)	1871	Carrickmacross	Magheross	Murder; suffocation
5.1039	Infant Child (female)	1872	Kinacloy	Monaghan	Possible murder; drowning
6.1040	Infant Child (male)	1872	Feragh	Monaghan	Natural causes
10.697	Infant Child (male)	1863	Skinnegin	Donagh	Unknown
6.557	Irwin, Eliza	1859	Carraghaduff	Donagh	Visitation of God
11.562	Irwin, Robert	1859	Clones	Clones	Head trauma, cart and horse accident
8.673	Jackson, Alexander	1862	Urbalkirk	Monaghan	Horse and cart accident
14.645	Jackson, Anne Jane	1861	Alagesh	Tedavnet	Visitation of God

Inquest	Name	Year	Townland	Parish	Verdict of Death
2.466	Jackson, Henry	1857	Rockcorry	Ematris	Intoxication; suffocation
10.1013	Jackson, Margaret	1871	Monaghan	Monaghan	Affection of the lungs
10.505	Jebbs, Mick	1858	Killes	Donagh	Visitation of God
8.459	Johnston	1857	Clonickney	Donagh	Suffocation; accidental?
	Johnston, Catherine	1856	Dyart (Nart)	Kilmore	Cholic
2.1021	Johnston, George	1872	Drumskelt	Aghnamullen	Cold, fatigue and old age
14.833	Johnston, George	1866	Drum	Currin	Falling; head injury
11.602	Johnston, Margaret	1860	Maghery	Clones	Mutilation of genitals during childbirth
	Johnston, Thomas	1857	Tullyglair (Ballytrain)		Heart disease
25.844	Kane, John	1867	Monaghan	Monaghan	Heart disease
5.519	Keelan, Isabella	1858	Monaghan	Monaghan	Internal disease accelerated by argument with husband
12.903	Keely, Edward	1868	Clones	Clones	Struck by train; accident
9.473	Keely, Susan	1857	Coolkill	Ematris	Burning
7.1089	Keenan, Bridget	1873	Drumscarore	Tedavnet	Natural causes
14.944	Keenan, Elizabeth	1869	Dandracgee	Clones	Drowning
22.486	Keenan, Mary	1857	Tandrugeeban	Monaghan	Drowning
7.538	Keenan, Peter	1859	Monaghan	Monaghan	Affection of the heart
5.429	Keith, William	1856	Listrekegency	Monaghan	Natural causes
	Kells, Francis	1856	Carin-Roe	Currin	Burning
12.1168	Kelly, Ann	1875	Derrykinard	Ematris	Dropsy
	Kelly, Male Child	1872	Newbliss	Killeevan	Burning
16.440	Kelly, Margaret	1856	Leitrim	Tyholland	Burning
1.931	Kelly, Mary	1869	Monaghan	Monaghan	Burning
5.416	Kelly, Mary	1856	Monaghan Jail	Monaghan	Dysentery
19.1125	Keough, Mary	1875	Monaghan	Monaghan	Suicide; drowning
12.1106	Kernan, Thomas	1874	Knockakerwin	Errigal Truagh	Visitation of the Almighty
20.764	Kerr, Francis	1865	Milltown	Ematris	Burning
16.1152	Kerr, John	1875	Monaghan	Monaghan	Crushed by a falling tree
19.763	Kerr, Mary Ann	1865	Milltown	Ematris	Burning
27.451	Kieff, William	1857	Monaghan	Monaghan	Crushed by a wagon; Railroad accident
10.901	Kiernan, Mary	1868	Coolnaeart	Currin	Heart disease
14.478	Kiernan, Michael	1857	Tullycolliff	Muckno	Accident with horse
3.734	Kiernan, Philip	1864	Clonfad	Killeevan	Cholic
7.898	Kilagher, John	1868	Cartaghert	Aghnamullen	Paralysis of the heart
15.717	Kirkpatrick, Edmond	1863	Clones	Clones	Burning; infections set in
7.1135	Kirley, John	1875	Eshanaglough	Tedavnet	Heart disease
21.951	Lamb, James	1870	Roosky	Monaghan	Serious apoplexy
16.806	Larkin, Patrick	1865	Faltagh	Aghabog	Accident; crushed by building
19.684	Lee, George	1863	Carravores	Ematris	Elderly neglect; starvation and exposure
9.629	Lee, Rebecca	1861	Monaghan	Monaghan	Great bodily prostration of health and strength
1.1023	Lemon, William	1872	Drumavale	Currin	Apoplexy
19.650	Lenon, Biddy	1862	Coolshanagh	Monaghan	Heart disease
18.982	Leonard, James	1870	Kiltubbert	Kilmore	Cerebral apoplexy
10.434	Leonard, Owen	1856	Mulnacross	Drumsnat	Apoplexy
3.1006	Leonard, Patrick	1871	Kiltubber	Kilmore	Heart disease
	Leslie, E. P.	1871	(Leslie) Demesne	Donagh	Unknown; 2 hours of illness
7.471	Linch, John	1857	Cladone	Clones	Railway accident; run over by a wagon
11.506	Lindsy, John	1858	Cornaglar	Kilmore	Visitation of God
24.988	Little, Archibald	1871	Tavenagh	Errigal Truagh	Drowning
	Little, Margaret	1871	Listillen (near Smithborough)		Burning
15.930	Livingston, Elisabeth	1869	Monaghan	Monaghan	Natural causes; Softening of the brain
17.682	Livingston, William	1862	Drumkeen	Aghabog	Murder; poisoned with arsenic
15.680	Livingston, William	1862	Rakeevan	Aghabog	Natural causes
15.979	Longmoore, George	1870	Drumbin	Tedavnet	Cirrhosis; fight

Inquest	Name	Year	Townland	Parish	Verdict of Death
1.965	Longmoore, John	1870	Drumbin	Tedavnet	Drowning
3.747	Loughran, Robert	1864	Monaghan	Monaghan	Head trauma; kicked by a horse
1.991	Lovet, Ann	1871	Clones Workhse	Clones	Rupture of a blood vessel
9.1104	Lowry, George	1874	Smithborough	Clones	Burning
2.1097	Lynch, Patrick	1874	Glenmore	Clones	Strangulated hernia
17.836	Mackey, John	1866	Annagalln	Tedavnet	Child birth
23.574	Macklin, Thomas	1860	Carronbawn	Drumsnat	Mill accident; arm shredded
5.824	Magee, Mary	1866	Clones	Clones	Murder; beaten to death
13.644	Maghath, Margaret	1861	Magheraharne	Ematris	Pemphagus; Lack of nourishment
4.534	Magin, Elizabeth	1859	Rockcorry	Ematris	Crushed by falling roof
17.441	Maguire, Catherine	1856	Kilgormly	Clones	Burning
8.539	Maguire, Felix	1859	Scotstown	Tedavnet	Disease of the heart accelerated by excessive drink
2.1064	Maguire, Mary	1873	Clones Workhse	Clones	Congestion of the lungs
7.1143	Maguire, Mary	1875	Clones	Clones	Murder; head trauma
8.752	Maguire, William	1864	Turrygaly	Tullycorbet	Drowning
11.676	Magwood, Mary	1862	Clones	Clones	Heart disease
22.1158	Magwood, William	1875	Scotstown	Tedavnet	Murder; head trauma
11.696	Malone, Margaret	1863	Tamah	Ematris	Congestion of the lungs; Heart disease
12.1046	Martin, Agnes	1872	Monaghan	Monaghan	Suicide; drowning
20.911	Martin, Elisabeth Ann	1869	Ballinode	Tedavnet	Burning; house fire
9.828	Martin, James	1866	Correvan	Aghabog	Heart disease
19.910	Martin, Margaret	1869	Ballinode	Tedavnet	Burning; house fire
4.706	Martin, Richard A.	1863	Correavern	Aghabog	Drowning
17.608	Martin, Rose	1860	Magherashogery	Currin	Death during childbirth
5.707	Martin, Thomas S.	1863	Carreaven	Aghabog	Drowning
6.671	Mathews, Mary	1862	Magherarny	Clones	Drowning
1.745	McAdam, James	1864	Legacurry	Tullycorbet	Head Trauma; Cart and horse accident
29.1165	McAdam, John	1876	Tiniscomfy	Donagh	Exposure to cold weather
2.1109	McAdoo, Jane	1874	Clones	Clones	Dropsy
	McAlair, Pat	1873	Drumhiller	Aghabog (Drumhillagh)	Burning
29.493	McAlier, Pat	1858	Drumcrew	Tedavnet	Burning
15.700	McAlier, Pat	1863	Shee	Tedavnet	Natural causes
17.512	McAlier, Thomas	1858	Monaghan	Monaghan	Accidental overdose of a narcotic
8.1089	McArdle, Arthur	1873	Stramore	Donagh	Alcohol poisoning
22.952	McArdle, Edward	1870	Corvoy	Tullycorbet	Hit by a cart
8.692	McArdle, Thomas	1863	Danunair	Monaghan	Crushed by heavy cart filled with manure
11.1118	McAree, Mary	1874	Ballyleck	Kilmore	Drowning
	McAtee, Rose	1858	Tonagh	Aghabog	Unknown
3.1025	McBride, James	1872	Magherakill	Donaghmoyne	Murder; Beaten to death
20.722	McCabe, Ann	1863	Clones	Clones	Hit by railway train
	McCabe, Bridget	1873	Liscumasky	Aghabog	Related to confinement
4.468	McCabe, Felix	1857	Scharvagh	Killeevan	Run over by a railway wagon
	McCabe, Infant	1873	Liscumasky	Aghabog	Premature birth
16.607	McCabe, James	1860	Guardihall	Killeevan	Natural causes
21.612	McCabe, John	1861	Monaghan	Monaghan	Crushed by falling stones at railway works
	McCabe, John	1856	Shevlin	Tyholland	Old age; heart attack
10.829	McCabe, Mary Ann	1866	Corrinshigoe	Currin	Burning
4.428	McCabe, Mathew	1856	Cortobar	Ematris	Drowning
22.913	McCabe, Patrick	1869	Clones	Clones	Falling down stairs
4.688	McCabe, Phillip	1863	Koolkill West	Ematris	Suicide; slashed own throat
4.1066	McCabe, Rose	1873	Caranure	Tullycorbet	Natural causes; heart disease
	McCabe, Son of James	1861	Nr Carrickmacross	Magheross	Died suddenly; under medical treatment for worms

Inquest	Name	Year	Townland	Parish	Verdict of Death
10.940	McCabe, Female Infant	1869	Mon. Infirm.	Monaghan	Drowning
12.1093	McCaffrey, Bridget	1873	Drumavare	Currin	Epilepsy
13.928	McCaffrey, James	1869	Clontask	Drummully	Visitation of God
13.744	McCaffrey, Thomas	1864	Lurganchamlough	Aghnamullen	Drowning
30.494	McCaffry, Edward	1858	Monaghan	Monaghan	Crushed by falling gravel
7.691	McCague, Phillip	1863	Milltown	Monaghan	Drowning
8.432	McCahey, Margaret	1856	Esker	Errigal Truagh	Internal haemorrhage
10.869	McCahey, Patrick	1867	Esker	Errigal Truagh	Bursting of blood vessel
10.974	McCall, Charles	1870	Corcreagh	Magheross	Choked to death
7.1114	McCann, Owen	1874	Latnamard	Aghabog	Suicide; drowning
9.1145	McCarney, Margaret	1875	Clones	Clones	Old age and infirmity
8.938	McCarole, Francis	1869	Killafaddy	Killeevan	Trampled by a horse
8.1030	McCarole, James	1872	Killeevan	Killeevan	Crushed in construction/ railway accident
7.797	McCarrell, Isabella	1865	Listellen	Killeevan	Apoplexy
8.885	McCarrole, Susan	1868	Feulkland	Donagh	Hit by train; accident
9.693	McCarron, John	1863	Killecran	Tedavnet	Apoplexy or disease of heart
10.1072	McCarron, Mary	1873	Rackelly	Errigal Truagh	Murder; heart trauma
23.1057	McCarron, Michael	1873	Tullyloan	Tedavnet	Heart disease
8.472	McCarron, Michael	1857	Monaghan	Monaghan	Native cholera
21.527	McCarron, Thadeus	1860	Coolnacart	Currin	Visitation of God
1.685	McCarter, John	1863	Drumkeen	Aghabog	Natural causes
	McCarvle, Mother of Pat	1875	Uscher (Urcher)	Kilmore	Sudden death
4.1099	McCarvle, Owen	1874	Corncuvelle	Killeevan	Visitation of the Almighty
23.447	McCarvle, Thomas	1857	Corlatt	Killeevan	Murder
8.798	McClave, Ellen	1865	Augherakeltan	Tedavnet	Apoplexy; falling into well
7.1069	McCleary, Susan	1873	Cornawall	Aghabog	Due to complications during confinement
4.735	McClelan, Sam	1864	Drumbreay	Aghabog	Natural causes
26.450	McCleland, John	1857	Drumliney	Aghabog	Burning
	McClery, James	1875	Mon. Asylum	Monaghan	Congestion of circulation
	McClusky, John	1875	Mon. Asylum	Monaghan	Diarrhoea
8.583	McClusky, Pat	1860	Drumsearer	Tedavnet	Natural causes
	McConkey, Infant	1870	Drumhirk		unknown
	McConnel, Bessy	1875	Mon. Asylum	Monaghan	Strumans disease of bowels
18.1052	McConnell, Francis	1872	Togan	Drumsnat	Attack of cramps
8.599	McConnell, James	1860	Drumshanny	Drumsnat	Drowned in bog-hole while playing with other children
1.791	McConnell, Joseph	1865	Derryrush	Aghnamullen	Suicide; hanging
8.972	McConnell, Robert	1870	Clones	Clones	Disease of the heart and brain; inebriate
	McConnor, Bridget	1874	Mon. Asylum	Monaghan	Consumption
7.960	McCormick, John	1870	Lisnagore	Killeevan	Heart disease
22.936	McCormick, Thomas	1871	Mon. Asylum	Monaghan	Epileptic fit; suffocation
7.672	McCoy, Robert John	1862	Lisguillen	Aghnamullen	Natural causes; bowel problems
21.765	McCracken, Mary A.	1865	Anaheagh	Monaghan	Burning
6.501	McCrarren, James	1858	Shamunlagh	Monaghan	Cart and horse accident;
19.721	McCrudden, Owen	1863	Corlatlatten	Errigal Truagh	Drowning; exposure
1.425	McCue, Charles	1856	Monaghan	Monaghan	Heart disease
6.851	McCullen, Owen	1867	Mon. Infirm.	Monaghan	Burning
	McCulloch, James	1865	Drummuck	Ballybay	Sudden death
26.990	McCullogh, Infant	1871	Cargathranna	Tullycorbet	Still birth
7.826	McDermot, Francis	1866	Doohat	Aghbog	Drowning
	McDermot, James	1860	Clones	Clones	Gout of the stomach
7.971	McDermot, John	1870	Carreskeen	Killeevan	Effusion of the brain
7.1102	McDonagh, William	1871	Mullen	Errigal Truagh	Drowning
12.1119	McDonald, Alice	1874	Smithborough	Clones	Inflammation of the bowels
9.1036	McDonald, Ann	1872	Mon. Poorhse	Monaghan	Burned/scalded by water; died as result of complications
4.654	McDonald, Bridget	1862	Garrin	Aghabog	Burning
10.524	McDonald, Rose	1858	Clones	Clones	Rupture of the heart

Inquest	Name	Year	Townland	Parish	Verdict of Death
9.939	McDonald, Terance	1869	Mon. Asylum	Monaghan	Nervous exhaustion
25.1161	McDowel, Revd Martin	1876	Creve	Aghnamullen	Apoplexy
10.630	McEleer, Michael	1861	Drumeroofoster	Tedavnet	Murder
	McElgum, Hugh	1875	Mon. Asylum	Monaghan	Consumption
5.469	McElmeel, Margaret	1857	Knocknagrave	Donagh	Burning
6.537	McElmeel, Terence	1859	Corgrunan	Errigal Truagh	Visitation of God
17.947	McElvy, Esther	1869	Knockatully	Monaghan	Spasmodic disease of stomach
16.530	McEnally, Bridget	1858	Saveagh	Tyholland	Arms crushed in flax mill accident
16.718	McEnally, James	1863	Corcahan	Kilmore	Drowning
2.633	McEnally, John	1861	Monaghan	Monaghan	Starvation; unable to eat
9.854	McEnally, Owen	1867	Drumcobready	Donagh	Drowning
9.433	McEnally, Peter	1856	Killelough	Tedavnet	Heart Disease
20.444	McEniff, Miles	1856	Monaghan Jail	Monaghan	Infirmity and old age
16.1022	McEnill, Mary	1874	Clones	Clones	Haemorrhage from bursting blood vessel
13.564	McEntee, Pat	1859	Sandhills	Currin	Visitation of God
15.606	McEntee, Patrick	1860	Monaghan	Monaghan	Burning
23.487	McGaghey, James	1857	Gotnanagh	Killeevan	Head trauma; crushed by the church bell
12.507	McGee, Michael	1858	Monaghan	Monaghan	Heart disease
18.762	McGillen, Edward	1864	Gingorry	Tyholland	Internal disease
8.628	McGinity, Owen	1861	Sheskin	Tedavnet	Drowning
3.653	McGinn, Catherine	1862	Glassdrummond	Killeevan	Burning
16.591	McGinn, Patrick	1860	Drumacree	Ematris	Drowned in bog-hole
	McGlone, Owen	1862	Scaravagh	Donagh	No cause of death
1.1020	McGlone, William	1872	Monaghan	Monaghan	Dropsy of the chest
2.1130	McGorman, Agnes	1875	Clones	Clones	Burning
28.1164	McGorman, Patrick	1876	Drumcrew-Dickson	Clones	Drowning
5.670	McGough, Patrick	1862	Alkill	Tyholland	Drowning
9.600	McGovern, Thomas	1860	Monaghan	Monaghan	Crushed by fll
	McGreanry, Catherine	1875	Mon. Asylum	Monaghan	Disease of neck vertebra
8.639	McGuiness, Biddy	1861	Skinegin	Tyholland	Crushed by roof falling in
	McGuiness, John	1866	Tappa	Tullycorbet	Beaten; Injuries from quarrel
28.1062	McGuiness, Mary	1873	Corcahan	Kilmore	Burning
12.543	McGuiness, Patrick	1859	Monaghan	Monaghan	Cart accident; head trauma
3.967	McGuirk, Mary	1870	Rockcorry	Ematris	Heart disease
14.699	McGurk, John	1863	Mon. Jail	Monaghan	Congestion of the lungs
13.698	McKee, William	1863	Carnahoo	Tullycorbet	Cart accident; drink
5.689	McKelvey, James	1863	Analoar	Clones	Suicide; hanging
3.822	McKenna, Bernard	1866	Monaghan	Monaghan	Effusion of the brain
8.827	McKenna, Biddy	1866	Mullashlanagh	Errigal Truagh	Peritonitis or inflammation of the bowels
11.742	McKenna, Bridget	1864	Killycarren	Errigal Truagh	Internal Pains
15.1018	McKenna, Catherine	1871	Monaghan	Monaghan	Fell down a ladder
3.467	McKenna, Charles	1857	Dirrinisell	Roslea	Neck injuries; fell out of cart
	McKenna, Ellen	1874	Edenmore	Donagh	Drowning
1.846	McKenna, Fole	1867	Moy	Errigal Truagh	Natural causes
6.921	McKenna, Hugh	1869	Derryvern	Donagh	Heart disease
1.1035	McKenna, James	1872	Monaghan	Monaghan	Disease of the stomach
7.502	McKenna, John	1858	Killicreen	Tedavnet	Apoplexy
15.759	McKenna, John	1864	Glenkeen	Errigal Truagh	Epileptic attack
17.876	McKenna, John	1868	Knockehalun	Tedavnet	Pains; Stroke
8.819	McKenna, John	1866	Kilnagullon	Errigal Truagh	Syncope; heart attack
17.788	McKenna, Margaret	1865	Mullaghgreenan	Aghabog	Drowning
10.585	McKenna, Mary	1860	Derrygasson	Donagh	Horse accident
6.417	McKenna, Mary Ann	1856	Emyvale	Donagh	Burning
11.830	McKenna, Owen	1866	Killyslievan	Errigal Truagh	Falling from heap of flax
1.954	McKenna, Pat	1870	Mullaless	Donagh	Cramps in bowels
8.1070	McKenna, Patrick	1873	Dernasell	Tedavnet	Murder/Head Trauma
2.746	McKenna, Peter	1864	Newbliss	Killeevan	Accidental suffocation

Inquest	Name	Year	Townland	Parish	Verdict of Death
3.880	McKenna, Peter	1868	Killyrean	Donagh	Exposure; alcohol poisoning
1.576	McKenna, Peter	1860	Aghadah	Tedavnet	Internal Pain
3.793	McKenna, Rose	1865	Glasmullagh	Errigal Truagh	Bursting of blood vessel
2.593	McKenna, Shibby	1860	Kilangeol	Errigal Truagh	Thrown down by cow
14.438	McKenna, Susan	1856	Derranalarra	Errigal Truagh	Epilepsy
19.514	McKenna, Thomas	1858	Skinnegin	Donagh	Drowned; fell in a well
18.510	McKenna, Thomas	1858	Killecurren	Tedavnet	Epilepsy
4.919	McKeown, Jane	1869	Monaghan	Monaghan	Neglect
5.1100	McKiever, Henry	1874	Bessmount Park	Tyholland	Accidental shooting; gunshot wound
15.439	McLoughlan, Ellen	1856	Monaghan	Monaghan	Apoplexy due to old age
10.1044	McMahon, Bernard	1872	Clones	Clones	Drowning
7.778	McMahon, Bridget	1865	Scotstown	Tedavnet	Accidental fall
3.414	McMahon, Elisabeth	1856	Clonreagh	Drummully	Burning
10.754	McMahon, John	1864	Newbliss	Killeevan	Burning
3.517	McMahon, John	1858	Dromore	Ematris	Fary or glanders
12.927	McMahon, John	1869	Adrumsee	Clones	Natural causes
	McMahon, Joseph	1859	Warrenpoint	Monaghan	Excessive drinking; fighting
1.878	McMahon, Mick	1868	Corfad	Tullycorbet	Alcohol poisoning
3.1098	McMahon, Peter	1874	Clonryce	Killeevan	Drowning
	McMahon, Peter	1865	Corfad	Tullycorbet	Unknown
9.973	McMahon, William	1870	Knockatown	Errigal Truagh	Murder; gunshot wound
22.446	McManus, Biddy	1857	Clones	Clones	Typhus fever
21.445	McManus, Infant Child	1857	Clones	Clones	Murder
12.643	McManus, Phillip	1861	Clones	Clones	Fell while working on a bridge
29.731	McMullen, John	1864	Monaghan	Monaghan	Heart disease
10.474	McMullen, Matilda	1857	Drollagh	Aghabog	Drowning
3.427	McMurrar, Francis	1856	Derraley	Donagh	Railway accident
5.850	McPhilips, Bridget	1867	Latnamard	Aghabog	Natural causes
11.755	McPhilips, Hugh	1864	Corravaghen	Ematris	Crushed by falling wall
	McPhillips, Hugh	1859	Carrivillah	Aghabog	Burning
5.814	McQuade, Ann	1856	Moy	Errigal Truagh	Visitation of God
9.711	McQuade, Arthur	1863	Glaslough	Donagh	Suffocation; fits
26.617	McQuade, Margaret	1861	Derryhallagh	Donagh	Old age and infirmity
	McQuade, Patrick	1863	Glaslough	Donagh	Long-standing illness
4.1132	McQuillen, John	1875	Monaghan	Monaghan	Fell to death at the cathedral
14.758	McRoberts, Thomas	1864	Emyvale	Donagh	Drowned in mill race
3.1131	Mehaffy, John	1875	Monaghan	Monaghan	Fell; concussion at the cathedral
5.625	Meighan, Anne	1861	Scotstown	Tedavnet	Natural effects of old age
4.635	Meighan, Bridget	1861	Descart	Aghabog	Heart disease
2.652	Meighan, John	1862	Clones	Clones	Destitution accelerated by internal disease
16.701	Meighan, Thomas	1863	Corshooe	Monaghan	Epileptic attack
15.906	Meighen, Ann	1868	Corcahan	Kilmore	Burning; Epilepsy
6.996	Meighen, Laurance	1871	Mon. Asylum	Monaghan	Suicide; hanging
2.861	Midcairne, John	1867	Coraclare	Errigal Truagh	Struck by lightning
1.621	Middleton, Mary Jane	1861	Clones	Clones	Disease of the heart
4.1086	Miller, Thomas	1873	Monaghan	Monaghan	Injuries from cart and horse accident
10.1105	Moan, Owen	1874	Clonkeen	Errigal Truagh	Visitation of the Almighty
1.703	Mohan, Margaret	1863	Crockcumberland	Clones	Heart disease
11.1014	Molloy, Edward	1871	Clones	Clones	Legs cut off by train
6.897	Molloy, John	1868	Drumgoone	Currin	Suffocation; accident
6.45	Molloy, Margaret	1856	Corrinargh	Currin	Drowning
	Monaghan, Bridget	1862	Mullacraunk	Tullycorbet	Beggar; died suddenly
8.899	Monaghan, Daniel	1868	Lissagarton	Clones	Heart disease
25.1059	Monaghan, James	1873	Eshloughfin	Tedavnet	Fell; cart and horse accident
	Monaghan, Philip	1876	Mon. Asylum	Monaghan	Consumption
12.942	Mooney, Ann	1869	Clones Poorhse	Clones	Broken Leg; Complications
2.453	Mooney, Ann	1857	Glaslough	Donagh	Rupture of blood vessels of the heart

Inquest	Name	Year	Townland	Parish	Verdict of Death
14.905	Mooney, John	1868	Castleshane	Monaghan	Swinepox; poisoned; negligence
10.1032	Mooney, Michael	1872	Curren	Aghabog	Murder; Stabbing
19.809	Mooney, Revd Thomas	1866	Monaghan	Monaghan	Congestion of brain resulting from retention of urine
27.1163	Moore, Anne	1876	Annakella	Clones	Epilepsy
2.622	Moore, Francis	1861	Mon. Infirm.	Monaghan	Shock to nervous system and depression at death of master, Mr Adams
25.449	Moore, James	1857	Monaghan	Monaghan	Exposure; drink related
22.105_	Moore, John	1872	Killinsah	Clones	Heart disease
20.1082	Moore, Margaret	1873	Killagoan	Monaghan	Bursting of a blood vessel; consumption
13.1120	Moore, William	1874	Mon. Asylum	Monaghan	Melancholia bronchitis
9.674	Moorhead, Andrew	1862	Lowertown	Clones	Cart and horse accident
17.548	Moorhead, Charles	1859	Golanduff	Killeevan	Struck by lightning
11.1092	Moorhead, Eliza	1873	Kernagal	Clones	Heart disease
11.1147	Moorhead, John	1875	Clones	Clones	Inflammation of the lungs
	Moorhead, Margaret	1871	Newbliss	Killeevan	Unknown; few days illness
21.409	Moorhead, Peter	1856	Calliagh	Aghabog	Drowning, drunk
7.458	Moreland, Mary	1857	Carsons	Ematris	Burning
6.970	Morris, John	1870	Clones	Clones	Burning
	Morrison, M.	1861	Clones	Clones	Rupture of blood vessel of the heart
17.981	Moyna, Mary	1870	Glaslough	Donagh	Heart disease
12.743	Moyna, Thomas J.	1864	Knocknacullion	Monaghan	Burning
6.470	Muldoon, Michael	1857	Clones	Clones	Murder; gunshot
11.801	Mullen, Mary	1865	Emyvale	Donagh	Bursting a blood vessel
13.1003	Mullen, William	1871	Monaghan	Monaghan	Attempted suicide; weakened constitution
11.888	Mulligan, Ann	1868	Leck	Kilmore	Drowning
14.509	Mulligan, Bridget	1858	Monaghan	Monaghan	General debility
13.424	Mulligan, Felix	1856	Kiltubbert	Kilmore	Visitation of God
23.1159	Mulligan, John	1875	Lisareark	Currin	Heart disease
4.415	Murdock, George	1856	Monaghan	Monaghan	Delirium tremors
8.961	Murdock, Jane	1870	Monaghan	Monaghan	Exposure to the cold
17.702	Murphy, Ann	1863	Mon. Jail	Monaghan	Brain fever
2.413	Murphy, Ann	1856	Monaghan	Monaghan	Burning
28.492	Murphy, Bridget	1858	Aughnacloghin	Donaghmoyne	Burning
1.1083	Murphy, Bridget	1873	Tullyard	Monaghan	Drowning
17.1153	Murphy, Charles	1875	Aghnaernid	Tedavnet	Heart disease
8.1144	Murphy, Ellen	1875	Cornapaste	Currin	Childbirth
24.1160	Murphy, John	1875	Skeholme	Currin	Effusion on the brain
7.817	Murphy, Michael	1866	Clones Poorhse	Clones	Heart disease
5.1112	Murphy, Michael	1874	Greagh	Tedavnet	Heart disease
4.595	Murphy, Mick	1860	Kernafeaghy	Clones	Fell out of cart; head injury
9.1043	Murphy, Owen	1872	Monaghan	Monaghan	Struck by Cart; Shock
3.993	Murphy, Thomas	1871	Clones	Clones	Drowning
19.1053	Murray, Ann	1872	Clones	Clones	Lung disease
	Murray, Patrick	1875	Mon. Asylum	Monaghan	Consumption
14.1048	Murray, Susan	1872	Annagore	Aghabog	Falling into a bog-hole
16.547	Murry, Owen	1859	Barrateetoppy	Tedavnet	Head trauma; horse and cart accident
6.750	Neill, Ann	1864	Moy	Errigal Truagh	Visitation of God
10.925	Nelson, James	1869	Longfield	Clones	Suicide; hanging
	Nesbitt, Mary	1869	Annagoes	Aghabog	Suspicious death; no inquest was held
9.1116	Nevill, Catherine	1874	Carrabrack	Donagh	Visitation of God
4.895	Niblock, Ann	1868	Aghaterny	Monaghan	Run over by jaunting cart; accident
5.958	Nikle, William	1870	Mullyglasson	Clones	Natural causes
	O'Donnell, Edward	1875	Mon. Asylum	Monaghan	Consumption

Inquest	Name	Year	Townland	Parish	Verdict of Death
7.418	O'Donnell, James	1858	Donagh	Donagh	Rupture of blood vessels of the heart
27.729	O'Hara, James	1864	Aghanartinton	Tedavnet	Drowning
7.431	O'Neil, Catherine	1856	Monaghan	Monaghan	Epilepsy due to intemperance
17.761	O'Neill, Mary	1864	Clones	Clones	Drowning
10.660	O'Neill, Rose	1862	Latlurkin	Monaghan	Suspicion of poisoning
2.1138	Orell, George	1875	Clones	Clones	Head trauma; hit with stone
13.678	Owen, Thomas	1862	Lisbane	Kilmore	Killed by the train
1.820	Pallate, Jane	1866	Tattynagall	Killeevan	Hanging; suicide
1.552	Paltate, Martha	1859	Cornaglar	Kilmore	Visitation of God
8.472	Paltate, Martha	1859	Cornaglar	Kilmore	Visitation of God
5.1027	Parks, Jane	1872	Monaghan	Monaghan	Accidental gunshot wound
7.657	Parr, Jacob	1862	Monaghan	Monaghan	Rupture of blood vessel in the heart
18.649	Phillip, Robert David	1862	Carraghan	Donagh	Internal injuries from drinking scalding hot tea
4.499	Phillips, Rebecca	1858	Rockcorry	Ematris	Natural causes
4.957	Prenter, Sally	1870	Mullaglassan	Clones	Natural causes; childbirth
17.807	Pringle, Sarah	1865	Tilleden	Donagh	Rheumatism in the stomach
18.720	Pritchard, Mary	1863	Terrntet	Tyholland	Drowning
17.1123	Prunty, Mary	1874	Corcreehey	Kilmore	Paralysis due to exposure
7.709	Prunty, Patrick	1863	Carchreechy	Kilmore	Suicide; hanging
5.935	Quigly, James	1869	Cossrea	Killeevan	Fell; inflammation of brain
13.803	Quinn, Peter	1865	Emyvale	Donagh	Heart disease
16.567	Raferty, Bernard	1859	Hill Hall	Donagh	Disease of heart and lungs
25.616	Raferty, Bridget	1861	Monaghan	Monaghan	Debility from refusing food
26.490	Raferty, John	1858	Anahagh	Tedavnet	General breakdown of strength
10.1117	Raferty, Margaret	1874	Mullen	Errigal Truagh	Heart Disease
27.618	Reburn, John	1861	Carrickmaclin	Magheross	Crushed by falling stone in Mr Shirley's Quarry
13.604	Reed, Rose	1860	Monaghan	Monaghan	Falling down stairs
17.1079	Reighall, Thomas	1873	Clones	Clones	Hit by a horse
21.1055	Reilly, Bernard	1872	Clones	Clones	Stupidly drunk
4.1007	Reilly, Hugh	1871	Clones	Clones	Drowning
10.675	Reilly, Margaret	1862	Clones	Clones	Fracture of skull; cart accident
	Reilly, Michael	1875	Mon. Asylum	Monaghan	Consumption
10.1000	Reilly, Patrick	1871	Clones Workhse	Clones	Internal haemorrhage
21.1157	Reilly, Sarah	1875	Tatinacake	Currin	Burning
26.1060	Reynolds, Mary	1873	Clones	Clones	Burning
17.568	Reynolds, Mary	1860	Clones Poorhse	Clones	Falling down stairs
5.596	Rice, Peter	1860	Monaghan	Monaghan	Continued drinking
1.732	Riddle, Mary Ann	1864		Ballybay	Burning
9.799	Rider, Ellen	1865	Drumrooghill	Ematris	Heart disease
7.937	Rinnock, Mary	1869	Legnakilly	Clones	Heart disease; rupture of a blood vessel
13.757	Robinson, John	1864	Mon. Jail	Monaghan	Natural causes
	Roe, James	1862	Ballitrain	Aghnamullen	Accidental gunshot wound
17.481	Ronaghan, Bridget	1857	Carren	Tyholland	Visitation of God
5.1141	Rooney, James	1875	Tornacrow (in Mullyash Mts)	Muckno	Drowning
	Rooney, P.	1868	Carn	Aghabog	Food poisoning
3.794	Rooney, Peter	1865	Cornanagh	Tullycorbet	Heart disease
5.995	Ross, Eliza	1871	Wieher	Ballybay	Burning
5.1087	Ross, John	1873	Clones	Clones	Heart disease
16.787	Ross, Mary	1865	Gortnawinney	Clones	Drowning
13.663	Ross, Susan	1862	Shee	Tedavnet	Natural causes; apoplexy?
	Rowen, Francis	1868	Cornawall (nr Newbliss/Smithborough)	Killeevan	Heart disease
15.805	Rudden, Biddy	1865	Mon. Jail	Monaghan	Diffusion on the brain
4.814	Rudden, Catherine	1866	Monaghan	Monaghan	Burning
21.912	Rudden, Patrick	1869	Clones	Clones	Heart disease

Inquest	Name	Year	Townland	Parish	Verdict of Death
9.504	Rully, Biddy	1858	Monaghan Jail	Monaghan	Natural causes
4.555	Rush, Patrick	1859	Monaghan	Monaghan	Wasting and weakness
18.877	Russell, Ann	1868	Shanmulla	Clones	Crushed by house falling down
9.640	Salmon, Thomas	1861	Monaghan	Monaghan	Cart and horse accident
	Scanlon, Merideth	1862	Fort Johnston	Donagh	Gunshot wound; accidental
10.781	Scott, Emily H.	1865	Skeagh	Drumsnat	Natural causes
2.497	Scott, Robert	1858	Clones	Clones	Visitation of God
9.886	Sewell, Jane	1868	Coravaghen	Drummully	Drowning
	Sewl, Elisabeth	1856	Newbliss		Drowning
15.510	Shannon, John	1858	Kilnaharvey	Ematris	Internal disease; heart disease?
12.751	Shanon, Robert	1864	Monaghan	Monaghan	Consumption
23.614	Shaw, James	1861	Baelderg	Donagh	Murder; gunshot wound
4.1038	Shaw, James	1872	Monaghan	Monaghan	Trampled by a horse
22.613	Shaw, Robert	1861	Balderg	Donagh	Murder
6.777	Sheridan, Ann	1865	Monaghan Jail	Monaghan	Attack of diarrhoea and an old sore
6.825	Sheridan, James	1866	Doohat	Aghabog	Drowning
	Sheriden, Ann	1876	Mon. Asylum	Monaghan	Struman's disease of bowels
6.1068	Sheriden, James	1873	Gormore	Drumsnat	Old age and infirmity
1.916	Sherlock, Bridget	1869	Stracollion	Tedavnet	Drowning
21.723	Sherry, Margaret	1863	Dromore	Errigal Truagh	Burning
1.1004	Sherry, Margaret	1871	Knockballyronan	Tedavnet	Drowning
20.950	Sherry, Pat	1870	Knockballyronan	Tedavnet	Inflammation of the bowels
6.1028	Sherry, Peter	1872	Mullenboy	Donagh	Head trauma; horse accident
3.848	Sherry, Susan	1867	Knockballyrooney	Donagh	Incipient dropsy
1.772	Shevling, Thomas	1865	Monaghan	Monaghan	Natural causes
	Shreenan, Ellen	1872	Latnamard	Aghabog	Apoplexy
3.812	Simpson, Edward	1866	Drumreenagh	Currin	Drowning, epilepsy
2.704	Skelton, Richard	1863	Monaghan	Monaghan	Disease of the heart
11.975	Slaven, Catherine	1870	Carrickmacross	Magheross	Heart disease
10.1144	Slievan (Slevin), Owen	1875	Coolderagh	Kilmore	Suffocation
	Sloan, Ann	1875	Drumchet		Apoplexy
13.872	Slowy, John	1867	Ballinode	Tedavnet	Visitation of God
	Smith, Anne	1874	Mon. Asylum	Monaghan	Debility and epilepsy
3.1065	Smith, Bridget	1873	Clones Workhse	Clones	Old age
22.573	Smith, Elisabeth	1860	Clones Workhse	Clones	Falling; previous wound on leg
14.679	Smith, George	1862	Coolshanagh	Monaghan	Effusion on the brain; head trauma
5.864	Smith, Henry	1867	Monaghan	Monaghan	Falling out of a window; Head trauma; suicide?
14.859	Smith, James	1867	Clones	Clones	Kicked by a horse
6.597	Smith, James	1860	Lisbrannon	Ematris	Natural causes
	Smith, Judith	1876	Mon. Asylum	Monaghan	Natural causes; exhaustion from mania
5.1067	Smith, Mary	1873	Rafreenan	Tedavnet	Heart disease
	Smith, Mary	1872	Cadah		Sudden death
18.569	Smith, Mick	1860	Aghadromdonagh	Currin	Cart and horse accident
12.831	Smith, Pat	1866	Monaghan	Monaghan	Murder
14.565	Smith, Patrick	1859	Cadagh	Tullycorbet	Burning; fell into the fire
5.456	Smith, Patrick	1857	Mulnacross	Drumsnat	Disease of the heart
	Smith, Patrick	1875	Mon. Asylum	Monaghan	General paralysis
4.1140	Smith, Patrick	1875	Curraghy	Clones	Inhaling gas from burning lime
8.1115	Smith, Patrick	1874	Tappa	Kilmore	Tubercular meningitis
10.1091	Smith, William	1873	Hilton Park	Currin	Falling from roof; shock; internal injuries
12.889	Smollen, James	1868	Monaghan	Monaghan	Hit by a stone
2.1036	Stalker, John	1872	Tully	Monaghan	Drowning
16.480	Steenson, Jane	1857	Monaghan	Monaghan	Drowning
6.520	Stewart, John	1858	Billis	Donagh	Visitation of God
1.515	Stewart, Samuel	1858	Aghereagh	Clones	Heart disease
7.1029	Stewart, Susan	1872	Kilnacloy	Monaghan	Heart disease

Inquest	Name	Year	Townland	Parish	Verdict of Death
18.442	Still, Susannah	1856	Tullyshelverly	Kilmore	Burning; house fire
2.1127	Stinson (Steen-), Richard	1875	Drumcall	Ematris	Extravasation and congestion of the brain
9.1071	Story, John	1873	Dawson's Grove	Ematris	Aneurysm of the heart
23.842	Story, Robert	1867	Aghagaw	Tedavnet	Injuries from a fall
24.488	Stowey, James	1858	Clones	Clones	Effusion of blood on chest;
23.725	Suellen, Ann	1863	Monaghan	Monaghan	Hit by a horse and cart
29.620	Sullivan, Mary	1861	Mulnahinchago	Tedavnet	Natural causes
	Sullivan, Mary Ann	1875	Mon. Asylum	Monaghan	Illness continued for one week previous to her disease
12.1015	Sullivan, Sarah	1871	Glen	Ematris	Emphysema; enlargement of the heart
11.713	Sunvill, James	1863	Drumbar	Tedavnet	Visitation of God
	Sweeney, Bessy	1874	Mon. Infirm.	Monaghan	Ordinary death
30.1166	Swift, James	1876	Curraghy	Clones	Effusion on the brain
14.1017	Tagert, John	1871	Emyvale	Donagh	Visitation of God
8.1011	Temple, James	1871	Cortlvin	Monaghan	Cart and horse accident; Concussion of the brain
16.835	Teucher, Mary	1866	Ballinode	Tedavnet	Drowning
22.724	Thomas, James	1863	Monaghan	Monaghan	Natural causes
11.586	Thompson, Catherine	1860	Classdaw	Aghabog	Burning
8.739	Thomson, Mary Ann	1864	Clonowlain	Currin	Drowning
8.779	Thomson, William	1865	Cortreane	Currin	Suicide, drowning
5.1008	Tierney, Owen	1871	Aughnakelton	Tedavnet	Natural causes
	Timlin, John	1867	Corsilage (near Rockcorry)		Unknown; in Swanzy's area
8.700	Todd, Margaret	1863	Emyvale	Errigal Truagh	Apoplexy arising from an attack of epilepsy
2.847	Tole (Toal), Catherine	1867	Smithborough	Drumsnat	Heart disease
24.448	Tole, John	1857	Meghararny	Clones	Head Injury; falling
10.712	Tole, Rachael	1863	Aughareagh	Currin	Crushed by roof of house falling in
	Torenan, Mathew	1875	Mon. Asylum	Monaghan	Consumption
	Torington, Mrs.	1874	Gornunah	Kilmore	Old and infirm
3.634	Treanor, Ann	1861	Maghery	Clones	Exposure
8.998	Treanor, Arthur	1871	Edenmore	Tedavnet	Visitation of God
4.968	Treanor, Bridget	1870	Cooldavnet	Tedavnet	Visitation of God
13.1149	Treanor, Catherine	1875	Killecarron	Errigal Truagh	Heart disease
23.914	Treanor, Fanny	1869	Roosky	Monaghan	Body found in water (canal)
7.638	Treanor, John	1861	Monaghan	Monaghan	Dropsy
11.642	Treanor, John	1861	Glenmore	Errigal Truagh	Epilepsy
3.1022	Treanor, John	1872	Monaghan	Monaghan	Impaled; fell off a roof
	Treanor, Mary	1875	Mon. Asylum	Monaghan	Old age, exhaustion, melancholia
5.736	Treanor, Michael	1864	Cloghfin	Errigal Truagh	Internal disease
15.945	Treanor, Philip	1869	Monaghan	Monaghan	Murder; forced drowning
2.553	Trimble, Elizabeth	1859	Monaghan	Monaghan	Burning
1.865	Twin Infant	1867	Deerpark (or Dunsirk)	Killeevan	Natural causes
1.866	Twin Infant	1867	Deerpark (or Dunsirk)	Killeevan	Natural causes
	Unknown Child (5 yrs)	1875			Death from eating tobacco
	Unknown Girl (15 yrs)	1875	Mon. Asylum	Monaghan	Consumption
19.790	Unknown Man	1865	Cortober	Ematris	Drowning
25.727	Unknown Man	1864	Monaghan	Monaghan	Drowning; either suicide or accidental
14.929	Unknown Man	1869	Clonkeelan	Drummully	Skeleton found in bog
1.1137	Waldrum, Ann	1875	Stonebridge	Clones	Chronic disease of the lungs
17.719	Wallace, Alexander	1863	Hill Hall	Donagh	Natural causes; apoplexy
	Wallace, Bridget	1875	Mon. Asylum	Monaghan	Epileptic fit
	Walsh, Rose	1875	Mon. Asylum	Monaghan	Mesenteric disease
	Ward, Catherine	1863	Cavanagarvan		Death during childbirth
4.624	Ward, James	1861	Drumacoose	Killeevan	Apoplexy
14.1094	Waters, John	1874	Lisdrumgormly	Clontibret	Suffocation; passed out drunk in a bog-hole

Inquest	Name	Year	Townland	Parish	Verdict of Death
	Watson, Jane	1875	Mon. Asylum	Monaghan	Old age and debility
9.868	Weilly, Margaret	1867	Annamartin	Drumsnat	Natural causes
14.716	Welsh, George	1863	Clones	Clones	Fall down the stairs; fight in the pub
12.476	Welsh, Mary Ann	1857	Clones Poorhse	Clones	Convulsions
14.1076	West, Eliza	1873	Lurgunbuoy	Currin	Crushed by roof falling in; suffocation
	Wetherell, John	1875	Mon. Asylum	Monaghan	Congestion of the lungs; Chronic bronchitis
11.475	Wheelen, William	1857	Glaslough	Donagh	Crushed by a fall of earth; railway accident
19.1081	White, Betty	1873	Dernasell	Clones	Decay of nature
3.1110	White, Patrick	1874	Durishrim (Scotstown)	Currin	Natural causes
13.832	Whitside, John	1866	Grimshaw	Clones	Drowning
13.544	Whitside, William	1859	Glaslough	Donagh	Epilepsy, rupture of blood vessel
6.581	Wiggit, John	1860	Derralidigan	Clones	Falling from horse
25.769	Willis, Mary Jane	1865	Aughadrumkeen	Ematris	Burning
2.792	Willis, Sarah	1865	Aghadrumkeen	Ematris	Heart disease; apoplexy
4.1026	Winslow, Sarah	1872	Clones Workhse	Clones	Congestion of the lungs
4.994	Winters, John	1871	Clanooney	Drummully	Drowning
14.464	Winters, John	1857	Kinturk	Killeevan	Rupture of blood vessels of the left lung
8.1103	Witherington, Martin	1874	Emyvale	Donagh	Heart disease
15.1151	Woods, John	1875	Monaghan	Monaghan	Choked to death
4.823	Woods, Margaret	1866	Bromvale	Drumsnat	Natural causes; effusion of the brain
9.924	Woods, Thomas	1869	Drumark	Aghabog	Killed by the train; accident
13.858	Wright, David	1867	Drumloo	Clones	Visitation of God
1.666	Wright, James	1862	Rafreenan	Tedavnet	Internal disease; heart disease?
2.686	Wright, Sarah	1863	Aghabog Churchyard	Aghabog	Natural causes
3.687	Wright, Thomas	1863	Aghabog Graveyard	Aghabog	Natural causes
13.904	Wright, William	1868	Drumber (Deun-)	Tedavnet	Natural causes
	Wylie [Wilde], Emily	1871	Drummaconner Hse	Drumsnat	Burning
	Wylie [Wilde], Mary	1871	Drummaconner Hse	Drumsnat	Burning

NOTES

Abbreviations: (NS) Northern Standard;
(PRONI) Public Record Office of Northern Ireland
(Clogher Record) Clogher Record Historical Journal

Chapter One (pp.15–70)
The Coroner and His Casebook

1 Coroner's Court, Dublin, The Role of the Coroner in Death Investigation, 2nd Ed (Dublin, 2001), p.24.

2 Department of Justice, Equality and Law Reform, Review of the Coroner Service: Report of the Working Group (Dublin, 2000), p.177.

3 Farrell, Dr Brian, Coroners: Practice and Procedure (Dublin, 2000), p.21.

4 Ibid.

5 Coroner's Act of 1836.

6 Waddell's region was North Monaghan; west of a line drawn from the Monaghan–Cavan border near Bawn to Castleblayney, and from there to the Armagh boarder in Truagh – as described in the Clogher Record.

7 Waddell had several tenants at Lisnaveane, including Michael Greenan, Mary Anne Caldwell, William McGuirk and Owen Gavan. Each had small homes and gardens. Another house and farm at Lisnaveane was leased to John Cowan. It was transferred to the Revd Mr Thomas Black in 1869, then split into two parts, given to Alexander Waddell and James Waddell, presumably W. C. Waddell's two brothers. Waddell also acted as a land agent for his relative, the Revd Mr C. Hope, managing his land and tenants.

8 Nesbitt, David, Full Circle: A Story of Ballybay Presbyterians (Ballybay, 1999), p.251.

9 Clogher Record articles 'The Great Famine in Monaghan: A Coroner's Account' by Brian Ó Mórdha; and 'Summary of Inquests Held on Currin, Co. Monaghan Victims 1846–1855' by Pilip Ó Mórdha, recorded some of these inquests and are the only known references to volume one of Waddell's records.

10 The original casebook of volume two is the property of Allister McCrory of Co. Down.

11 In Melancholy Madness, inquires are just a brief mention of death, not a full inquest, but have been recorded by the author as such in order to keep a full and accurate count of the deaths recorded by W. C. Waddell.

12 Inquest no. 27.491, Phillip Coyle, Cooldarragh, Drumsnat Parish, January 1858.

13 Farrell, Dr Brian, p.21.

14 Coroner's Court, Dublin, p.13.

15 Foster, Jeanne Cooper, Ulster Folklore (Belfast, 1951), pp.22–23.

16 'Death of W. C. Waddell, Esq. Coroner', NS, 11 May 1878.

17 Information on John Frederick Hodges, MD, PhD, JP (1815–1899) is furnished from research performed, collected and written by Professor Richard S. J. Clarke, MD, PhD, FRCA, Honorary Archivist of the Royal Hospital and Queen's University, Belfast. Hodges' career was quite impressive, he did not practise medicine but was essentially a chemist. He was a professor of chemistry, RBAI, 1848–9; lecturer in medical jurisprudence at Queen's College, Belfast 1848–99; professor of agriculture 1849–99; public analyst for Co. Armagh 1879; director of the Chemico–Agriculture Society of Ulster and editor of its journal; one of the founders of the Royal Society of Chemistry, London; honoured by many European countries and wrote many books and papers including The First Book of Lessons in Chemistry in its Application to Agriculture of the Farm (1862); president of the Belfast Natural History and Philosophical Society 1874–77; government analyst and analyst for Belfast, JP for Co. Antrim; and he was the first president of the Belfast Hospital for Diseases of the Skin, Glenravel Street, founded in 1873.

18 Inquest no. 26.845, William Harvison, Monaghan Jail, 13 February 1867.

19 Inquest no. 22.936, Thomas McCormick, Monaghan Asylum, January 1871.

20 NS, 3 November 1855.

21 Inquest no. 22.573, Elizabeth Smith, Clones Workhouse, January 1860.

22 Inquiry, Mary Nesbitt, Annagose, Aghabog Parish, March 1869.

23 Inquest no. 20.950, Pat Sherry, Knockballyroney, Tedavnet Parish, January 1870.

24 Inquest no. 15.590, Judith Fox, Lattacrossan, Currin Parish, June 1860.

25 Inquest no. 1.412, Thomas Hughes, Sillis, Donagh Parish, February 1856. Hughes' body was exhumed from the Tynan churchyard in Co. Armagh. Hughes' death was recorded prior to the exhumation and investigation in Inquest no. 22.410.

26 Inquest no. 2.466, Henry Jackson, Rockcorry, Ematris Parish, August 1857.

27 Inquest no. 4.499, Rebecca Phillips, Rockcorry, Ematris Parish, February 1858.

28 Inquest no. 5.519, Isabella Keelan, Monaghan, Monaghan Parish, July 1858. (Note: the name Keelan appears predominately in the parish of Magheross, and it is likely that Waddell was covering a case for Swanzy.)

29 Inquest no. 19.684, George Lee, Corragore, Ematris Parish, February 1863.

30 Inquest no. 23.447, Thomas McCarvle, Corlat, Killeevan Parish, January 1857.

31 Inquest no. 10.1032, Michael Mooney, Carn, Aghabog Parish, June 1872.

32 Inquest no. 21.409, Peter Moorehead, Calliagh, Aghabog Parish, January 1856.

33 'Death Under Suspicious Circumstances', NS, 5 February 1875

34 Extravasate: to force out or cause to escape from a proper vessel or channel; to pass by infiltration or effusion from a proper vessel or channel (as a blood vessel) into surrounding tissue (Merriam-Webster Dictionary).

35 Inquest no. 2.1127, Richard Stinson [Steenson], Drumcall, Ematris Parish, February 1875.

36 Medical Jurisprudence (London, 1932), p.491.

37 A shed or barn.

38 Inquest no. 8.867, Elisabeth Crawley, Carrickmacross, Magheross Parish, October 1867.

39 Stevens, Serita Deborah, Klarner, Anne, Deadly Doses: A Writer's Guide to Poisons (Ohio, 1990), p.7.

40 Inquest no. 10.660, Rose O'Neill, Latlorcan, Monaghan Parish, 18 April 1862.

41 Medical Jurisprudence (London, 1932), p.500.

42 Inquiry, John McCabe, Shelvins, Tyholland Parish, October 1856.

43 Inquiry, Pat Clarken, Annaghybane, Ematris Parish, November 1860.

44 Inquiry, Margaret Curley, Rossnaglogh [East], Aghabog Parish, September 1857.

45 Inquiry, Dunlop (likely William Dunlop, a member of the Drumkeen Presbyterian Church), Killygragy, Aghabog Parish, July 1862.

46 The inquests when exhumations took place were as follows, in chronological order: 1] Inquest no. 1.412, Thomas Hughes, 25 February 1856, accidental drowning/possible homicide; 2] Inquest no. 24.488, James Slowey, 6 January 1858, effusion of blood on the chest/suspected foul play; 3] Inquest no. 10.660, Rose O'Neill, 18 April 1862, unknown causes/suspected poisoning to induce abortion; 4] Inquest no. 17.682, William Livingston, 19 January 1863, arsenic poisoning/suspected poisoning with laudanum; 5] Inquest no. 1.685, John McCarter, 16 February 1863, natural causes/suspected poisoning; 6] Inquest no. 2.686, Sarah Wright, 23 February 1863, natural causes/suspected poisoning; 7] Inquest no. 3.687, Thomas Wright, 28 February 1863, natural causes/suspected poisoning; 8] Inquest no. 15.945, Philip Treanor, 1 December 1869, murder/forced drowning. (Phillip Treanor's body was exhumed after it was determined that another post-mortem needed to be conducted to try to achieve a more accurate cause of death); 9] Inquest no. 7.1143, Mary Maguire, 4 September 1875, beaten/head injuries.

47 Inquest no. 15.680, William Livingston, Rakeevan, Aghabog Parish, 2 January 1863.

48 Inquest no. 17.682, William Livingston, Drumkeen Graveyard, Aghabog Parish, 19 January 1863.

49 'Inquest – Case of Poisoning', NS, 14 February 1863.

50 Inquest no. 3.687, Thomas Wright, Aghabog Graveyard, February 1863 and Inquest no. 2.686, Sarah Wright, Aghabog Graveyard, February 1863; Inquest no. 1.685, John McCarter, Drumkeen Graveyard, Aghabog Parish, February 1863.

51 Glanders is a malignant disease that can be contracted from a horse; characterised by a bloody discharge from the nose and tumours in different parts of the body. Dr Phelps O. Brown, author of *The Complete Herbalist* (1878) states that, 'The body finally exhales a fetid odour, the mind wanders, delirium and coma follow, and by the end of the second week, or during the third, it generally proves fatal, if not arrested sooner in its course. It is very rare; and attendants upon a horse affected with glanders should be very careful that they do not com ein contact with the virus. The affected horse should be shot, as the disease is very seldom cured.'

52 Records of Death for Ann and Tabitha McCarter, North-Eastern Health Board, Registrar's Office, Rooskey, Monaghan.

53 PRONI, Belfast, Church of Ireland, Aghabog Parish, MIC/1/131. McQuag is referred to as McQuey in *Griffith's Valuation of Ireland* (Aghabog, 1860).

54 John McCarter of Rakeevan appears as John McArthur in Griffith's Valuation of 1860.

55 Inquest no. 16.907, William Foster, Drumbrean, Aghabog Parish, November 1868.

56 'The Coroners' Bill', NS, 5 March 1875.

57 'Monaghan Assizes, Salary of Co. Coroners', NS, 20 July 1867.

58 'The Coroners' Charges', NS, 11 March 1876.

59 Rose, Lionel, *The Massacre of the Innocents: Infanticide in Britain 1800–1939* (London, 1986) p.59.

60 Ibid, p.58.

61 Inquest no. 14.545, Infant Child, Monaghan, May 1859.

62 'Coroners Inquest', NS, May 1872.

63 Inquest no. 9.1036, Ann McDonald, Kilnacloy, Monaghan Poorhouse, Monaghan Parish, June 1872.

64 Inquest no. 12.831, Pat Smith, Monaghan, Monaghan Parish, October 1866.

65 Inquest no. 13.1014, Letitia Andrews [or Letitia Noble], Clones, Clones Parish, November 1871.

66 Inquest no. 9.640, Thomas Salmon, Monaghan, October 1861.

67 Inquest no. 3.414, Elizabeth McMahon, Clonrye, Drummully Parish, March 1856.

68 'Death of W. C. Waddell, Esq., Coroner', NS, 11 May 1878.

69 Inquest no. 13.644, Margaret Maghath, Magheraharne, Ematris Parish, December 1861.

70 Davitt, Michael, *1846–1906, The Fall of Feudalism in Ireland: The Story of the Land League Revolution* (Harper & Brothers, 1904).

71 King's Inns Admission Papers 1607–1867 (Dublin, 1982), p.470.

Chapter Two (pp.71–108)
Infanticide

1 Showalter, Elaine, *The Female Malady: Women, Madness and English Culture, 1830–1980* (London, 1987), p.59.

2 Cullen, Mary, 'Breadwinners and Providers: Women in the Household Economy of Labouring Families 1835–6' in Cullen, Mary, Luddy, Maria (eds) *Women, Power and Consciousness in Nineteenth-Century Ireland* (Dublin, 1995), p.113.

3 Sherry, Brian (ed), *Along the Black Pig's Dyke: Folklore from Monaghan and South Armagh* (Castleblayney, 1993) pp.70–71.

4 Inquest no. 10.940, Unknown Child [child of a woman aka Mary McCabe], Monaghan Infirmary, Monaghan Parish, October 1869.

5 'Monaghan Assizes, MURDER', NS, 9 April 1870, p.2.

6 Rose, Lionel, *The Massacre of the Innocents: Infanticide in Britain 1800–1939* (London, 1986) p.30.

7 Wilde, Sir William, 'A Short Account of the Superstitions and Popular Practices relating to Midwifery and some of the Diseases of Women and Children in Ireland' in *Monthly Journal of Medical Science*, May 1849, No. 35, pp.711–726.

8 Rose, Lionel, p.86.

9 Although the Eight Tates is a reference to an area in Tyholland Parish, a contradictory reference to Master John Crow(e)'s residence is the townland of Cordevlis, Barony of Dartry, which might suggest the townland was located in the parish of Aughnamullen. There are several townlands with the name of Cordevlis. A John Crowe was listed in the Griffith's Valuation in the townland of Cordevlis, Aughnamullen Parish.

10 Hearn, Mona, 'Life for Domestic Servants in Dublin 1880–1920' in Luddy, Maria, Murphy, Cliona (eds) *Women Surviving: Studies in Irish Women's History in the 19th and 20th Centuries* (Dublin, 1990), p.166.

11 Inquest no. 10.660, Rose O'Neill, Latlurkin, Monaghan Parish, 18 April 1862.

12 Wilde, Sir William, pp.711–726.

13 Inquest no. 19.443, Infant Child (female), 22 December 1856.

14 Scroggy's Bridge or Scroggs Bridge is a reference to a bridge extending over the canal in or near Monaghan town. The Irish word *scroigeach* pronounced 'scraggy' is an adjective for something thin, sparse, threadbare (*scáinte*); or stringy, wiry, lanky (*reangach*). Scroggy's Bridge is mentioned in two separate inquests in the casebook. Perhaps Scroggy is the last name of a person or family living nearby the bridge.

15 Inquest no. 6.690, Infant Child (female), Monaghan, Monaghan Parish, April 1863.

16 Inquest no. 3.454, Infant Child (female), Newbliss, Killeevan Parish, March 1857.

17 Rose, Lionel, pp.88–89.

18 Inquest no. 6.1040, Infant Child (male), Soraghan, Feragh, Monaghan Parish, 30 July 1872.

19 McLoughlin, Dympna, 'Workhouses and Irish Female Paupers 1840–70' in Luddy, Maria, Murphy, Cliona (eds) *Women Surviving: Studies in Irish Women's History in the 19th and 20th Centuries* (Dublin, 1990) p.141.

20 Inquest no. 3.454, Infant Child (female), Newbliss, Killeevan, March 1857.

21 Inquest no. 18.1080, Infant Child, Corclare, Errigal Truagh Parish, June 1873.

22 Inquest no. 12.662, Infant Child, Derrynahesco, Tedavnet Parish, May 1862.

23 Rose, Lionel, p.66.

24 Rose, Lionel, p.39.

25 Inquest no. 5.749, Infant Child Hoey, Srananny, Donagh Parish, September 1864.

26 Rose, Lionel, p.40.

27 The reference made here refers to Inquest no. 19.443, Infant Child (female), December 1856 and Inquest no. 26.770, Infant Child (female), February 1865.

28 Several persons I have spoken to in Co. Monaghan relayed stories to me that female servants in the 'big houses' in Co. Monaghan were rumoured to have been raped by the master or other male relatives and bore illegitimate children. They also stated that those women who dared speak of the circumstances of the conception, were committed to the Monaghan lunatic asylum.

29 Inquest no. 12.1074, Infant Child (male) Goodfellow, Kilmore East, Ematris Parish, May 1873.

30 'Infanticide in Rockcorry', NS, 6 May 1873, p.2.

31 'Concealment of Birth', NS, 12 July 1873, p.2.

32 Inquest no. 24.615, Essy Kells, Derrins, Currin Parish, January 1861.

33 Inquest no. 1.1096, Infant Child (female) Kelly, Cormeen [Aughnamullen], Ematris Parish, March 1874.

34 Inquest no. 10.541, Infant Child Croarken, Kilcorran, Clones Parish, April 1859.

35 'CHILD MURDER: Sentence of Death', NS, 13 December 1882.

36 Elizabeth Smith (alias Lee), GPB, PEN 1890, National Archives, Dublin.

37 Connoly, S. J., *Priests and People in Pre-Famine Ireland 1870–1845* (Dublin, 2001) pp.188, 190.

38 The practice of churching in Co. Monaghan has been described as 'A practice of puri-fication, whereby after a woman had a baby she had to go a certain amount of time to church, and be "churched". This meant going up to the altar rails and the priest prayed over her. All the women did it. I think it was a sexual reason. It was forbidden to have (sexual) relations until it was done. It was very important and urgent as well. The men didn't have to do any purification practice. I think it stopped around the 1950s.' (Garry Carville, Annyalla, in Brian Sherry's Along the Black Pig's Dyke, p.45). Another description continues 'Churching was blessing them (women) and bringing them back to purity after having gone through the conception. It was after mass. Well, I never agreed with it because I thought if a woman was married decently and became pregnant, that was part of the programme. There was no call in taking her up to the altar and making a show of her. And there was people didn't like it. Sure ye'd nearly think the elder people would think she did something wrong.' [Gene McCann, Castleblayney, in Brian Sherry's Along the Black Pig's Dyke, p.45].

39 Ibid, p.179.

40 'Coroner's Inquest', NS, 3 August 1872, p.2.

41 Inquest no. 5.1039, Infant Child (female), Kilnacloy, Monaghan Parish, August 1872.

42 Inquest no. 7.997, Infant Child, Cloncaw, Donagh Parish, April 1871.

43 Wilde, Sir William, pp.711–726.

44 Oral stories related by several residents of Monaghan town.

45 O'Connor, Anne, Child Murderess and Dead Child Traditions: A Comparative Study, FF Communications (Helsinki, 1991) Vol. cvii2, No. 249.

46 Ibid, p.69.

47 Ibid, p.70.

48 Inquest no. 5.556, Infant Child, Monaghan, Monaghan Parish, September 1859.

49 Inquest no. 12.526, Infant Child, Monaghan, Monaghan Parish, September 1858.

50 Inquest no. 11.525, Infant Child, Monaghan, Monaghan Parish, September 1858.

51 Inquest no. 18.683, Infant Child, February 1863.

52 Inquest no. 5.578, Infant Child, Clonamully, Tedavnet Parish, March 1860.

53 Rose, Lionel, p.61.

54 Only January and February were recorded in 1876; the coroner's casebook ends there.

55 Langan-Egan, Maureen, Galway Women in the Nineteenth Century (Dublin, 1999), p.67.

56 Inquest no. 7.1143, Mary Maguire, Clones, Clones Parish, September 1875.

57 Record of marriage of Peter Maguire and Margaret Kelaghan, 1 May 1875 from Births, Deaths and Marriages, Registrar's Office, North-Eastern Health Board, Rooskey.

58 'Alleged Murder of a Child, From Our Reporter', NS, 10 September 1875, p.2.

59 'Clones Special Petty Sessions, Alleged Murders', NS, 1 October 1875, p.2.

60 Martha Reilly was a peddlar who was in the Maguire's house at 11a.m. on the morning of 31 August. She only stated that she asked Margaret Maguire how the child was, and that the mother stated 'the child was well'.

61 Informations: the evidence and testimony.

62 'Monaghan Spring Assizes, Alleged Child Murder', NS, 11 March 1876, p.2.

63 Langan-Egan, Maureen, p.62.

64 'Alleged Child Desertion', NS, 28 May 1875, p.2.

65 Inquest no. 3.498, Infant Child McGrayons, July 1858.

66 Luddy, Maria, 'Prostitution and Rescue Work in Nineteenth Century Ireland' in Luddy, Maria, Murphy, Cliona (eds) Women Surviving: Studies in Irish Women's History in the 19th and 20th Centuries (Dublin, 1990) pp.51–84.

67 McLoughlin, Dympna, 'Workhouses and Irish Female Paupers 1840–70' in Luddy, Maria, Murphy, Cliona (eds) Women Surviving: Studies in Irish Women's History in the 19th and 20th Centuries (Dublin, 1990) p.121.

68 Langan-Egan, Maureen, p.63.

69 Sarah Browne, GPB, PEN 1890/48, National Archives, Dublin.

70 Luddy, Maria, 'Prostitution and Rescue Work in Nineteenth Century Ireland' pp.51–84.

71 'Found Drowned', NS, March 1876, p.2.

72 Elisabeth Finnegan, GPB, PEN 1885/99, National Archives, Dublin.

73 Inquest no. 3.1025, John McBride, April 1872.

74 'Co. Monaghan Assizes, Crown Court', NS, 13 July 1872, p.2.

75 Rose, Lionel, p.85.

76 Inquest no. 7.1069, Susan McCleary, Cornawall, Aghabog Parish, March 1873.

77 Inquest no. 17.608, Rose Martin, Magherashaghry, Currin Parish, December 1860.

78 Inquiry, Mrs Robert Clarke, Caddagh/Dromore, Tullycorbet Parish, March 1857.

79 Inquest no. 11.620, Mrs Margaret Johnston, Clones, Clones Parish, October 1860.

80 Edmund Hayes: the fourth son of William Hayes of Millmount near Banbridge in Co. Down; born 1804; appears at the Belfast Academical Institute; matriculated in Dublin University in 1820; graduated as bachelor of arts and entered Gray's Inn 1825; was called to the Irish bar, and proceeded to doctor of laws 1832; went for a time on the north-east circuit and afterwards the home circuit; joint author of *Reports of Cases in the Court of Exchequer in Ireland 1830–4*; married Grace Maryanne, daughter of John Shaw of St Doulagh's in Co. Dublin in 1835; lectured on constitutional and criminal law; published *Crimes and Punishments or a Digest of the Criminal Statute Law of Ireland* in 1843; was a conservative in politics; became a Queen's Counsel in 1852; married his second wife, Harriett Trenchall, widow of James Shaw; became solicitor-general 1858; appointed a justice of the Queen's Bench in 1859; resigned 1866; died at Crinkenhouse in 1867. From Elrington Ball, J., *The Judges in Ireland 1221–1921* (New York, 1927), Vol. 1 and 2.

81 'Monaghan Spring Assizes', NS, 2 March 1861, p.2.

82 Ibid.

83 Wilde, Sir William, pp.711–726.

84 Inquest no. 8.1144, Ellen Murphy, Cornapaste, Currin Parish, September 1875.

85 'Sudden Death', NS, 10 September 1875, p.1.

86 Inquest no. 22.446, Bridget (Biddy) McManus, Clones Fever Hospital, Clones Parish, January 1857.

87 Foster, Jeanne Cooper, 'Women in childbirth used to have a knife by the bed. This was believed to prevent fairies or witches from injuring the mother or child.' *Ulster Folklore* (Belfast, 1951), p.47.

88 Inquest no. 21.445, Infant Child (female) McManus, Clones Fever Hospital, Clones Parish, January 1857.

89 *Merriam-Webster Online Collegiate Dictionary* (http://www.m-w.com).

90 Showalter, Elaine, *The Female Malady: Women, Madness and English Culture 1830–1980* (New York, 1987) pp.58–59.

91 Lawless-Murphy, Jo, *Reading Birth and Death: A History of Obstetric Thinking* (Cork, 1998), p.120.

Chapter Three (pp.109–138)
Mansions of Despair

1 Cockerham, William C., *The Sociology of Mental Disorder* (London, 1972), pp.176–84.

2 'Monaghan District Asylum', NS, 22 May 1869.

3 Arsenberg, C. M. and Kimball, S. T., *Family and Community in Ireland* (2nd Ed, Cambridge, Mass, 1968) p.3.

4 Scheper-Hughes, Nancy, *Saints, Scholars and Schizophrenics: Mental Illness in Rural Ireland* (California, 1979), pp.53–69.

5 'Found Drowned', NS, 23 September 1871.

6 Inquest no. 6.1009, John Brown, Glasdrummand, Clontibret Parish, September 1871.

7 For more information refer to Elaine Showalter's *The Female Malady: Women, Madness and English Culture 1830–1980* (New York, 1987).

8 Inquest no. 1.991, Ann Lovett, Clones Workhouse, Clones Parish, 16 February 1871.
9 Inquest no. 6.637, Mary Hearty, Monaghan Jail, September 1861.
10 Finnane, Mark, *Insanity and the Insane in Post-Famine Ireland* (London, 1981), p.183.
11 Ibid, p.183.
12 'Determined Suicide', NS, 15 November 1873.
13 Robins, Joseph, *Fools and Mad: A History of the Insane in Ireland* (Dublin, 1986), p.78.
14 Kelleher, Michael, J., *Suicide and the Irish* (Dublin, 1996).
15 Finnane, Mark, p.150.
16 Robins, Joseph, p.109.
17 Inquest no. 11.1033, Jane Divine, June 1872.
18 Death certificate of Jane Divine, Registrar's Office, North-Eastern Health Board, St Davnet's, Monaghan.
19 NS, 15 June 1872.
20 Finnane, Mark, pp.161–162
21 Ibid, p.165.
22 Ibid, p.167.
23 'Weekly Petty Sessions, "A Lunatic"', NS, 15 January 1875.
24 Coroner Inquiry, John McCluskey, June 1875.
25 O'Dowd, Anne, *Spalpeens and Tattie Hokers, History and Folklore of the Irish Migratory Agricultural Worker in Ireland and Britain* (Dublin, 1991), p.59.
26 Malcolm, Elizabeth, *Medicine, Disease and the State in Ireland 1650–1940* (Dublin, 2000), p.181.
27 'Homicide by a Lunatic', NS, 12 April 1873.
28 Inquest no. 10.1072, Mary McCarron, Rakelly, Errigal Truagh Parish, 10 April 1873
29 'Monaghan Summer Assizes: Murder', NS, 12 July 1873, p.2.
30 Ó Gráda, Cormac, *Ireland before and after the Famine: Explorations in Economic History, 1800–1925* (Great Britain, 1988), pp.156, 180.
31 Connell, K. H., *Irish Peasant Society* (Blackrock, 1996) p.116.
32 Ibid, p.118.
33 Ó Gráda, Cormac, p.166.
34 Inquest no. 5.636, Nathanial Beatty, August 1861.
35 For more information, see O'Connor, Anne, *Child Murderess and Dead Child Traditions: A Comparative Study*, FF Communications, (Helsinki, 1991) Vol. CVII2, No. 249.
36 Inquest no. 7.521, Jane Boylan, Monaghan, Monaghan Parish, August 1858.
37 Conley, Carolyn, *Melancholy Accidents: The Meaning of Violence in Post-Famine Ireland* (Lexington, 1999), p.125.
38 Inquest no. 24.988, Archibald Little, Tavanagh, Errigal Truagh Parish, January 1871.
39 Malcolm, Elizabeth, p.177.
40 Arsenberg, C. M. and Kimball, S. T., p.3.
41 Malcolm, Elizabeth, p.186.
42 Inquest no. 7.709, Patrick Prunty, Corcreeghy, Kilmore Parish, August 1863.
43 Inquest no. 4.775, David Hill, Cordoolough, Tullycorbet Parish, 27 February 1865.
44 'Attempt to Commit Suicide', NS, 17 June 1871. (Note: The brewery was closed in 1857).
45 Inquest no. 13.1003, William Mullen, Monaghan, Monaghan Parish, June 1871.
46 Robins, Joseph, p.115.
47 Strahan, S. A., *Suicide and Insanity* (London, 1894), pp.111–112.
48 Inquest no. 14.891, Michael Duffy, Monaghan, Monaghan Parish, June 1868.
49 Robins, Joseph, p.117.
50 Ibid.
51 Inquest no. 11.782, Bernard Daly, Monaghan Jail, Monaghan Parish, April 1865.
52 Inquest no. 16.1019, Elizabeth Heasty, Monaghan, Monaghan Parish, December 1871.
53 Death Certificate of Elizabeth Heasty, Monaghan Civil Records Office.
54 'Melancholy Suicide', NS, 30 December 1871.
55 Showalter, Elaine, p.7.

56 Luddy, Maria & Murphy, Cliona, 'Life for Domestic Servants in Dublin 1880–1920' in Luddy, Maria & Murphy, Cliona (eds) *Women Surviving: Studies in Irish Women's History in the 19th and 20th Centuries* (Dublin 1990) pp.148–170.
57 Black, Eugene C., *Victorian Society and Culture* (London, 1973), p.211.
58 Luddy, Maria & Murphy, Cliona, 'Life for Domestic Servants in Dublin 1880–1920', pp.148–170.
59 Inquest no. 12.1046, Agnes Martin, Monaghan, Monaghan Parish, September 1872.
60 Bascom, William R., 'Folklore and Anthropology' in Dundes, Alan, *The Study of Folklore* (Englewood Cliffs, NJ, 1965) pp.25–33.
61 Livingstone, Peadar, *The Monaghan Story* (Enniskillen, 1980), pp.248–249.
62 Pauline, Sister Mary, *God Wills It: Centenary Story of the Sisters of St Louis* (Dublin, 1859), p.122.
63 Death Record, Mary Keough, January 1875, Registrar's Office, North-Eastern Health Board, St Davnet's, Monaghan.
64 'Suicide of a Nun in the Convent of St Louis', NS, 8 January 1875.
65 Inquest no. 19.1125, Mary Keough, Monaghan, Monaghan Parish, January 1875.
66 McCann-Skeath family, Mullaghcroghery, Co. Monaghan.

Chapter Four (pp.139–186)
Behind Closed Doors

1 *Ordnance Survey Memoirs of Ireland, Counties of South Ulster* (Dublin, 1998), p.93.
2 *Ordnance Survey Memoirs of Ireland*, Parish of Ematris, p.118.
3 Vaughan, W. E., *Landlords and Tenants in Mid-Victorian Ireland* (Oxford, 1994), p.120.
4 Ibid, p.122.
5 Inquest no. 8.639, Biddy McGuiness, Skinnagin, Tyholland Parish, October 1861.
6 Inquest no. 10.712, Rachel Tole, Aghareagh, Currin Parish, October 1863.
7 'Singular and Fatal Occurrence', NS, 22 January 1875
8 Inquest no. 19910 and 20.911, Margaret and Elizabeth Ann Martin, Bellanode, Tedavnet Parish, January 1869.
9 Inquest no. 14.785, Mary Dawson, Drumcaw, Aghabog Parish, May 1865.
10 Inquest no. 4.654, Bridget McDonald, Garran, Aghabog Parish, March 1862.
11 Inquest no. 22.486, Mary Keenan, Tandergeebane, Monaghan Parish, December 1857.
12 Inquest no. 23.842, Robert Storey, Aghagaw, Tedavnet Parish, February 1867.
13 Inquest no. 8.692, Thomas McArdle, Dunsinare, Monaghan Parish, April 1863.
14 A tramp is a large haycock which is tramped with the feet to make it more compact.
15 Inquest no. 7.598, Felix Began, Calliagh, Aghabog Parish, September 1860.
16 Inquest no. 27.1061, James Duffy, Lislynchahan, Ematris Parish, January 1873. Mortification (synonym Gangrene) is the death and decay of tissue in a part of the body, usually a limb, due to injury, disease or failure of blood supply. Erysipelas is an infectious disease characterised by a deep red inflammation of the skin or mucous membranes causing a rash.
17 Inquest no. 2.593, Shane (Shibby) McKenna, Kilnageer, Errigal Truagh Parish, July 1860.
18 Inquest no. 19.684, George Lee, Corravacan, Ematris Parish, February 1863.
19 Inquest no. 12.1002, Rose Ginely, Kilnaclay, Drumsnat Parish, June 1871.
20 'Inquest', NS, 17 June 1871.
21 Inquiry, Phillip Donaghy, Edenaferkin, Tullycorbet Parish, March 23, 1857.
22 Inquest no. 23.953, John Christy, Golanmurphy, Killeevan Parish, March 1870.
23 Lady Wilde, *Ancient Legends: Mystic Charms and Superstitions of Ireland* (London, 1887), p.119.
24 Steiner-Scott, Elizabeth, 'To Bounce a Boot Off Her Now and Then; Domestic Violence in Post-Famine Ireland' in Gialannella-Valiulis, Maryanne, O'Dowd, Mary (eds) *Women & Irish History* (Dublin, 1997) pp.124–143.

25 Ibid.

26 For more information, *see* Diane Urquhart's *Women in Ulster Politics 1890–1940* (Dublin, 2000).

27 Inquest no 5.824, Mary Magee, Clones, Clones Parish, September 1866.

28 Death Record, Mary Magee, 8 September 1866, Registrars Office, Monaghan.

29 'Inquest', NS, 15 September 1866.

30 O'Dowd, Anne, *Spalpeens and Tattie Hokers: History and Folklore of the Irish Migratory Agricultural Worker in Ireland and Britain* (Dublin, 1991).

31 For more information *see* O'Dowd, Mary.

32 Inquest no. 16.718, James McEnally, November 1863. In the townland of Corcahan in the parish of Kilmore, an inquest was held on view of the body of James McEnally on 25 November 1863. Catherine Cavenagh deposed that deceased had been her nephew; she saw him last on 28 October past when he assisted in getting some turf. He was a lad of about 7 years of age. 'About 1 o'clock he said he would look for a rod. He did not returning when expected, I looked for him but, learning that a little boy had gone down the road, I thought he had gone to his grandmother's which he one day said he would do. I rested satisfied of his safety and having to go to Scotland, I went on the 2nd November and remained about 2 weeks.' Still thinking he was at his grandmother's she was satisfied and heard nought of him 'till this day when she heard he was drowned when he was brought home dead. Art McGuiness deposed to having to 'turn some cattle out of one of my fields this day and coming back from having done so, on passing a pool of water, I observed a bundle floating on the surface which, looking carefully at for some time, concluded 'twas a human body. I gave the alarm, which brought several persons and some of the police when the body was removed and at the time quite dead.' Sergeant McDonald of the Stranooden police confirmed the above. Dr Reid deposed to having examined the deceased body, which 'presents every appearance of having come to his death by suffocation from drowning'. The verdict was death from falling accidentally into a pool of water from off a narrow pass and in which he was found 25 November 1863.

33 O'Dowd, Anne, 'Women in Rural Ireland in the Nineteenth and Early Twentieth Centuries: How the Daughters, Wives and Sisters of Small Farmers and Landless Labourers Fared', *Rural History*, 1994, Vol. 5, No. 2, pp.171–83.

34 Foster, Jeanne Cooper, *Ulster Folklore* (Belfast, 1951), p.11.

35 Inquest no. 6.457, Susan Barkey, Carnbane, Drumsnat Parish, 22 April 1857.

36 Foster, Jeanne Cooper, p.120.

37 Inquest no. 14.565, Patrick Smith, Caddagh, Tullycorbet Parish, December 1859.

38 Inquest no. 19.763 and 20.764, Mary Ann and Francis Kerr, Milltown, Ematris Parish, January 1865.

39 Wilde, Lady Jane, *Ancient Legends of Ireland* (London, 1887), pp.72, 370.

40 Sherry, Brian (ed), *Along the Black Pig's Dyke: Folklore from Monaghan and Cavan* (Castleblayney, 1993), p.23.

41 Ibid.

42 Foster, Jeanne Cooper, *Ulster Folklore* (Belfast, 1951) p.24.

43 Wilde, Lady Jane, *Ancient Legends: Mystic Charms and Superstitions of Ireland* (London, 1887), p.119. Story after story depicts a changeling being held over a fire or being threatened with fire in order to bring the healthy child back to the family. 'The Fairy Child' describes a woman whose husband did not believe that their first-born child was his. When he began to beat his wife, two women appeared, called 'the Avengers'. They first beat up the man and then took the child to the fairies. The end result of the story goes: 'So we made the fire. Then the tailor shut the door, and lifted the unlucky little wretch out of the cradle, and sat it on the fire. And no sooner had the flames caught it, than it shrieked aloud and flew up the chimney and disappeared. And when everything was burned that belonged to it, I knew you would come back to me with our own fine boy. And now let us name the name of God and make the

Sign of the Cross over him, and ill luck will never again fall on our house – no more forever.'

44 Sherry, Brian, p.23.

45 Bourke, Angela, *The Burning of Bridget Cleary* (Great Britain, 1999), p.30.

46 Ibid, p.38.

47 'Letters to the Editor', NS, 27 October 1855.

48 Inquest no. 13.477, Hugh Croarken, Shanroe, Clones Parish, October 1857.

49 'Painful Case of Manslaughter', NS, 12 July 1884; 'Manslaughter of a Pauper Child', NS, 18 December 1884.

50 Charles Robert Barry was the eldest son of James Barry of Limerick, solicitor; born 1823; matriculated in Dublin University 1840; entered Lincoln's Inn 1843; bachelor of arts 1845; was called to the Irish bar 1848; married Kate, daughter of David Fitzgerald of Dublin and sister of Lord Fitzgerald 1855; was in religion a Roman Catholic and in politics a liberal; became a Queen's Counsel 1859; master of arts 1862; became third sergeant 1866; solicitor-general 1868, and attorney-general 1870; was appointed a justice of the Queen's Bench 1872; became a lord justice of appeal 1883; resided in Dublin in Fitzwilliam Square; died 1897. (From Elrington Ball, J., *The Judges in Ireland 1221–1921* (New York, 1927).

51 Patrick McCabe, GPB, PEN 1884/929, National Archives, Dublin.

52 Conley, Carolyn, *Melancholy Accidents: The Meaning of Violence in Post-Famine Ireland* (Lexington, 1999), pp.81–82.

53 Sherry, Brian, p.86.

54 Inquest no. 5.655, William Gibson, Cornasoo, Kilmore Parish, March 1862.

55 Inquest no. 18.649, Robert David Phillips, Carrigans, Donagh Parish, January 1862.

56 Inquest no. 24.1058, Mary Finley, Drumbin, Tedavnet Parish, January 1873.

57 Inquiry, Corly, Female Child, Rossnaglogh, Aghabog Parish, September 1857.

58 Inquest no. 21.1157, Sarah Reilly, Tattincake, Currin Parish, December 1875.

59 Inquest no. 25.769, Mary Jane Willis, Aghadrumkeen, Ematris Parish, February 1865.

60 Children who died from disease were not recorded in the coroner's casebook. This appears to have been because there was no suspicion of the cause of death.

61 Inquest no. 8.559, Susan Donaghy, Corduff, Aghabog Parish, September 1859.

62 Inquest no. 16.1078, Hugh Calaghan, Creeve, Monaghan Parish, May 1873.

63 Sherry, Brian, p.87.

64 Inquest no. 9.886, Jane Sewell, Corrawillin, Drummully Parish, April 1868.

65 Inquest no. 16.440, Margaret Kelly, Leitrim, Tyholland Parish, November 1856.

66 Inquest no. 13.588, Ellen Brides, Knocks West, Currin Parish, May 1860.

67 Inquest no. 13.744, Thomas McCaffrey, Lurgachamlough, Aghnamullen Parish, June 1864.

68 Inquest no. 4.706 and 5.707, Richard Alexander Martin and Thomas Samuel Martin, Corevan, Aghabog Parish, August 1863.

69 Inquest no. 8.752, William Maguire, Terrygeely, Tullycorbet Parish, September 1864.

70 Inquest no. 6.796, Mary Hughes, Dundonagh, Donagh Parish, August 1865.

71 Inquest no. 16.591, Patrick McGinn, Drumacreeve, Ematris Parish, June 1860.

72 'Fatal Accident', NS, 1 October 1875.

73 Inquest no. 10.1144, Owen Slievan [Slevin], Cooldarragh, Kilmore Parish, September 1875.

74 Possibly pronounced to the coroner as 'yockin': a term used to describe a spell of work at the plough.

75 Inquest no. 10.421, Mary Cushlan, Urbalkirk, Monaghan Parish, May 1856.

76 Inquest no. 5.689, James McKelvey, Anaclar, Clones Parish, March 1863.

77 Guy, William, *Principles of Forensic Medicine* (London, 1868), pp.325–326.

78 Inquest no. 17.548, Charles Moorehead, Golanduff, Killeevan Parish, May 1859.

79 Inquest no. 18.549 and 19.550, Jane Carson and William Carson, Milltown, Monaghan Parish, May 1859.

80 Inquest no. 20.551, John Dodson, Clones Parish, July 1859.

81 Inquest no. 2.861, John McCarn (Medecurne), Corclare, Errigal Truagh Parish, July 1867.
82 Casey, Daniel J., Rhodes, Robert E. (eds) *Views of the Irish Peasantry 1800–1916* (Connecticut, 1977), p.45.
83 Sherry, Brian, p.22.
84 Sherry, Brian, p.93.
85 Inquest no. 10.754, John McMahon, Newbliss, Killeevan Parish, October 1864.
86 Inquest no. 15.834, James Hearse (Hearst), Killycreen, Clones Parish, November 1866.
87 Inquest no. 2.1130, Agnes McGorman, Clones, Clones Parish, March 1875.
88 'Death from Burning in Clones – Inquest', NS, 5 March 1875.

Chapter Five (pp.187–212)
Death By Misadventure

1 *Merriam-Webster's Online Collegiate Dictionary* (http://www.m-w.com).
2 Inquest no 6.970, John Morris, Clones, Clones Parish, July 1870.
3 Inquest no. 9.420, Thomas Corbitt, Corrinshigo, Currin Parish, May 1856.
4 One perch = 5 ¹/₂ yards or 16 ¹/₂ feet.
5 Inquest no. 11.586, Catherine Thompson, Closdaw, Aghabog Parish, May 1860.
6 Inquest no. 6.417, Mary Ann McKenna, Emyvale, Donagh Parish, April 1856.
7 Sherry, Brian (ed) *Along the Black Pig's Dyke: Folklore from Monaghan and South Armagh* (Castleblayney, 1993), p.154.
8 Inquest no. 8.599, James McConnell, Drumsheeney, Drumsnat Parish, October 1860.
9 Inquest no. 2.1138, George O'Reilly, Clones, Clones Parish, 31 July 1875.
10 Inquest no. 12.889, James Smollen, Monaghan, Monaghan Parish, May 1868.
11 Evans, E. Estyn, 'Peasant Beliefs in the Nineteenth Century' in Casey, Daniel J., Rhodes, Robert E. (eds), *Views of the Irish Peasantry 1800–1916* (Connecticut, 1977), p.50.
12 'Melancholy Accident', NS, 9 May 1868, p.2.
13 Inquest no. 6.825 and Inquest no. 7.826, James Sheridan & Francis McDermott, Doohat, Aghabog Parish, August 1866.
14 Inquest no. 1.810, John Caulfield, Killynenagh, Currin Parish, March 1866.
15 Inquest no. 5.958, William Nikle [Nichol], Mullaglasson, Clones Parish, April 1870
16 Inquest no. 30.494, Edward McCaffrey, Monaghan, Monaghan Parish, February 1858.
17 Inquest no. 15.874, Foster Dunwoody, Tully, Monaghan Parish, January 1868.
18 'Melancholy Accident – Death from Incautious Use of Firearms', NS, 25 January 1868.
19 Inquest no. 5.1027, Jane Parks, Ardgonnell, Tynan Parish, Co. Armagh, 12 April 1872.
20 'Fatal Accident to a Girl', NS, 13 April 1872.
21 Inquiry, Merideth Scalon, Fort Johnston, August 1862. For more information on the Johnstone family, *see* C. L. Johnstone's *A History of the Johnstones 1191–1909* (London, 1909).
22 Inquest no. 18.482, Elinor Dinny, Aughnacloy, Drumsnat Parish, November 1857.
23 Inquest no. 11.661, William Doran, Cornawall, Ematris Parish, May 1862.
24 Carolyn Conley reviewed all the Outrage papers (at the National Archive) in the post-famine years and, within the context of that collection, found that much of the violence occurring was of a 'recreational nature', part of Irish social culture. For more information *see* her book, *Melancholy Accidents: The Meaning of Violence in Post-Famine Ireland* (Lexington, 1999).
25 Inquest no. 21.1055, Bernard Reilly, Clones, Clones Parish, November 1872.
26 Inquest no. 14.716, George Welsh, Clones, Clones Parish, October 1863.
27 Inquiry, Joseph McMahon, Monaghan, Monaghan Parish, August 1859.
28 Inquest no. 20.484, John Byers, Carrigans, Donagh Parish, December 1857.
29 'Melancholy Accident', NS, December 1857.
30 'Accidental Death', NS, 19 October 1861.
31 Inquest no. 9.640, Thomas Salmon, Monaghan, Monaghan Parish, October 1861.

32 Inquest no. 1.931, Mary Kelly, Monaghan Town, August 1869.

33 Inquest no. 3.993, Thomas Murphy, Clones, Clones Parish, March 1871; the death was also reported in NS, March 1871.

34 Inquest no. 10.561, Francis Halfpenny, Gibraltar, Tyholland Parish, November 1859.

35 Inquest no. 5.864, Henry Smith, Monaghan Town, October 1867.

36 Inquest no. 7.691, Phillip McCague, Milltown, Monaghan Parish, April 1863.

37 Inquest no. 5.580, James Andrews, Clones, Clones Parish, March 1860.

38 Inquest no. 13.508, Francis Cumiskey, Point, Kilmore Parish, April 1858.

39 'Death from Drowning', NS, 24 April 1858.

40 Inquest no. 24.915, James Graham, Smithborough, Clones Parish, February 1869.

41 Inquest no. 19.790, Unknown Man, Cortober, Ematris Parish, June 1865.

42 It is not James McCaffrey who describes Patrick Smith as a 'wild Arab of society', but instead it is the coroner who adds that comment. All descriptions about the man appear to provide a description of someone who is either a beggar or a traveller.

43 Inquest no. 4.1140, Patrick Smith, Corraghy, Clones Parish, August 1875.

44 Inquest no. 13.977, John Holdsworth, Carrickmore, Clones Parish, September 1870.

45 Inquest no. 2.1036, John Stalker, Tully, Monaghan Parish, July 1872.

46 'Death from Accidental Drowning', NS, 9 June 1872.

47 Inquest no. 14.929, Unknown Man, Clonkeelan, Drummully Parish, June 1869.

48 'Discovery of the Remains of a Human Body in Clonkeelan Bog, Near Clones', NS, 19 June 1869.

49 Wilson, T. G., *Victorian Doctor: Being the Life of Sir William Wilde* (London, 1942), p.338.

50 The girls' surname was entered in the coroner's report book as 'Wylie'. It appears that it was either yet another attempt at diverting attention from the famous name or just a mistake made by the coroner in several instances. He does correctly enter the name as Wilde when referring to a letter he received from Sir William. *See* Chapter One for more information.

51 Yeats, J. B., *Letters to his son W. B. Yeats and Others 1869–1922* (London, 1983), p.296.

52 Inquiry, Emily Wylie [Wilde], 9 November 1871; Inquiry, Mary Wylie [Wilde], 21 November 1871.

53 Melville, Joy, *Mother of Oscar, The Life of Jane Francesca Wilde* (London, 1994).

Chapter Six (pp.213–250)
Death in the Workplace

1 Inquest no. 26.720, Mary Benner, Seaveagh, Tyholland Parish, January 1864.

2 For more information on acts within industry in Ireland, *see* Greer, Desmond, Nicolson, James W., *The Factory Acts in Ireland, 1802–1914* (Dublin, 2001).

3 This information was gathered in April 2003 from an interview with William Joyce Topley and Thomas Norman Topley, the grandsons of William Taggert.

4 Inquest no. 11.1014, Edward Molloy, Clones, Clones Parish, November 1871.

5 Armstrong, David L., *The Growth of Industry in Northern Ireland: The Story of the Golden Age of Industrial Development 1850–1900* (Oxford, 1999), pp.322–323.

6 Hogg, William E., *The Millers and the Mills of Ireland of about 1850* (Dublin, 2000), p.301.

7 Inquest no. 11.830, Owen McKenna, Killyslavin, Errigal Truagh, November 1866.

8 Inquest no. 4.748, Samuel Caruth, Skinnahergna, Errigal Truagh, August 1864.

9 Inquest no. 22.410, Thomas Hughes, Sillis, Donagh Parish, February 1856.

10 Greig, William, *General Report on the Gosford Estates in Co. Armagh* (1821).

11 Inquest no. 16.806, Patrick Larkin, Faltagh, Aghabog Parish, December 1865.

12 Inquest no. 17.719, Alexander Wallace, Hillhall, Donagh Parish, December 1863.

13 Gribbon, H. D., *The History of Water Power in Ulster* (Belfast, 1969), p.103.

14 Armstrong, David L., p.329.

15 Greig, William.

16 Inquest no. 16.530, Bridget McEnally, Seaveagh, Tyholland Parish, December 1858.
17 Inquest no. 26.728, Mary Benner (Bannon?), Seaveagh, Tyholland Parish, January 1864.
18 Inquest no. 23.574, Thomas Macklin, Carnbane, Drumsnat Parish, January 1860.
19 Inquest no. 19.1155, Ellen Bready, Listellan, Killeevan Parish, December 1875.
20 Armstrong, David L., p.322.
21 'Mill Accidents', NS, 20 April 1872.
22 Inquest no. 11.964, William Bailie, Dunraymond, Kilmore Parish, June 1870.
23 Inquest no. 1.576, Peter McKenna, Aghagaw, Tedavnet Parish, March 1860.
24 Gribbon, H. D., p.18.
25 Inquest no. 14.758, Thomas McRoberts, Emyvale, Donagh Parish, November 1864.
26 Inquest no. 16.835, Mary Tierney, Bellanode, Tedavnet Parish, December 1866.
27 Inquest no. 16.647, Patrick Goodwin, Carneys-Island, Clones Parish, 11 January 1862
    and Inquest no. 17.648, Alice Goodwin, Carneys-Island, Clones Parish, 20 January
    1862.
28 'Inquest at the Monaghan Poorhouse', NS, 15 June 1872.
29 Inquest no. 9.1036, Ann McDonald, Monaghan Poorhouse, Monaghan, June 1872.
30 Inquest no. 2.453, Ann Mooney, Glaslough, Donagh Parish, February 1857.
31 Inquest no. 11.1014, Edward Molloy, Clones, November 1871.
32 Inquest no. 2.426, Bernard Clarken, Mullaloughan, Donagh Parish, July 1856.
33 Inquest no. 9.460, Michael Crolly, Clones, May 1857.
34 Inquest no. 12.643, Phillip McManus, Clones, November 1861.
35 Inquest no. 12.603, Christopher Anderson, Coolnacarte, Currin Parish, October 1860.
36 Inquest no. 4.468, Felix McCabe, Scarvy, Killeevan Parish, August 1857.
37 Inquest no. 27.451, William Kieff (Keefe), Monaghan, Monaghan Parish, February 1857.
38 Inquest no. 7.471, John Linch, Cladowen, Clones Parish, August 1857.
39 Patterson, E. M., *The Great Northern Railway of Ireland* (Surrey, 1962), p.85.
40 *Irish Railway Collection* (Ulster Folk and Transport Museum, 1993), p.32.
41 Inquest no. 13.527, William Heartly, Srananny, Donagh Parish, November 1858.
42 Inquest no. 12.903, Edward Keely, Clones, Clones Parish, October 1868.
43 *Irish Railway Collection.*
44 'Fatal Accident on the Irish North-Western Railway, Clones', NS, 19 January 1867.
45 Inquest no. 21.840, John Finegan, Clones, January 1867.
46 Inquest no. 2.821, William Hewlett (Heazlett), Monaghan, Monaghan Parish, July 1866.
47 'Fatal Railway Accident', NS, 28 July 1866.
48 'Melancholy Railway Accident, Newbliss', NS, Thursday, 8 May 1869.
49 Inquest no. 9.924, Thomas Woods, Drumhirk, Aghabog Parish, May 1869.
50 Inquest no. 12.677, George Alford, November 1862.
51 Inquest no. 25.844, John Kane, Monaghan, Monaghan Parish, February 1867.
52 Inquest no. 4.1132, John McQuillen, Monaghan, Monaghan Parish, March 1875.
53 Inquest no. 3.1131, John Mehaffy, Monaghan, Monaghan Parish, March 1875.
54 'The Late Fatal Accident at the New Cathedral – Inquest', NS, 26 March 1875.
55 'Fatal Accident at the Cathedral – Two Persons Killed', NS, 19 March 1875.
56 'Fatal Accident at the Roman Catholic Cathedral,' NS, 3 December 1875.
57 Inquest no. 18.1154, Thomas Cunningham, Monaghan, December 1875.
58 Inquest no. 23.487, James McGaghey, Gortnana, Killeevan Parish, December 1857.
59 'Frightful Accident', NS, 27 January 1872.
60 Inquest no. 3.1022, John Treanor, Monaghan, Monaghan Parish, January 1872.
61 Inquest no. 10.1091, William Smith, Hilton Park, Currin Parish, December 1873.
62 'Melancholy and Fatal Accident', NS, 22 March 1862.
63 Ibid.
64 Inquest no. 6.656, John Hetherington, Monaghan, March 1862.
65 'The Late Accident in the Courthouse: To the Editor of *The Northern Standard*, A letter
    written by Jonathan Fleming', NS, 29 March 1862.
66 'Fatal Accident – A Man Killed by the Fall of a Tree', NS, 26 November 1875, p.2.

67 Inquest no. 16.1152, John Kerr, Monaghan, Monaghan Parish, November 1875.
68 'The Late Fatal Accident at Rossmore Park', NS, 17 December 1875, p.2.
69 Inquest no. 27.1061, James Duffy, Monaghan Infirmary, Monaghan Town, January 1873.
70 Inquest no. 8.938, Francis McCarole, Killyfuddy, Killeevan Parish, August 1869.
71 Inquest no. 7.1010, Edward Cusack, Clones Workhouse, Clones, September 1871.
72 Inquest no. 17.1079, Thomas Reighall, Clones, Clones Parish, May 1873.

Chapter Seven (pp.251–312)
With Intent to Kill

1 Conley, Carolyn, *Melancholy Accidents: The Meaning of Violence in Post-Famine Ireland* (Lexington, 1999), p.1.
2 Ibid. p.40.
3 Carolyn Conley calculated that Monaghan had a 28.6% conviction rate for homicides and Ulster had a 39.6% conviction rate. (*See Melancholy Accidents: The Meaning of Violence in Post-Famine Ireland*).
4 For example, an article about dog licences appeared in *The Northern Standard* in April 1878 stating: 'A number of persons who had neglected taking out licence within the proper time were summoned by the police. As all the cases were reported to the constabulary, the persons offending were fined the mitigated penalty, 1s each, and directed to take out licences forthwith.'
5 Vaughan, W. E., *Landlords and Tenants in Mid-Victorian Ireland* (Oxford, 1994), p.144.
6 *See* Carolyn Conley, p.1.
7 Vaughan, W. E., p.145. In a table entitled 'Deaths caused by Gunshot Wounds', Vaughan calculates percentages based upon all agrarian outrages lodged in the National Archives. 30% of gunshot wounds occurred within families, 40% between neighbours and 74% occurred when the source of the dispute was between landlords and tenants.
8 Vaughan, W. E., p.143.
9 Fitzpatrick, David, 'Class, Family and Rural Unrest in Nineteenth-Century Ireland' in *Irish Studies*, 1982, Vol. 2, p.59.
10 'Fatal Consequences of a Family Dispute', NS, 25 May 1861.
11 A colig/colligeen/callig is an earwig. In Irish, *cuileog an lín* means literally 'insect of the flax'.
12 Inquest no. 10.630, Michael McEleer, Drumcoofoster, Tedavnet Parish, May 1861.
13 'Monaghan Spring Assizes, Manslaughter', NS, 8 March 1862.
14 Valuation Office, Land Records, OS5 Drumcoo (Foster).
15 Inquest no. 10.1032, Michael Mooney, Carn, Aghabog Parish, June 1872.
16 David Richard Pigot was the only son of John Pigot, a physician of Kilrush in Co. C born in 1796; he first appears at school in Fermoy; matriculated in Dublin Unive 1814; studied medicine in Edinburgh; entered the Middle Temple 1818; grad bachelor of arts 1819; married Catherine, eldest daughter of Walter Page of A mills in Co. Cork, 1821; studied law in London; was called to the Irish bar 182(on the Munster circuit; proceeded master of arts 1832; was in religion a Rom tholic and in politics a liberal; became a King's Counsel 1835; was appointe tor-general 1840; retired on the fall of the ministry 1841; was appointed Chi of the Exchequer 1846; received university degree of doctor of law *honoris co* died 1873; was buried at Kilworth.
17 'Co. Monaghan Assizes, "Murder"', NS, July 1872.
18 *The Impartial Reporter and Fermanagh Farmers Journal*, 10 January 1861.
19 'Murder of the Brothers Shaw', NS, 12 January 1861.
20 Vaughan, W. E., p.145.
21 'Court of Queen's Bench', NS, 29 November 1862.
22 Francis McCann (or Muckian) is listed in the Griffith's Valuation and in

cords held at the Valuation Office in Dublin as leasing land at Corcullioncrew and Corgullionglish in the Donaghmoyne Parish, Co. Monaghan. The family is referred to by several spellings including McCann, Muckian, Muckean, McKian, etc.

23 'Fratricide in Castleblayney', NS, 20 August 1870.

24 'Charge of Murder', NS, 25 February 1871

25 'The Verdict – The Murder Case – The Sentence', *Dundalk Democrat*, 4 March 1871.

26 James McKian; GPB, PEN 1888/49, National Archives, Dublin.

27 Land Records, Castleblayney Town, Co. Monaghan, Valuation Office, Dublin.

28 Inquest no. 15.566, James Farrell, Monaghan, Monaghan Parish, 29 December 1859.

29 Inquest no. 23.447, Thomas McCarvle, Corlatt, Killeevan Parish, January 1857.

30 Conley, Carolyn, p.149.

31 Doherty, James, *Armagh Prison 1822–1877*, Masters Dissertation for Queen's College Belfast (September 1992), p.93.

32 Malcolm, Elizabeth, *Ireland Sober, Ireland Free* (Dublin, 1986), p.328.

33 Malcolm, Elizabeth, p.333.

34 Doherty, James, p.68.

35 *See* Tobias, J. J., *Nineteenth-Century Crime: Prevention and Punishment* (Newton-Abbot, 1972)) for more information on Victorian contemporary views on the causation of crime.

36 Inquest no. 3.1025, John McBride, Maghernakill, Broomfield District, Donaghmoyne Parish, April 1872.

37 'Castleblayney Quarter Sessions', NS, 20 April 1872.

38 'Co. Monaghan Assizes, Crown Court', *Dundalk Democrat*, 20 July 1872.

39 Luddy, Maria, 'Abandoned Women and Bad Characters: Prostitution in Nineteenth-Century Ireland' in Hayes, Alan, Urquhart, Diane (eds), *The Irish Women's History Reader* (London and New York, 2001) pp.87–94.

40 Name-calling often preceded such 'recreational fighting'. Indian meal was the replacement food for potatoes used by the most destitute families of the country. 'Black blanket carriers' is likely to be a reference to Protestantism used in a derogatory manner. For example, 'black men' were members of the Imperial Grand Black Chapter of the British Commonwealth, a Protestant organisation formed in 1797; open only to members of the Orange Order. Most references to someone being called 'black' are Roman Catholics referring to someone devoted to the Protestant cause. (*Concise Ulster Dictionary*, Oxford, 1996).

41 Conley, Carolyn, p.169.

42 'Murder on St. Patrick's Night', NS, 24 March 1866.

43 For more information on the Gray family of Ballybay, *see* James and Peadar Murnane's *At the Ford of the Birches: The History of Ballybay, its People and Vicinity* (Monaghan, 1999).

44 Inquest no. 2.811, Owen Fox, Lisgillan, Aghnamullen Parish, March 1866.

45 Inquest no. 3.1037, David Gorman, Derryveen, Donagh Parish, July 1872.

46 Inquest no. 4.1038, James Shaw, Monaghan, Monaghan Parish, July 1872.

47 'Melancholy Accident', NS, July 1872.

48 Beames, M. R., 'The Ribbon Societies: Lower Class Nationalism in Pre-Famine Ireland' in Philpin, Charles, H. E. (ed) *Nationalism and Popular Protest in Ireland* (Cambridge, 1987) p.128

49 Keenan, Mel, 'The Armagh Five: Irish Ribbonism in Tasmania 1840–1850' in *The Electronic Journal of Australian and New Zealand History*, ISSN 132–5752 (5 June 1996).

50 PRONI, Belfast, Mic. 371.

51 Inquest no. 1.892, Thomas Hughes, Monaghan, July 1868.

52 *The Impartial Reporter*, 23 July 1868.

53 This entry was recorded in the minute notes from a meeting of the Orange Order in Monaghan by Christopher McGimpsey. *See* his article 'Border Ballads and Sectarian Affrays' in *Clogher Record* (Enniskillen, 1982).

54 Inquest no 17.900, James Clarke, Monaghan, Monaghan Parish, November 1868.
55 'Coroner's Inquest into the Cause of Death of James Clarke', NS, 12 December 1868.
56 Christopher McGimpsey's article 'Border Ballads and Sectarian Affray' in *Clogher Record* (Enniskillen, 1982) asks this very same question. Having looked at the evidence of the inquests, the trials of both Baird and McKenna and detailing the political and religious events taking place in Co. Monaghan at that time, he concluded that Mc-Kenna killed Clarke in retaliation for the murder of Hughes.
57 This report was from *The London Times* as researched by Christopher McGimpsey.
58 'Monaghan Assizes', NS, 10 July 1869.
59 Ibid.
60 Ibid.
61 O'Daly, E. E., *The History of the O'Dalys* (1937), pp.348–349.
62 Hanratty is also referred to in newspapers articles as 'O'Hanlon'.
63 'The Patriotic Brotherhood in Armagh and Monaghan', NS, 7 October 1882.
64 Joseph Daly, GPB, PEN 1890, National Archives, Dublin.
65 Ibid.
66 'Coroners Inquest', NS, 15 March 1873.
67 Inquest no. 8.1070, Patrick McKenna, Dernasell East, Tedavnet Parish, March 1873.
68 'Monaghan Summer Assizes', NS, 12 July 1873.

Chapter Eight (pp.313–330)
Matters of Life and Death

1 Jervis, Sir John (1802–1856) *Jervis on the office and duties of Coroners: with forms and precedents*, 11ed (London, 1993), p.3.
2 Inquest no. 12.751, Robert Shannon, Monaghan, Monaghan Parish, October 1864.
3 Inquest no. 15.439, Ellen McLoughlin, Monaghan, Monaghan Parish, November 1856.
4 Inquest no. 22.841, Robert Connolly, Corragore, Ematris Parish, January 1867.
5 Inquest no. 1.425, Charles McCue, Monaghan, Monaghan Parish, July 1856.
6 Inquest no. 1.465, Margaret Maguire, Emy, Donagh Parish, July 1857.
7 Inquest no. 11.1014, Edward Molloy, Clones, November 1871.
8 Inquest no. 5.655, William Gibson, Cornasoo, Kilmore Parish, March 1862.
9 Inquest no. 9.659, Samuel Benson, Garran, Clones Parish, April 1862.
10 Inquest no. 12.1119, Alice McDonald, Smithborough, Clones Parish, October 1874.
11 Inquest no. 4.428, Matthew McCabe, Cortober, Ematris Parish, August 1856.
12 Inquest no. 4.455, Thomas Crawford, Clonnagore, Drummully Parish, April 1857.
13 Johnson, James Rawlins, *A Treatise on the Medicinal Leech* (London, 1816).
14 Ibid.
15 Buchan, Dr William, *Domestic Medicine or the Family Physician*, 2nd Ed (London, 1785).
16 Inquest no. 1.533, Robert Campbell, Crumlin, Tyholland Parish, February 1859.
17 Felter, Dr Harvey and Lloyd, John Uri, *Kings American Dispensatory* (1898).
18 Inquest no. 12.1034, Michael Coyle, Maghill, Drumsnat Parish, June 1872.
19 Inquest no. 5.469, Margaret McElmeel, August 1857.
20 Inquest no. 9.473, Susan Keely, Coolkill, Ematris Parish, August 1857.
21 Inquest no. 3.734, Philip [Mc]Kiernan, Clonfad, Killeevan Parish, March 1864.
22 Inquest no. 10.781, Emily Scott, Skeagh, Drumsnat Parish, April 1865.
23 Inquest no. 14.905, John Mooney, Castleshane, Monaghan Parish, October 7, 1868.
24 'Co. Monaghan Spring Assizes – Charge of Manslaughter', NS, 6 March 1869.
25 Buchan, Dr William, *Domestic Medicine or the Family Physician* (London, 1785).
26 Inquest no. 17.512, Thomas McAlier, Monaghan, Monaghan Parish, May 1858.
27 Inquest no. 4.1099, Owen McCarvle, Corravilla, Killeevan Parish, April 1874.
28 Inquest no. 6.557, Eliza Irwin, Corraghduff, Donagh Parish, September 1859.
29 Inquest no. 13.564, Pat McEntee, Sandhills, Currin Parish, December 1859.

MELANCHOLY MADNESS

Appendix One (p.333)
Coroner's Reports

1 This list was compiled and first appeared in Dr Brian Farrell's book, *A History of the Coroner in Ireland* (Dublin, 1999).
2 In 1999, the National Archives accessioned a large quantity of coroner's papers from Cork Circuit Court Office but these papers have not yet been arranged and listed.

Appendix Two (pp.334–339)
Recording Death During the Famine

1 McDonald, Brian, *Clogher Record*, (Enniskillen, 2000), Vol. XVI, No. 1, p.8.
2 Ó Mórdha, Pilip, 'Summary of Inquests Held on Currin, Co. Monaghan Victims, 1846–1855' in *Clogher Record*, (Enniskillen, 1995), Vol. XV, No. 2, pp.90–100.
3 Ibid.
4 Ó Mórdha, Brian, 'The Great Famine in Monaghan: A Coroner's Account', *Clogher Record*, (Enniskillen, 1960–61), Vol. IV, Nos 1 and 2, pp.29–41.
5 Ó Mórdha, Pilip, pp.90–100.
6 Ó Mórdha, Brian, pp.29–41

Appendix Three (p.340)
Listing of Doctors

1 Mr Bernard McKenna of Emyvale was referred to by all in the vicinity as 'Dr McKenna' as he regularly attended patients; however, he was not a medically trained doctor.

Also available from
Mercier Press

THE LEGACY OF HISTORY
Martin Mansergh

The value of looking back is to understand where we are and why; to honour that which was noble; to acknowledge and try to correct what went wrong. Ireland's history has had a profound influence on the Irish as a people and it has certainly shaped the character of the State. *The Legacy of History* helps to flesh out and put into perspective the background to the problems with which we have had to deal, as well as highlighting what remains to be done.

THE COURSE OF IRISH HISTORY
Edited by T. W. Moody and F. X. Martin

A revised and enlarged version of this classic book provides a rapid short survey, with geographical introduction, of the whole course of Ireland's history. Based on a series of television programmes, it is designed to be both popular and authoritative, concise but comprehensive, highly selective but balanced and fair-minded, critical but constructive and sympathetic. A distinctive feature is its wealth of illustrations.

THE GREAT IRISH FAMINE
Edited by Cathal Póirtéir

This is the most wide-ranging series of essays ever published on the Great Irish Famine and will prove of lasting interest to the general reader. Leading historians, economists, geographers – from Ireland, Britain and the United States – have assembled the most up-to-date research from a wide spectrum of disciplines, including medicine, folklore and literature, to give the fullest account yet of the background and consequences of the Famine.